REAL LIFE WITH
Celiac Disease

Troubleshooting and Thriving Gluten Free

Melinda Dennis, MS, RD, LDN, and Daniel A. Leffler, MD, MS

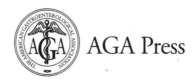

AGA Press

Real Life with Celiac Disease

Disclaimer

This publication provides accurate information on the subject matter covered. The publisher is not providing legal, medical, or other professional services. Reference herein to any specific commercial products, procedures, or services by trade name, trademark, manufacturer, or otherwise does not constitute or imply endorsement, recommendation, or favored status by the AGA Institute. The views and opinions of the author(s) expressed in this publication do not necessarily state or reflect those of the AGA Institute, and they shall not be used to advertise or endorse a product.

Printed in the United States of America

13 12 11 10   1 2 3 4 5 6

ISBN 978-1-60356-008-5

Library of Congress Control Number: 2010902343

For additional copies or information on licensing or translating this content, please contact:

AGA Press
4930 Del Ray Avenue
Bethesda, MD 20814-2513
www.gastro.org/publications

*To all of our patients, who provide us with the inspiration and
drive to keep learning and improving.*

*To my wonderful parents, who took turns going with me to
my first celiac conferences, and to my friends, who care as much about
cross-contamination as I do.*
Melinda

For Ryn and for Vayla
Panta rhei.
Dan

CONTENTS

THE GLUTEN-FREE LIFE: Solutions and Strategies 73

My Celiac Disease Journey

Marge Benham-Hutchins, PhD, RN

My diagnosis of celiac disease changed my life, for the better. This may sound odd to some of you, but others who have traveled the same path I have will understand. Years of misdiagnosis led to increasingly poor health and discouragement. Finally being diagnosed opened the door to both medical and self-management of the disease.

I had lived with more than 25 years of symptoms. There were numerous tests and vague explanations, such as "irritable bowel" or "nervous stomach" from health care providers. Then I read about celiac disease and immediately made the connection—and my own diagnosis. When I approached my primary care provider with this information, he responded, "You don't want to have celiac disease." This response totally confused me. Of course I did not want to have a disease! But I did want some answers and hopefully a way to treat and manage the symptoms that were influencing every aspect of my life. While I was pondering his response, he changed the topic to my turning 50 years old and my need for a screening colonoscopy. Quick thinking on my part resulted in a negotiation. I would get the colonoscopy if I could have a referral to a gastroenterologist specialist for my other problems. This negotiation led to both a colonoscopy and an upper endoscopy (EGD), which revealed severe villous atrophy—a classic change to my small intestine caused by celiac disease.

As I was waking up from the procedures, the gastroenterologist informed me that, even visually, I had the classic celiac changes to my small intestine and the degree of abnormality was suggestive of long-term untreated celiac disease. He urged me to make a follow-up appointment and informed me that I would need to follow a gluten-free diet for life. A few minutes later, I was offered a choice between graham crackers and saltines (both contain gluten)! Looking back, I realize that this was the first of many challenges. Challenges have included educating not only myself, my family, and my friends about gluten-free living but also a lot of my health care providers.

My first steps were healing from the physical effects of a late diagnosis while simultaneously learning the gluten-free diet. Having celiac disease influences almost all aspects of my life, as it certainly must yours. It requires day-to-day self-management, for life.

As anyone who has tried it knows, eliminating gluten from your diet is no easy task. One cannot ignore the fact that eating is a social activity, and we who have celiac disease are by necessity forced to be detailed and selective about what we eat. Gluten is hidden in many foods; even those naturally gluten free may be processed in such a way that gluten is added.

Healing physically was also a challenge. Because I had undiagnosed celiac disease for so long, I had developed a number of secondary problems, including thyroid disease, hair loss, depression, chronic anemia, lymphocytic (microscopic) colitis, and small intestinal bacterial overgrowth (SIBO). Although these were all explained by the diagnosis, they still required both short- and long-term treatment and management.

Although the biopsies taken during my EGD confirmed very active celiac disease, my celiac blood tests were only mildly elevated. My doctors, who did not have a lot of experience with celiac disease, could not explain this discrepancy to me. Shortly after my diagnosis, I volunteered to participate in a research study. In return for a blood sample, I would be provided with my celiac antibody (tTG) levels. This time my tTG level was 42 units (less than 20 units is normal), even higher than at diagnosis! Despite what I thought was strict adherence to the gluten-free diet, my levels stayed above normal for another year.

At that time, I moved to Boston and became a patient at the Celiac Center at Beth Israel Deaconess Medical Center (BIDMC) and saw both Daniel Leffler and Melinda Dennis. Being treated by health care providers who specialize in celiac disease was another turning point for me. I was aware of the Celiac Center and attended a patient-centered conference there just before seeing Dr. Leffler for the first time. It was amazing to see the number of people (just like me) trying to navigate the confusing path to diagnosis and major life changes.

As a health care informatics researcher and registered nurse, I often felt as if I had to find answers to my own questions. That all changed when I met Dr. Leffler and later dietitian Melinda Dennis; their knowledge and empathy increased my confidence and hope—confidence in their expertise and hope for my future. Being a patient, I was viewed as an active and participating member of the health care team.

For example, my tTG level had remained at 42 units despite what I thought was meticulous dietary management. Ms. Dennis taught me to look carefully for hidden gluten and gluten cross-contamination, and Dr. Leffler led treatment for my SIBO and possible concurrent Crohn's disease. We approached my chronic anemia using the same team process—with me at the center of the team—and worked together to combine diet, vitamins, and oral iron supplements. A year later, my anemia has resolved, and I am very happy to report that on follow-up endoscopy, my intestine is completely healed.

The importance of family support cannot be overlooked. Perhaps you are a family member reading this book. Celiac disease management influences the day-to-day lives of your family members. For example, running out for a "quick bite to eat" becomes much more difficult and cross-contamination with gluten-containing foods is a daily concern. The support, encouragement, and often advocacy of my husband and daughter have been crucial components of my healing and living with celiac disease.

Discouragement and depression are common problems with any chronic disease. For me, active involvement in my own healing, volunteering for celiac disease research, and educating those new to celiac disease, as well as other health care providers, has provided me with a sense of purpose.

Having the care of knowledgeable and informed health care providers has provided me with the most support. Second only to this is the support that's come from learning from others with celiac disease. When I was first diagnosed, I joined a support group in North Texas. These dedicated volunteers produce a monthly newsletter, provide frequent email updates, and work with local restaurants to develop procedures to ensure safe gluten-free dining. In addition, they hold monthly educational meetings, including "Celiac Disease 101." It was there that I learned how to read food labels, which local stores stocked gluten-free products, and how to eat out safely.

Even before I moved to Boston, I contacted the local celiac disease support group, appropriately named Healthy Villi (www.healthyvilli.org). In short order, a member contacted me to see how they could be of assistance. I had a lot of questions about where to shop and dine in Boston, and I also signed up for their newsletter. The first educational offering I attended included a cooking demonstration, food vendors, and presentations by celiac disease specialists from BIDMC on topics ranging from research updates to diagnosis to dietary guidelines. Because I subscribe to the national Celiac Listserv,* I receive online information and support. This is an excellent way that people with celiac disease can share information and resources with others all over the world.

Navigating the complex path to both diagnosis and living with celiac disease requires that you have reliable information and guidance from both knowledgeable professionals and support groups. This book fills the need for a comprehensive text that supports both individuals with celiac disease and their families as they navigate the often complicated road from symptoms to recovery.

* To subscribe, send an email to celiac@listserv.icors.org, leaving the subject line blank; as your email message, write sub celiac, your first name, and your last name.

ACKNOWLEDGMENTS

We are grateful to the following for their support.

The many dedicated leaders of the celiac support and advocacy organizations, and especially our colleagues and the members of the New England–based Healthy Villi, who devote their time and energy to furthering the cause.

All of Melinda's dietitian colleagues and friends who have chosen to specialize in celiac disease and tirelessly work together on behalf of their patients and clients to promote awareness and education in the medical and nutrition fields and the food service industry.

Peter Green, who gave Dan his start in the world of celiac disease.

Helen Shields, an inspirational educator and clinician and long-time mentor to both of us.

Patt Samour, Director of Nutrition at BIDMC, who is always just at the end of the phone line, giving support and counsel on challenging cases, and who is a champion for the field of dietetics.

Carol Parrish, one of Melinda's key mentors in nutritional care in gastroenterology.

Javed Sheikh, our constant source of expertise and guidance in the worlds of allergy and immunology.

Christine Charlip, our fearless editor, who guided us through the creation of our first book.

Detlef Schuppan, who is constantly pushing the boundaries of our understanding of celiac disease.

In particular, we are both indebted to Ciaran Kelly for his perpetual good-natured mentorship and wisdom.

Melinda Dennis, MS, RD, LDN (*right*), was diagnosed with celiac disease 20 years ago. She is the Nutrition Coordinator and a founding member of the Celiac Center at Beth Israel Deaconess Medical Center in Boston, Massachusetts. Melinda is the author of

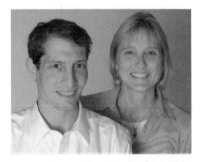

several journal articles and has lectured nationally on the nutritional management of celiac disease and optimizing nutritional health. She serves on the American Dietetic Association's Evidence Analysis Library Task Force for Celiac Disease and on the American Gastroenterological Association Press Advisory Board. She is the founder, former chairperson, and current Nutrition Advisor to the Healthy Villi Greater Boston Celiac/DH Support Group, the nation's largest celiac disease–related support group. Melinda offers dietitian coaching, lecturing, consulting,

Photo: Oran Barber BIDMC

gluten-free classes, shopping tours, and health adventure retreats for those following the gluten-free diet through her nutrition consulting service Delete the Wheat, LLC (www. DeletetheWheat.com).

Daniel A. Leffler, MD, MS, is the Director of Clinical Research and also a founding member of the Celiac Center at Beth Israel Deaconess Medical Center, Boston, Massachusetts. Dr. Leffler has spearheaded multiple studies evaluating clinical outcomes in celiac disease and investigating potential therapies for celiac disease and leads initiatives to improve patient care. His current focus is clinical and translational research in celiac disease, including factors that influence dietary adherence; clinical outcomes in celiac disease; development of novel noninvasive tests of celiac disease activity; and creation of disease-specific survey tools to assess diet adherence, symptoms, and quality of life. He lectures on both research aspects and clinical care of celiac disease nationally and internationally and has published numerous articles and book chapters on celiac disease. Dr. Leffler serves as a medical advisor to both the Healthy Villi and National Foundation for Celiac Awareness. Dr. Leffler is also active in medical education at Harvard Medical School, where he has received recognition for excellence in tutoring and mentoring.

Life with a Gluten-Related Disorder

Melinda Dennis, MS, RD, LDN, and Daniel A. Leffler, MD, MS

There has been no better time in history to have celiac disease.

Melinda's Story

My story may sound familiar to some of you. I woke up one morning 20 years ago with an itchy, blistering rash on my elbows and knees. I thought I had contracted a rash from the yoga studio but, in fact, I was diagnosed by a dermatologist with dermatitis herpetiformis. An endoscopy and a really useless nutrition consultation followed. The next thing I knew, my mom and I were walking dejected through the grocery aisles, looking for food. One cereal. One bag of rice cakes. Shock and frustration. Mom was holding back tears, certain that her genes were the cause of my condition. At that moment, I decided that I would master my condition and not be controlled or beaten by it. I never looked back. Years later, I changed careers, earned a Masters degree in nutrition and health promotion, and became a dietitian specializing in celiac disease here at Beth Israel Deaconess Medical Center (BIDMC).

Back when I was diagnosed, barely anyone knew about celiac disease. We have come such a very long way, and I am grateful to be riding this wave of rising interest and awareness. I like to use the term *graceful assertiveness* when I think about what it takes to voice our dietary needs in the world. Some patients don't like to make a fuss or draw attention to themselves, and I understand that feeling completely, having experienced it myself. But the reality is that we all deserve and are entitled to available, affordable, and nutritious gluten-free food and specialized medical and dietary care.

Dan's Story

Before medical school, my interests focused on how nutrition can impact health. This led me to study nutrition at Columbia University, where I completed a Masters degree and had the good fortune to first learn about celiac disease from Dr. Peter Green. Throughout the years that followed in medical school, celiac disease continued to stand out as a unique example of how food and health interact. Although nutrition is a key factor in many diseases, celiac disease is a model for how individuals can dramatically improve their health through diet alone. I continued to follow the field of celiac disease closely and was fortunate to be able to work as a medical resident with Dr. Ciaran Kelly, an internationally renowned celiac gastroenterologist, at BIDMC.

The Path Forward

We stayed at BIDMC and, together with Dr. Kelly, created the Celiac Center. The mission of the center is to enhance the health and well-being of those with celiac disease and other gluten-related disorders through excellence in medical care, education, and research. Over the last six years since we founded the Celiac Center at BIDMC, we've seen more than 2,000 people for celiac disease and other gluten-related disorders. People come for all sorts of reasons; their exact diagnoses may be unclear, they may have not been responding as expected to treatment, or they may just be coming in for routine testing. However, uniting all these visits is the need for accurate information and answers to all their questions.

Although, with the right care and treatment the vast majority of people with gluten-related disorders thrive, many patients, like Marge whom you met in the Foreword, experience a wide variety of obstacles between diagnosis and optimal health. Most patients lack access to the medical and nutrition expertise on celiac disease that is available at a specialized celiac center. People with celiac disease should be proactive and educate themselves about their condition so they can ask for and receive proper testing and care.

In *Real Life with Celiac Disease,* we have drawn from the experience of nearly 20 combined years of working with celiac disease to focus on the most common and important questions and issues that our patients with celiac disease present to us. Although not every question or problem has a clear solution, driven by patients, the field of celiac disease is evolving rapidly. We have brought together leading experts in celiac disease from all around the world to provide answers and information that we believe is comprehensive and clear and represents the most up-to-date information available.

Although we traveled very different paths to come to work in celiac disease, we both agree on this central point: Celiac disease happens to be one of the best understood and most common autoimmune disorders in the world. The rate of diagnosis is increasing faster than any other gastrointestinal disorder, and new discoveries are being made all the time that are helping us understand who is at risk for celiac disease; how to improve diagnosis; and how to optimize nutritional health, monitoring, and treatment.

Despite the great leaps forward made by clinicians and scientists, many of whom have contributed chapters to this book, we are all too aware that these advances have remained out of reach for many people with celiac disease and gluten-related disorders. We hear all the time from patients how hard it was to get to this point, frustration that no one recognized their symptoms and put the story together for them, and disappointment that the dietitian they were referred to knew less about the gluten-free diet (GFD) than they did, in short, "that they had to do it themselves."

For decades, celiac disease was not thought to be a common disorder, especially in the United States. Thankfully, this error in vision is changing. However, generations of physicians have yet to integrate this knowledge into clinical practice. For this reason, although we have been very involved in educating clinicians, it remains crucial that people with gluten-related disorders have the background, resources, and understanding to advocate for themselves on all levels, from getting diagnosed to advocating for research. Even for those fortunate enough to receive care at a specialized celiac center or from a clinician who has made the effort to acquire greater knowledge about celiac disease, there can be many important unanswered questions.

We wrote *Real Life with Celiac Disease* to answer many of the most commonly voiced questions and concerns. How do I take my supplements? How much gluten can I "get away" with? How did I get celiac disease? What is the chance that my children will get it? What lab tests should I be requesting, and why? What's the difference between gluten intolerance and celiac disease? What are these itchy bumps all over my arms? Why did it take so long to get diagnosed? How do I interpret the disclaimers I see all over food labels? If my blood tests return to normal, why can't I start eating gluten again?

Important Terminology

Agreeing on a definition of celiac disease is probably a good place to start. Currently, celiac disease is broadly agreed to be "a heightened immune responsiveness to gluten and related proteins leading to autoimmune enteropathy (small intestinal damage), often with systemic manifestations."

There is a lot of information in that sentence, so let's break it down.

A heightened immune responsiveness to gluten. This simply means that the immune system, the part of the body that is responsible primarily for fighting off infections, begins to recognize gluten as a threat and becomes active.

Gluten and related proteins. Every grain seed is made of three main parts (Figure 1). The bran is the outer protective layer or husk, which contains fiber, iron, and B vitamins. The germ is the inner part, which is the earliest form of the future plant; it contains minerals, B vitamins, and vitamin E. The bran and the germ are lost when grains are refined to make white flour instead of whole wheat flour. The endosperm is the middle layer, which contains the proteins and sugars the plant will need to grow until it can make its own energy from the sun by photosynthesis. Much of the protein in the endosperm is gluten. Gluten specifically

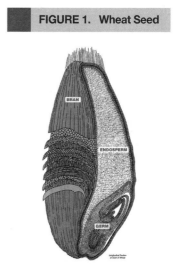

FIGURE 1. Wheat Seed

From http://www.wheatfoods.org/ HighResolution-Kernel-of-Wheat-Diagram.64.8.htm?ld2=14&~. Accessed February 10, 2010.

is the protein from wheat, but other grains, including rye, barley, spelt, and triticale, are very closely related to wheat and the proteins in their seeds are similar enough to gluten to cause a reaction in people with celiac disease.

Autoimmune. For many years, it was not clear if celiac disease was an allergy or an autoimmune disease. In an allergy, the body makes antibodies (immune system proteins) that attach to food or other environmental molecules. When antibodies attach to their target, they cause the release of inflammatory chemicals from specific immune system cells called *mast cells.* These chemicals can have a variety of effects, including swelling, rashes, and tissue damage. In an allergy, the target is the foreign substance that has entered the body, and the body is an innocent bystander. In an autoimmune disease, on the other hand, the body itself is the target. Although in celiac disease gluten starts and perpetuates the reaction, the attachment of antibodies to gluten does not cause injury and inflammation, and mast cells are not involved. Instead, people with celiac disease make antibodies that attach to tissue transglutaminase, an important natural enzyme in your body. The development of antibodies that attach to parts of your own body, rather than to foods or other foreign substances, plus the lack of involvement of mast cells proves that your immune system is targeting your own body. Therefore, celiac disease is an autoimmune disorder rather than an allergy.

Enteropathy (small intestinal damage). This refers to the celiac disease–related damage in the small intestine, in particular, damage to the fingerlike projections called *villi* that line the intestine (Figure 2). The villi, and the microvilli that cover the villi like hairs, greatly increase surface area for absorption of nutrients. In fact, if the intestine were only a simple tube, it would spread out to be 2 square feet in area, but with the folds and villi, it would cover an entire tennis court! In addition, the villi hold many of the enzymes needed to digest and absorb nutrients. You can see why it requires a biopsy and microscopic examination to determine the extent of damage to the small intestine.

In active celiac disease, the first and mildest change is an increase in villi white blood cells, known as *intraepithelial lymphocytes* (Figure 3). Damage to the connections between intestinal cells known as *tight junctions* and deposits of tissue transglutaminase antibody may be seen even earlier, but the importance of these problems is unclear, and they are difficult to measure. As inflammation continues, the villi become damaged, and the crypts deepen as they try to produce new cells quickly to replace the damaged villi. Soon the intestine cannot keep up with repairs, and the villi begin to shorten. With enough damage, they can be completely lost. Fortunately, the intestine has incredible regenerative ability and in most cases, if you can remove the inflammation, the villi will heal back to normal.

Systemic manifestations. For decades, celiac disease has been considered a disease of gastrointestinal symptoms. Only recently has it been recognized that most people with celiac disease have symptoms that are primarily not gastrointestinal. Symptoms can range from bone damage to infertility to trouble with balance. Failure to recognize the manifestations of celiac disease that occur away from the gastrointestinal tract is a major reason why so many individuals are not diagnosed.

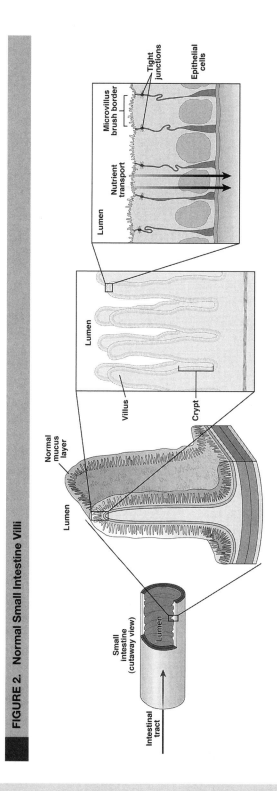

FIGURE 2. Normal Small Intestine Villi

Intestinal tract

Small intestine (cutaway view)

Lumen

Lumen

Normal mucus layer

Villus

Crypt

Lumen

Microvillus brush border

Tight junctions

Nutrient transport

Epithelial cells

FIGURE 3. Normal and Damaged Villi

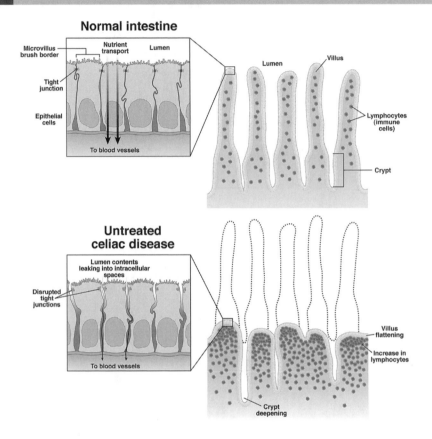

Within celiac disease there are a number of categories.

Classic or typical celiac disease refers to celiac disease presenting primarily with gastro-intestinal or nutritional problems.

Nonclassic or atypical celiac disease refers to celiac disease that is primarily causing problems outside of direct gastrointestinal or nutritional concerns.

Silent celiac disease refers to celiac disease that occurs in the absence of any related symptom or nutritional deficiency. Individuals with silent celiac disease are typically found through screening.

Latent celiac disease is a condition in which an individual is positive for celiac antibodies (either endomysial antibody or tissue transglutaminase antibody) but has a normal intestinal biopsy. Management of those with latent celiac disease is controversial, and the decision of whether to start a GFD or simply watch for problems needs to be made on an individual basis.

Gluten intolerance does not have a single, widely agreed upon definition, but most leaders in the field use it to refer to a condition in which people develop symptoms when exposed to gluten but lack a significant immune reaction. In other words, ingesting gluten makes people with gluten intolerance feel unwell but they have no damage to the intestine and the accurate celiac blood tests, endomysial antibody or tissue transglutaminase antibody, are normal. Symptoms of gluten intolerance can be just as severe as symptoms of celiac disease, but there is no evidence of the complications seen with untreated celiac disease such as anemia or bone disease.

Gluten sensitivity is a broad category that includes all of the above disorders as well as a variety of other less common gluten-related disorders such as gluten ataxia.

The Unique Nature of This Book

Although there are a variety of excellent clinical and lifestyle books about celiac disease, this book is different. We believe *Real Life with Celiac Disease* will help you improve your well-being and that you will relate to many of the patients whose stories are here. We hope that you will carry this book with you to your health care provider to discuss your problems and create a treatment approach that works for you. You can use this book to explain to friends and family why you need to avoid gluten—all gluten, not just some or when it's convenient. You will understand how important it is to eat more nutritiously to regain health and reach an optimal weight. You may find the reason for your continued symptoms and the resources you need to advocate for yourself.

Real Life with Celiac Disease: Troubleshooting and Thriving Gluten Free will help you if:

- You have celiac disease and want to be educated to the fullest about maximizing your health and minimizing risks.
- You want to support a friend or family member who has celiac disease.
- You suspect that you or someone you know may have celiac disease.
- You want to understand the difference between gluten intolerance and celiac disease.
- You find the food labeling laws confusing.
- You are following the GFD and are still experiencing symptoms.
- You want to know more about lab tests, follow-up care, balancing your diet, supplements, and the potential complications of untreated celiac disease.
- You are a vegetarian or have diabetes or want to lose weight *and* maximize your nutritional health.
- You need ideas for traveling and dining out safely.
- You are a clinician who needs information *now* to help the increasing number of patients coming to see you with concerns about celiac disease.

Taking an active role in educating yourself is the first step toward better health. Life with celiac disease can be a learning and empowering process. We hope that the practical knowledge in this book will benefit you and the people in your life. We are heartened by each person who comes to understand celiac disease and related gluten disorders, because you are out there helping the many undiagnosed people get the care they need, too.

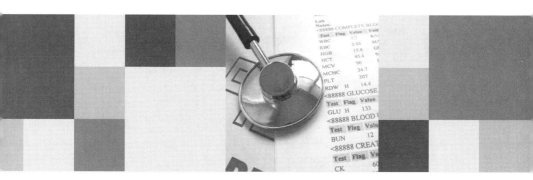

THE BASICS:
DEFINITIONS AND DIAGNOSIS

This section reviews the history of celiac disease, where it is found, and how the disease announces itself. Chapters examine the various tests used to diagnose celiac disease, including blood tests, endoscopy, and genetic testing. This will allow you to have a good understanding of what celiac disease is and how it is diagnosed.

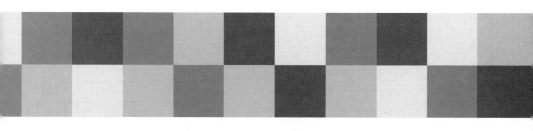

CHAPTER 1

A Global Disease: The Iceberg Dilemma

Ahmet Aybar, MD, and Alessio Fasano, MD

Once upon a time, 10,000 years ago, gluten was not a part of the human diet, and therefore, there was no celiac disease. Eight thousand years passed after the introduction of gluten into the human diet before celiac disease surfaced and came to medical attention. Over the following centuries, physicians came to believe that this was a rare disorder mainly affecting children of European origin. However, the epidemiology of celiac disease has been entirely rewritten during the past few decades, changing a series of paradigms and preconceptions. Unfortunately, many health care professionals and policy makers continue to perceive celiac as a rare condition of childhood.

From the Incidence to the Prevalence of Celiac Disease

The methods we use to measure how often celiac disease occurs have changed over the years. Early investigations reported the *incidence* of celiac disease, which is the number of new diagnoses in the study population during a given period. At first, diagnosis was entirely based on the detection of typical gastroenterological symptoms and confirmation by small intestine biopsy.[1] One of the first epidemiological studies conducted in 1950 established that the cumulative incidence of the disease in England and Wales was 1 in 8,000, but an incidence of 1 in 4,000 was detected in Scotland. At that time, diagnosis was difficult because of differing symptoms and was confirmed by nonspecific tests such as blood counts, certain vitamin levels, and symptomatic response to the gluten-free diet. Awareness of the disease greatly increased in the 1960s when more advanced tests such as intestinal biopsy became available. Consequently, in the mid 1970s, the incidence was reported to be 1 in 450–500 in studies from Ireland, Scotland, and Switzerland.[1]

In the 1980s, highly sensitive and specific screening tools first emerged. We began to measure blood antigliadin antibodies (AGA) first, and later the endomysial (EMA) and tissue transglutaminase (tTG) antibodies. These tests showed that many people had unsuspected celiac disease: Either they were without symptoms or they had symptoms that did not seem to be related to celiac disease. This made it apparent that we could not simply count the number of diagnosed cases to understand the epidemiology of celiac disease, because most atypical cases had escaped diagnosis. To determine the overall frequency with which celiac disease was occurring, we would need to screen a target population using a sensitive blood test. This is the way in which disease prevalence is measured, using the ratio between the number of affected individuals and the sampled population.

With this new approach, it has been well established that the prevalence of celiac disease throughout the world is similar in many regions.[2] Furthermore, these screening tests showed that celiac disease is one of the most common genetically based diseases, occurring in 1 of 130 to 300 people in the European population.[1,2] Another interesting observation is that despite similar genetic backgrounds and environmental factors, the clinical presentation of celiac disease may vary greatly in neighboring countries. This led researchers to incorrect conclusions. One example of this is Denmark, where the incidence of celiac disease was thought to be 1 in 10,000—almost 10-fold less than in Finland and 30-fold less than in Sweden, countries where the inhabitants share similar genetic backgrounds. More recent studies suggested that celiac disease was actually as frequent in Denmark as other Scandinavian countries, with a prevalence of 1 in 500 and that most cases in Denmark were undiagnosed because of the lack of typical symptoms. Factors such as type of cow's milk formulas, breast feeding, age at gluten introduction, quantity of gluten, and quality of cereals may all influence the type of symptoms that individuals develop.[1]

These results are not all that surprising, because celiac disease is the result of interactions between genetic (both human leukocyte antigen [HLA]- and non–HLA-associated genes) and environmental (gluten-containing grains) factors that would be shared in common among many European countries. It is also not surprising that recent epidemiological studies performed in regions such as North and South America, North Africa, the Middle East, and Asia, where celiac disease was traditionally considered rare despite the coexistence of the two risk factors (genes and gluten-containing grains), showed that the disease was under-diagnosed there as well.[2] As already seen in Europe, the symptoms of celiac disease in these countries varies greatly, which may explain the difference in prevalence previously reported. This difference stems from the fact that celiac disease with typical gastrointestinal symptoms and findings (in the intestine) is 15 times less common than celiac disease with atypical findings (effects outside of the intestine), which makes the diagnosis more challenging. These new findings also revealed that celiac disease contributes substantially to childhood illness and mortality in developing countries.[2]

The Celiac Iceberg

The epidemiology of celiac disease is easy to visualize using the iceberg model (Figure 1).[1] The prevalence of celiac disease can be seen in the overall size of the iceberg. Prevalence is influenced not only by the predisposing genes in the population but also by the pattern of gluten consumption. In countries where a large part of the population is of Caucasian origin, the prevalence of celiac disease is in the range of 0.5–1% of the general population. Most of these cases are properly diagnosed because of the patients' complaints, such as chronic diarrhea,

FIGURE 1. Celiac Iceberg

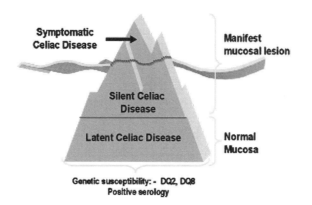

unexplained iron deficiency anemia, or for other reasons, such as a family history of celiac disease. These cases make up just the visible part of the celiac iceberg—the tip of the iceberg—which is what represents the incidence of the disease.

In developed countries, for each diagnosed case of celiac disease, an average of 5–10 cases remain undiagnosed, which is represented by the submerged part of the iceberg. Celiac disease is usually undiagnosed because of atypical, minimal, or even absent symptoms or complaints. These people with undiagnosed celiac disease remain untreated and are, therefore, at risk for long-term complications. The water line, namely the ratio of diagnosed to undiagnosed cases, mostly depends on the physician's decision to request blood tests for celiac disease markers when symptoms don't necessarily suggest it, so this hinges on the physician's awareness of the many possible manifestations of celiac disease. This is the reason that celiac blood testing, usually to measure immunoglobulin A tTG, is ordered whenever celiac disease is felt by the patient or clinician to be a possibility.

Some of the cases that are undiagnosed because of lack of symptoms can emerge later when the individual's health deteriorates. This "dynamic" aspect of the celiac disease iceberg has been clearly shown by a recent Finnish study of 3,654 schoolchildren.[3] When blood samples were collected in 1994, no cases of celiac disease were found in the study group. When the same group was tested seven years later, in 2001, 56 participants were positive for celiac antibodies and 27 participants were diagnosed with celiac disease by biopsy. Interestingly, 10 of the 56 who were positive for tTG antibodies had been diagnosed between 1994 and 2001 because they developed abdominal complaints.

How to deal with the celiac iceberg is currently a matter of debate in the scientific community.[4,5] At first glance, there seem to be good arguments in favor of mass screening:

- Celiac disease is a common disorder that causes significant illness in the general population.
- Early detection is often difficult because the symptoms of celiac disease are so diverse.

- Sensitive and simple screening tests are available, specifically the tTG antibody test.
- If left unrecognized and untreated, the disease can manifest with severe complications that are difficult to manage, such as infertility, osteoporosis, and lymphoma.
- There is an effective treatment—the gluten-free diet.

However, the cost of public screening efforts may not be worthwhile; this is an area that needs further clarification. Although it is well established that people with untreated celiac disease develop complications, the natural history of undiagnosed or untreated celiac disease, particularly the so-called silent form, remains unclear. Until we know more about this, we hesitate to suggest a gluten-free diet as a sort of blanket treatment because it can strongly interfere with quality of life, especially in adults. Also, despite the high sensitivity of the celiac disease blood markers, their predictive value decreases when applied to the general population. Furthermore, we don't know the appropriate age to begin screening for celiac disease. For all these reasons, the best approach to the iceberg of undiagnosed celiac disease seems to be to focus on at-risk groups, which minimizes costs and is ethically appropriate.[6] Recent data confirm that primary care physicians with increased awareness of the many diverse symptoms of celiac disease, coupled with a willingness to perform the celiac blood tests, can uncover a large portion of the submerged celiac disease iceberg.[6]

SELF-MANAGEMENT TIPS

☐ Celiac disease is equally common throughout most of North America, Europe, the Middle East, North Africa, and India.

☐ Most people who are diagnosed with celiac disease have typical gastro-intestinal symptoms. However, many people with celiac disease do not have these symptoms, and so diagnosis may be delayed or never made.

☐ Currently, screening the general population for celiac disease is not feasible.

☐ Improving awareness of celiac disease among primary care physicans is the best way to improve diagnostic rates and shorten the time to diagnosis and treatment.

References

1. Fasano A, Catassi C. Current approaches to diagnosis and treatment of celiac disease: an evolving spectrum. *Gastroenterology* 2001;120:636–51.
2. Fasano A, Araya M, Bhatnagar S, Cameron D, Catassi C, Dirks M, Mearin ML, Ortigosa L, Phillips A, Celiac Disease Working Group, FISPGHAN. Federation of International Societies of Pediatric Gastroenterology, Hepatology, and Nutrition consensus report on celiac disease. *J Pediatr Gastroenterol Nutr* 2008;47:214–19.

3. Mäki M, Mustalahti K, Kokkonen J, Kulmala P, Haapalahti M, Karttunen T, Ilonen J, Laurila K, Dahlbom I, Hansson T, Höpfl P, Knip M. Prevalence of celiac disease among children in Finland. *N Engl J Med* 2003;348:2517–24.
4. Fasano A. Should we screen for coeliac disease? Yes. *BMJ* 2009 Sep 17;339:b3592. doi: 10.1136/bmj.b3592.
5. Evans KE, McAllister R, Sanders DS. Should we screen for coeliac disease? No. *BMJ* 2009 Sep 17;339:b3674. doi: 10.1136/bmj.b3674
6. Catassi C, Kryszak D, Louis-Jacques O, Duerksen DR, Hill I, Crowe SE, Brown AR, Procaccini NJ, Wonderly BA, Hartley P, Moreci J, Bennett N, Horvath K, Burk M, Fasano A. Detection of celiac disease in primary care: a multicenter case-finding study in North America. *Am J Gastroenterol* 2007;102:1454–60.

Ahmet Aybar, MD, is a pediatric gastroenterology Fellow in the Department of Pediatrics, University of Maryland School of Medicine, Baltimore. **Alessio Fasano, MD,** is Professor of Pediatrics, Medicine, and Physiology, and Director, Mucosal Biology Research Center, University of Maryland School of Medicine, Baltimore.

CHAPTER 2

What Causes Celiac Disease, and Where Did It Come From?

Z. Myron Falchuk, MD

Celiac disease is a sensitivity to the protein gluten, which is found in some grains, most notably wheat. Ingestion of gluten results in great damage to epithelial cells that line the surface of the small intestine and is often associated with other negative effects throughout the body. Having healthy epithelial cells is crucial to the function of the small intestine. This type of cell is responsible for active digestion and absorption of sugars, fats, and proteins, which is accomplished with the help of enzymes located in the microvillus brush border of the epithelial cells (Figure 2, page 5). In addition, epithelial cells play a role in transporting digested nutrients from the intestine into the blood and lymphatic system for delivery to other parts of the body. When intestinal epithelial cells are damaged, digestion and absorption of nutrients are impaired, resulting in malabsorption (Figure 3, page 6). The effects of malabsorption range from trivial to severe. At one end of the spectrum are individuals who cannot absorb one dietary element, such as iron, so they develop anemia. At the other extreme are those who are unable to absorb any nutrients, including fats, sugars, carbohydrates, and trace minerals and vitamins, particularly fat-soluble vitamins. They develop severe diarrhea and malnutrition. In between these two extremes are individuals with many different presentations and symptoms, including those who are obese or whose primary complaint is constipation.

Celiac disease is not a new disease. What is new is our understanding that the disease is much more prevalent than we originally thought—about 1 in 3,000 people. Today we believe that 1 in 130 individuals has celiac disease. What created this change? Medical detective work. For many years, physicians have understood that disease in the small intestine and other digestive organs could produce diarrhea. In 1888, Samuel Gee published a report on the "Coeliac Affection." (The word *coeliac* came from the ancient Greek word *koeliac,* which referred to chronic diarrhea, more than 2,000 years ago.) Gee described patients with diarrhea and malnutrition and attributed the problem to dietary causes. He had no clue that gluten was the culprit. Over the years, much attention was paid to diarrheal diseases in children because malnutrition has such serious effects in this age group. Early in the last century, there was a prevalent condition known as *intestinal infantilism* that frequently resulted in children with failure to grow and even death. It is probable that this condition was actually celiac disease.

The earliest treatments involved elimination diets whose success was almost always one of chance. Bananas were extensively recommended, and some physicians even felt a magical power in this fruit, attributing some of its success to the presence of a special enzyme capable of hydrolyzing starches and sugars. The shortage of bananas during World War II created a panic in mothers treating their celiac babies with bananas. A big breakthrough in understanding celiac disease came in 1951 when Willem Dicke published the results of his observations that, during World War II, Dutch children with diarrheal disease improved dramatically with reduced wheat rations, and then worsened again once the grain supply returned to normal. His observations resulted in his understanding that gluten caused celiac disease and that the only effective treatment was a gluten-free diet.

Progress came quickly with the introduction of devices, first the Crosby capsule and later endoscopy, that allowed easy sampling of the small intestine lining (mucosa) for damage. Postmortem studies had shown major damage to the mucosa of patients who had died with celiac disease. The Crosby capsule allowed physicians to identify the classic damage in celiac disease: flattening of the absorptive villi and severe damage to the epithelial cell lining (Figure 3, page 6) as well as the presence of round cell inflammation. Being able to distinguish patients with celiac disease from others with unrelated diarrheal conditions made possible more targeted treatment with gluten-free diets.

The original theory was that celiac disease resulted from a missing but crucial enzyme that breaks down protein. The absence of this enzyme resulted in the inability to digest gluten as well as the production of toxins that damaged epithelial cells. Although many experiments confirmed the absence of such enzymes in the intestines of those with celiac disease, none of these deficiencies ever proved to be the source of the disease. Once these individuals were treated with the gluten-free diet, there were no more enzyme deficiencies, indicating that the absence of these enzymes was a consequence, not the cause, of the disease.

Current theories are based on an immunological cause for celiac disease: that gluten interacts with white blood cells in the lining of the intestine. White blood cells are vital to immune system function, but the interaction with gluten results in inflammation and production of immune chemicals and antibodies that damage the small intestine. The initial evidence to support this theory was circumstantial and included the observation of abnormally large numbers of white blood cells in the lining of the intestine. Other evidence to support a role for the immune system came from blood testing showing the presence of antigliadin antibodies (gliadin is the component of gluten that is injurious to the intestine) in those with celiac disease. Also, when treated with cortisone, which works to reduce immune reactions, people with celiac disease improved.

Our understanding of the role of genetics in immunologically related diseases such as celiac disease is growing in detail (see Chapter 6 on genetics). Studies showing that little pieces of small intestinal tissue can produce antigliadin antibodies outside of the body suggested that the inflammation was in the intestine rather than elsewhere in the body. A major breakthrough in our study of celiac disease came from the demonstration that tissue transglutaminase (tTG) antibody is present in more than 90% of people with celiac disease. tTG is central to the development of celiac disease. In the lining of the small intestine, tTG acts on gluten and changes to a form that is much more inflammatory. In the process, the body makes antibodies to tTG in the same way that gliadin antibodies are produced. Because it is almost always abnormal to make antibodies against parts of your own body, antibodies to tTG are very accurate for celiac disease testing (see Chapter 4 on celiac blood testing). Small bowel biopsy plus tTG testing are key in making the diagnosis and have allowed us to identify many previously undiagnosed people with celiac disease. In fact, the majority of people with celiac disease do not have diarrhea and malabsorption but a myriad of signs and symptoms (see Chapter 3 on uncommon presenting features).

Since Dicke's discovery, treatment for celiac disease has remained a strict gluten-free diet. Eliminating the symptoms and decreasing the risk of intestinal cancer and lymphoma are the main reasons for treating even those with minimal symptoms. Although efforts to produce wheat without some types of gliadin have been successful through genetic engineering, the presence of other gliadins in wheat prevents it from being included in the diet of someone with celiac disease. There must be total removal of gluten to control celiac disease. Celiac disease remains a unique disease that has helped us understand how environment, genetics, and immunology can interact in creating disease. Unraveling this puzzle over the last 130 years has been very gratifying.

Further Reading

- Abel E. The rise and fall of celiac disease in the United States. *J Hist Med Allied Sci* 2010;65:81–105.
- Falchuk M, et al. An in vitro model of gluten-sensitive enteropathy. *J Clin Invest* 1974;53:487–500.
- Falchuk M, et al. Predominance of histocompatibility antigen HL-A8 in patients with gluten-sensitive enteropathy. *J Clin Invest* 1972;51:1602–605.
- Falchuk M, et al. Gluten-sensitive enteropathy influence of histocompatibility type on gluten sensitivity in vitro. *J Clin Invest* 1980;66:227–33.

Z. Myron Falchuk, MD, is a gastroenterologist and Chief of Clinical Gastroenterology at the Celiac Disease Center, Beth Israel Deaconess Medical Center, and Associate Professor of Medicine, Harvard Medical School, Boston, Massachusetts.

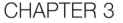

CHAPTER 3

Common and Uncommon Presentations of Celiac Disease

Ciaran P. Kelly, MD

Sanjeev, 65, was always tired. When his friends and family got together for parties and holiday gatherings, he learned to periodically hide in a quiet room to rest and regain his strength while the party carried on. A short nap on the couch was his first priority after getting home from work—dinner could wait. When his physician discovered, during a routine physical, that his liver blood tests were abnormal, Sanjeev feared the worst: incurable viral hepatitis, end-stage cirrhosis, or liver cancer. The diagnosis that ultimately was made by the liver specialist surprised everyone. Sanjeev had celiac disease!

He started a gluten-free diet (GFD) with mixed emotions. He was happy to have a treatable condition but mourned the loss of so many of his favorite foods. Within two weeks, his attitude changed. It seemed miraculous; he was enjoying a level of energy that he could only have dreamed of. He also enjoyed a sense of health and well-being that was new to him.

His digestive system also changed. He thought his intestines had been working fine, but now he could enjoy food in a whole new way. He had always been underweight but on the GFD he gained energy, strength, and pounds like never before. To cement his newfound devotion to the GFD, Sanjeev discovered that mistakes in the diet, usually caused by his eating a meal outside his own home, resulted in a brief but unwelcome return to his former lethargy, malaise, and digestive woes. Now, if anyone ever says he's tired, Sanjeev advocates immediate celiac antibody testing.

Recognizing Celiac Disease

Almost all systems and parts of the body may be affected by celiac disease. As a result, celiac disease has a reputation for being a clinical chameleon that wears many disguises. It presents or manifests in the body in many different ways. Unfortunately, this leads to delays in diagnosis and mistaken diagnoses, such as irritable bowel syndrome (IBS), lactose intolerance, and even imagined illness (somatization disorder).

A broad spectrum of symptoms (problems experienced by patients and reported to their health care provider, such as abdominal discomfort) and signs (problems directly observed by a health care provider, such as the skin rash of dermatitis herpetiformis) can occur in celiac disease. It can present in ways that are easier to recognize (called *typical*) or ways that are more difficult to recognize (called *atypical*). The typical and atypical presentations are described below. Although these descriptions are widely used and accepted, their use is open to question because the so-called atypical presentations may actually be as common as those that are called typical.

People with undiagnosed celiac disease can be found in almost any medical specialty clinic, from dermatology to neurology to orthopedic surgery to obstetrics and gynecology. The broad spectrum of symptoms highlights three needs for health care providers:

- to be on the lookout for celiac disease
- to be aware of the many types of clinical presentation
- to make good use of current, accurate diagnostic testing

Whether typical or atypical, none of the many symptoms and signs of celiac disease are unique to the disorder. In fact all are "nonspecific," which is to say they can also occur in many other conditions. This is why it is common for people to recognize their own symptoms in the long list of celiac-associated problems. If you have some of the symptoms and signs, you probably need to ask your physician about being tested for celiac disease by blood work and, if indicated, intestinal biopsy. These are the tests that can accurately diagnose celiac disease. It is not wise to guess at a diagnosis and start treatment with a GFD based on symptoms and signs alone. As often as not, the diagnosis is incorrect and this often leads to ineffective and unnecessary dietary restrictions, and leaves the real cause of the problem undiscovered.

Typical Manifestations of Celiac Disease

Gastrointestinal

As might be expected, the most common symptoms and signs of celiac disease are gastrointestinal. However, it is important to highlight the fact that many of those with untreated celiac disease have minimal or no gastrointestinal symptoms.

Diarrhea, abdominal bloating, and abdominal discomfort are the most common intestinal symptoms. Weight loss is less common and usually occurs in more severe cases. In fact, celiac disease is increasingly being diagnosed in overweight individuals. Diarrhea may be associated with urgency (having to rush to the bathroom) or even episodes of fecal incontinence (soiling accidents). Abdominal cramping can be severe, especially before and during the passage of a bowel movement. Stool may be abnormally loose and watery, of high volume, and contain undigested fat that floats in the toilet bowl. Diarrhea in celiac disease has two major causes. First, the injured small intestine becomes leaky and fluid secretion overtakes normal absorption (called *secretory diarrhea*). Second, components of the diet are not absorbed as they normally should be, and these malabsorbed nutrients hold water within the intestine, leading to worsening of diarrhea (called *osmotic diarrhea*). Diarrhea is often worse after meals but can also continue even when you have not eaten and awaken you in the middle of the night. Constipation is less common but does occur in a minority of those with untreated celiac disease, especially in childhood.

These gastrointestinal symptoms and signs are similar to those seen in IBS, and so it is important to check for the possibility of celiac disease before making the IBS diagnosis. The symptoms of lactose intolerance are also similar, with the important exception that celiac symptoms do not respond completely to treatment with lactase enzyme supplements or with a lactose-free diet.

Malabsorption and Nutritional Deficiencies

The damage to the small intestine that occurs in celiac disease leads to incomplete and inadequate absorption of nutrients from the diet. In addition to making diarrhea worse, malabsorption can lead to loss of protein, calories, vitamins, and minerals. When severe, protein and calorie malabsorption leads to muscle and weight loss.

The specific nutrient that most commonly becomes deficient in celiac disease is iron. This leads to iron deficiency anemia, which is now a very common initial presentation for celiac disease. Women who are menstruating (and lose iron through bleeding) or pregnant and growing children are the most susceptible to iron deficiency. In the past, folic acid deficiency was the second most common cause of anemia in celiac disease, but many foods now are fortified with folate, making deficiency far less common. Vitamin B_{12} deficiency is a third and important cause of anemia in untreated celiac disease. Importantly, vitamin B_{12} deficiency can also lead to disorders of the brain, spinal cord, and nerves in the arms and legs. This nerve injury may not reverse completely with vitamin B_{12} therapy, so early recognition and prevention are especially important.

Vitamin D is important in regulating calcium absorption from the gut as well as the "deposits and withdrawals" of calcium from the calcium bank in the bones (see Chapter 47 on bone disease). Vitamin D concentrations in the blood are commonly low in the U.S. population, especially in those living in northern climes where sun exposure is limited and less vitamin D is generated in skin. As a result, thinning of the bones, called *osteopenia* when it is mild and *osteoporosis* when it is more severe, is common in newly diagnosed celiac disease. In severe cases, calcium concentrations in the blood may fall, leading to muscle spasms (tetany). Over the long term, the body's practice of taking calcium from the bones to support blood calcium concentrations can lead to fractures in the spine and long bones that occur spontaneously or with minimal trauma.

Vitamin D is a fat-soluble vitamin whose absorption from the gut depends on fat absorption. Fat malabsorption in untreated celiac disease leads to vitamin D deficiency and, less often, to deficiencies of the other three fat-soluble vitamins, A, E, and K. Deficiency of vitamin A causes night blindness, whereas vitamin K deficiency leads to faulty blood clotting and excess bleeding. Vitamin E is an antioxidant that helps to protect cells against injury in situations of stress.

Other vitamin and mineral deficiencies in untreated celiac disease are less common and usually only seen in those with longstanding and untreated severe diarrhea, significant weight loss, and malnutrition.

Atypical Manifestations of Celiac Disease

The typical and atypical symptoms and signs of untreated celiac disease are listed in Table 1, organized by body system and according to whether they are likely to respond to treatment with a GFD. The resulting list is long and somewhat complex, which reflects the multiple, varied, and complex presentations of celiac disease.

A note of caution is warranted. Whether typical or atypical, none of the many manifestations of celiac disease are unique to the disorder and each can also occur in conditions other than celiac disease. If you or your physician recognize your symptoms within the long list of celiac-associated problems, this should prompt testing for celiac disease by blood work (Table 2) and, if indicated, intestinal biopsy. However, it is not wise to presume a diagnosis

TABLE 1. Celiac Disease Manifestations and Associations

Body System	Usually Responds to GFD Treatment	Sometimes Responds to GFD Treatment	Associated Conditions (Not Expected to Respond to GFD Treatment)
Typical presentations			
Gastrointestinal	Diarrhea Fecal urgency or incontinence Excess gas production Abdominal discomfort Abdominal bloating Constipation Fat in stool	Lactose intolerance Fructose malabsorption Heartburn Microscopic colitis	Inflammatory bowel disease Small intestinal bacterial over-growth

Nutritional deficiencies (oral supplements are often needed until intestine heals on GFD; see Chapter 14 on supplements)	Protein/calories
	Iron
	Vitamin B$_{12}$
	Folic acid
	Fat-soluble vitamins:
	   Vitamin D
	   Vitamins A, E, and K
	Calcium and other minerals
	Zinc and other trace elements		

Atypical presentations			
Immune system		Reduced function of the spleen	IgA deficiency Sarcoidosis Lupus (SLE)

TABLE 1. Celiac Disease Manifestations and Associations (*Continued*)

Body System	Usually Responds to GFD Treatment	Sometimes Responds to GFD Treatment	Associated Conditions (Not Expected to Respond to GFD Treatment)
Brain and nerves		Fatigue Depressed mood Poor concentration	Poor coordination (cerebellar ataxia) Tingling and numbness of hands and feet (peripheral neuropathy) Seizure disorder
Skin and hair	Dermatitis herpetiformis	Alopecia (hair loss) Follicular keratosis	Patches of depigmentation (vitiligo)
Mouth	Canker sores (aphthous ulcers) Angular cheilitis (cracks at the corners of the mouth)	Dental enamel loss	
Liver	Abnormally high liver enzymes on blood testing		Primary biliary cirrhosis Autoimmune hepatitis
Bones and joints		Short stature Thinning of the bones (osteoporosis and osteopenia) Joint pains	Rheumatoid arthritis
Blood	Anemia from deficiency of: Iron Vitamin B_{12} Folic acid		
Reproductive		Reduced fertility (men and women) Recurrent miscarriages	

(*continued*)

TABLE 1.   Celiac Disease Manifestations and Associations (*Continued*)

Body System	Usually Responds to GFD Treatment	Sometimes Responds to GFD Treatment	Associated Conditions (Not Expected to Respond to GFD Treatment)
Endocrine glands			Type 1 diabetes Thyroid disease Addison's disease
Kidney			IgA nephropathy
Lung			Fibrosing alveolitis Pulmonary hemosiderosis Lung cavities

and start treatment with a GFD based on symptoms and signs alone. As often as not, the diagnosis is incorrect and can lead to ineffective and unnecessary dietary restrictions while leaving the real cause of the problem undiagnosed and untreated.

If you have symptoms and signs from multiple categories, that is an even stronger indication that you need to be tested. The cost of a missed or delayed diagnosis can be substantial in terms of your suffering and unnecessary testing and treating for other disorders. Conversely, the cost of blood testing for celiac disease using the tissue transglutaminase antibody assay (or the newer deamidated gliadin peptide test) is modest, and the test is easy to perform and widely available. The bottom line is that the best approach is simple: If you think that celiac disease is a possibility, get tested for it. Testing is easy and accurate.

TABLE 2.   Common Situations Where Testing for Untreated Celiac Disease Is Appropriate

- Chronic or recurrent gastrointestinal symptoms, including
  - Symptoms suggesting irritable bowel syndrome
  - Symptoms suggesting lactose intolerance that do not resolve on a lactose-free diet
- Unexplained iron deficiency anemia
- Unexplained, marked vitamin D deficiency
- Unexplained osteoporosis
- Unexplained vitamin B_{12} deficiency
- Unexplained weight loss (or failure to gain weight in children)

SELF-MANAGEMENT TIPS

☐ The most typical symptoms and signs of celiac disease result from intestinal injury with malabsorption and include gastrointestinal problems and nutritional deficiencies.

☐ Many people with untreated celiac disease have no gastrointestinal symptoms or nutritional deficiencies but instead have a wide and varied range of problems affecting many different organ systems.

☐ Because of the varied and nonspecific nature of celiac disease manifestations, it's important that
  – patients and health care providers watch out for celiac disease
  – patients and health care providers learn more about the many types of presentation
  – individuals receive accurate diagnostic testing before starting treatment with a GFD

Ciaran P. Kelly, MD, is Medical Director, Celiac Disease Center, Beth Israel Deaconess Medical Center, and Professor of Medicine, Harvard Medical School, Boston, Massachusetts.

CHAPTER 4

Blood Tests in Celiac Disease

Daniel A. Leffler, MD, MS, and Detlef Schuppan, MD, PhD

Beth is a 27-year-old woman who has had "stomach problems" on and off since high school. She had read about gluten sensitivity in a magazine article and decided that she would like to be tested for this condition. She discussed this with her physician, who was not familiar with celiac disease, but after discussing it they decided to get "the works" and sent Beth's blood samples off for a number of tests for celiac disease (Table 1). Beth went home and spent some time on the Internet, then decided to pursue some further testing on her own. The results of all these tests are shown in Table 1. Beth and her primary care physician are now trying to sort out whether she has celiac disease.

An Overview of Celiac Testing

Contemporary tests for celiac disease are more accurate than nearly any other blood test used to detect or monitor inflammatory or autoimmune disorders. Each test relies on the identification of specific antibodies that are produced at higher levels in people with active celiac disease. They are often called *serologic tests,* which refers to identification of antibodies in serum, the fluid portion of blood.

Blood testing in celiac disease has had a checkered past. Earlier generations of tests were not very accurate. However, the past decade has seen remarkable growth in the number and quality of these tests, which is the main reason why so many people are now being correctly diagnosed with celiac disease. Yet, the number of tests available also results in significant confusion for both patients and physicians about which test to order and how to interpret the results. The majority of the following discussion applies equally to adults and adolescents, although there are some differences in very young children that are noted. Also, all celiac tests are expected to normalize on a gluten-free diet (GFD), so their use for diagnosis depends on you continuing to eat gluten.

Antigliadin Antibodies

The first serologic test developed for use in celiac disease was antigliadin antibodies (AGA), which began to be used in the early 1980s. This was a major step forward; before AGA

TABLE 1. Tests for Celiac Disease

Test*	Normal Range	Beth's Result	Comments
IgA antigliadin antibody (IgA-AGA)	<20 units†	18 units	Inferior to IgA-tTG in most cases; should not be routinely ordered
IgG antigliadin antibody (IgG-AGA)	<20 units†	46 units	High false positive rate; may be ordered in people with IgA deficiency if IgG-DGP is not available
IgA tissue transglutaminase (IgA-tTG)	<20 units†	12 units	Test of choice in most cases because of accuracy and cost
Endomysial antibody (EMA)	<1:20	1:5	Very accurate but less sensitive than IgA-tTG, which has replaced this as the test of choice in most areas
Total IgA	70–400 mg/dL	126 mg/dL	Should be ordered in all initial celiac testing to rule out IgA deficiency
IgA deamidated gliadin peptide (IgA-DGP)	<20 units†	14 units	Nearly as accurate as IgA-tTG or IgA-EMA
IgG deamidated gliadin peptide (IgG-DGP)	<20 units†	16 units	Test of choice in IgA-deficient individuals
IgA/IgG deamidated gliadin peptide (IgA/IgG-DGP)	<20 units†	12 units	Test of choice in IgA-deficient individuals
RAST (radio-allergosorbent test) allergen testing for wheat	<0.35: undetectable† 0.35–0.70: low 0.71–3.50: moderate 3.51–17.5: high >17.5: very high	0.78 kU/L	RAST tests for levels of IgE antibody (IgE antibody is involved in most allergic disorders) to specific proteins/allergens. If RAST is highly positive to a particular food, it is likely that you have allergic antibodies to that food. Unfortunately, 20–30% of people with a negative RAST can still have an allergic reaction and many people with a positive RAST (especially in the moderate range) have no reaction. So, both negative as well as positive findings could be misleading. If the RAST to a particular food is nonreactive, skin testing to that food must be performed.

TABLE 1. Tests for Celiac Disease (*Continued*)

Test*	Normal Range	Beth's Result	Comments
Immunocap wheat IgE	<0.35: undetectable[†] 0.35–0.70: low 0.71–3.50: moderate 3.51–17.5: high >17.5: very high	1.18 kU/L	Similar to RAST testing, Immunocap tests for allergen specific IgE antibodies and is useful in the diagnosis of some allergic disorders
Skin prick	<4 mm mark: normal 5–10 mm mark: mild sensitivity 10–15 mm mark: moderate sensitivity >15 mm mark: high sensitivity	No significant reaction to wheat	Skin tests are performed by exposing a tiny area of scratched skin to the food being evaluated. A positive skin test results in a mosquito-bite–like reaction at the site of the test. Skin prick testing is usually done when RAST is negative but a particular allergen is suspected. False positives and negatives are common; however, if skin testing to fresh food extract is negative, there is a 95% chance that the food can be eaten without an allergic reaction.
Saliva AGA test[‡]	§	29	Nonvalidated test; should not be routinely used; unclear how to interpret results in the absence of published studies. Appears to have high false positive rate.
Saliva tTG/EMA test[‡]	§	11	See comments for saliva AGA test.
Stool AGA test	§	36	See comments for saliva AGA test.
Stool tTG/EMA test	§	20	See comments for saliva AGA test.

IgA, immunoglobulin A; IgG, immunoglobulin G; IgE, immunoglobulin E.
*Tests are performed on blood unless otherwise noted.
[†]Normal range may vary in different labs.
[‡]Note that this refers to salivary antibody testing, not the salivary genetics testing discussed in Chapter 6 on genetic testing.
§Normal ranges not well established.

testing was available, only clinical suspicion and duodenal biopsy were available for celiac testing. Both immunoglobulin A and G (IgA and IgG) class antibodies can be tested for and are considered to provide similar accuracy. AGA tests are about 80% accurate. Although that may sound good at first, it really means that most people with a positive test do not have celiac disease.[1,2] This is significantly lower than any of the more recently developed tests, and for this reason, AGA testing has largely fallen out of favor. They may, however, still be useful for testing young children and suspected gluten-related neurological disorders.

The one advantage of AGA testing that has ensured its survival over the past decades is the availability of an IgG-based test for use in people with IgA deficiency (see Chapter 7 on diagnostic dilemmas). However, in the past few years, other tests based on IgG have been developed that are, in general, superior to IgG-AGA in terms of accuracy. For these reasons, AGA testing is not routinely needed or recommended these days.

Endomysial Antibodies

Endomysial antibody (EMA) testing was developed in the mid-1980s and found to be significantly more accurate that AGA testing. However, the EMA test is less commonly performed because it is more expensive and more technically difficult than other newer tests. Nevertheless, in centers with significant experience with EMA, this still may be the test of choice but its sensitivity is lower than that of the IgA tissue transglutaminase (IgA-tTG) test. There seems to be little benefit to testing both EMA and IgA-tTG simultaneously, because the agreement rate of these tests is very high, and individuals testing positive for either test should be referred for endoscopy.

Tissue Transglutaminase

In 1997, Detlef Schuppan's research group identified tTG as the target to which the auto-antibodies react in the EMA test.[3] This allowed for the creation of a test that essentially measures the same thing as EMA but is much easier to perform, more sensitive, and more cost effective. Early tTG assays used transglutaminase derived from guinea pig liver. Most assays now use human recombinant tTG, which is more accurate. As with EMA, you must be certain to measure total IgA level along with IgA-tTG to check for selective IgA deficiency. Someone with IgA deficiency will have a false negative result for IgA-tTG; their tests need to measure IgG antibodies.

In addition to standard laboratory-based tTG assays, tTG-based fingerstick testing has sensitivity similar to standard tTG assays but lower specificity.[4] The benefits of this test include ease of interpretation (positive or negative), no laboratory processing, and results within minutes, all of which aid in clinical decision making. Another major limitation, however, is that it does not provide a measure of the amount of antibodies, which is necessary for following an individual's response to the GFD over time.

Deamidated Gliadin Peptide

The most recently developed test is for deamidated gliadin peptide (DGP). Gluten in its normal form does not cause much inflammation in most adults. However, tTG changes (deamidates) gluten into a much more inflammatory protein. For this reason, antibodies to deamidated gliadin are a much more accurate measure of the reaction to gluten than antibodies to native gluten (AGA antibodies) and almost as accurate as IgA-tTG testing.[5] The major advantage of DGP is that the IgG-DGP test is better than any of the other IgG tests, so IgG-DGP or a combined IgA/IgG-DGP is now the best test to use in people who are IgA deficient.

Celiac Testing in Young Children

As for adults, IgA-tTG is the test of choice for most children.[6] Data suggest, however, that all serologic tests become less sensitive in children who are under the age of 2. Early reports suggested that AGA was better than EMA in very young children,[7] however, newer data suggest that IgA-tTG and IgA-DGP testing is as good as or more accurate than AGA testing even in children under the age of 3.[8,9]

Serologic Testing for Celiac Disease Monitoring

Serologic testing for diagnosis of celiac disease is highly accurate. Unfortunately, these tests are not very useful for monitoring either how closely someone is following a GFD or whether the small intestine is healing.[10,11] Testing for tTG, EMA, or DGP will not reliably indicate whether someone is eating gluten free and is less accurate than simply asking if you are avoiding gluten and how you are doing it.[12,13]

Other Tests

Allergen Testing for Wheat
Allergic reactions to foods occur in the following conditions:

- an individual has IgE antibodies that recognize and attach to a particular food component; these IgE antibodies attach to the surface of specific immune system cells called *mast cells*
- the individual eats the food component that is recognized by the IgE antibodies; the food component (usually a protein) then causes the mast cells to release histamine and other chemicals that cause an allergic reaction

Allergic reactions to foods have the following characteristics, which help to distinguish allergic reactions from other types of adverse food reactions:

- small amounts of the food can cause an allergic reaction
- reactions usually occur every time the food is eaten
- reactions occur rapidly after eating the food: most within 30 minutes and nearly all within 4 hours

Any food can cause an allergic reaction, but 90% of all allergic reactions are related to one of the following eight foods: eggs, fish, milk, peanuts, shellfish, soy, tree nuts, and wheat.

A blood test for IgE to specific foods, called *RAST* (radio-allergo-sorbent test, named after the original method used for the test), is useful in screening for allergies, especially when there has been a reaction that was severe or life-threatening but had no clear cause. The test is specific when results are highly positive, so if your RAST is significantly positive to a particular food, it is likely that you have allergic antibodies to that food. However, many people with moderately positive RAST results will not have a noticeable reaction to that food. Unfortunately, the test also lacks sensitivity. This means that in 20–30% of cases when the RAST to a particular food is nonreactive, there could still be IgE specific to that food throughout the body that would react if the food were eaten. Therefore, both negative and positive findings could be misleading. If the RAST to a particular food is negative but allergy is still suspected, skin testing to that food can be performed to confirm results.

Stool and Saliva Tests

A variety of tests for celiac disease, gluten sensitivity, and other inflammatory disorders are available through commercial laboratories. Although it is possible that these categories of tests may provide some useful information beyond what is available through standard blood testing for celiac disease, there have been few published studies of these tests, so it is difficult for most physicians to interpret or use the results. However, these few studies suggest that saliva and stool tests are inferior to equivalent blood tests.[14,15] Although it is understandably attractive to obtain results without having to have blood drawn, most people with known or suspected celiac disease require other blood tests, such as a complete blood count or iron levels, so there is little to be gained from routinely performing saliva or stool tests.

What Beth Decided

After puzzling over her results for some time (Table 1), Beth and her physician decided that, with no family history of celiac disease or other autoimmune disorders and no abnormalities on her blood tests (she was not anemic and had no apparent vitamin deficiencies), her probability of having celiac disease with a normal IgA-tTG level was quite low. Because her symptoms were mild and chronic, she decided not to pursue further testing or to consult a gastroenterologist but would follow up with her primary care physician on a regular basis.

SELF-MANAGEMENT TIPS

- ☐ Blood tests for celiac disease are simple and accurate.
- ☐ IgA-tTG is currently the test of choice in most settings because it is highly accurate, reliable, inexpensive, and easy to interpret. It's important also to measure total IgA to be sure that the result will be reliable.
- ☐ EMA and DGP testing also provide accurate results depending on regional expertise.
- ☐ AGA testing is not as reliable and should not be routinely used for celiac disease diagnosis, with the possible exception of young children and gluten-related neurologic disorders.
- ☐ All celiac antibodies normalize on a GFD. Therefore, testing for diagnosis is accurate only if you are eating gluten.
- ☐ Your test should be repeated over the first two years of treatment with the GFD to check for improvement in levels of antibodies.

References

1. Rostom A, Murray JA, Kagnoff MF. American Gastroenterological Association (AGA) Institute technical review on the diagnosis and management of celiac disease. *Gastroenterology* 2006;131:1981–2002.

2. Hill ID. What are the sensitivity and specificity of serologic tests for celiac disease? Do sensitivity and specificity vary in different populations? *Gastroenterology* 2005;128:S25–32.

3. Dieterich W, Ehnis T, Bauer M, Donner P, Volta U, Riecken EO, Schuppan D. Identification of tissue transglutaminase as the autoantigen of celiac disease. *Nat Med* 1997;3:797–801.

4. Raivio T, Korponay-Szabo I, Collin P, Laurila K, Huhtala H, Kaartinen T, Partanen J, Maki M, Kaukinen K. Performance of a new rapid whole blood coeliac test in adult patients with low prevalence of endomysial antibodies. *Dig Liver Dis* 2007;39:1057–63.

5. Lewis NR, Scott BB. Meta-analysis: deamidated gliadin peptide (DGP) antibody and tissue transglutaminase (tTG) antibody compared as screening tests for coeliac disease. *Aliment Pharmacol Ther* 2010;31(1):73–81.

6. Hill ID, Dirks MH, Liptak GS, Colletti RB, Fasano A, Guandalini S, Hoffenberg EJ, Horvath K, Murray JA, Pivor M, Seidman EG. Guideline for the diagnosis and treatment of celiac disease in children: recommendations of the North American Society for Pediatric Gastroenterology, Hepatology and Nutrition. *J Pediatr Gastroenterol Nutr* 2005;40:1–19.

7. Burgin-Wolff A, Dahlbom I, Hadziselimovic F, Petersson CJ. Antibodies against human tissue transglutaminase and endomysium in diagnosing and monitoring coeliac disease. *Scand J Gastroenterol* 2002;37:685–91.

8. Holding S, Abuzakouk M, Dore PC. Antigliadin antibody testing for coeliac disease in children under 3 years of age is unhelpful. *J Clin Pathol* 2009;62:766–67.

9. Basso D, Guariso G, Fogar P, Meneghel A, Zambon CF, Navaglia F, Greco E, Schiavon S, Rugge M, Plebani M. Antibodies against synthetic deamidated gliadin peptides for celiac disease diagnosis and follow-up in children. *Clin Chem* 2009;55:150–57.

10. Dickey W, Hughes DF, McMillan SA. Disappearance of endomysial antibodies in treated celiac disease does not indicate histological recovery. *Am J Gastroenterol* 2000;95:712–14.

11. Tursi A, Brandimarte G, Giorgetti GM. Lack of usefulness of anti-transglutaminase antibodies in assessing histologic recovery after gluten-free diet in celiac disease. *J Clin Gastroenterol* 2003;37: 387–91.

12. Vahedi K, Mascart F, Mary JY, Laberenne JE, Bouhnik Y, Morin MC, Ocmant A, Velly C, Colombel JF, Matuchansky C. Reliability of antitransglutaminase antibodies as predictors of gluten-free diet compliance in adult celiac disease. *Am J Gastroenterol* 2003;98:1079–87.

13. Leffler DA, Edwards George JB, Dennis M, Cook EF, Schuppan D, Kelly CP. A prospective comparative study of five measures of gluten-free diet adherence in adults with coeliac disease. *Aliment Pharmacol Ther* 2007;26:1227–35.

14. Baldas V, Tommasini A, Santon D, Not T, Gerarduzzi T, Clarich G, Sblattero D, Marzari R, Florian F, Martellossi S, Ventura A. Testing for anti-human transglutaminase antibodies in saliva is not useful for diagnosis of celiac disease. *Clin Chem* 2004;50:216–19.

15. Halblaub JM, Renno J, Kempf A, Bartel J, Schmidt-Gayk H. Comparison of different salivary and fecal antibodies for the diagnosis of celiac disease. *Clin Lab* 2004;50:551–57.

Detlef Schuppan, MD, PhD, is Professor of Medicine at Harvard Medical School, Boston, Massachusetts, and the University of Munich, Germany. He is Director of Research at the Celiac Center at Beth Israel Deaconess Medical Center and serves on the board of multiple international gastroenterology associations. He has been a leader in the field of celiac disease for many years and was responsible for first identifying the role of tissue transglutaminase in celiac disease. Dr. Schuppan has published more than 300 papers, and his current work focuses on the immune mechanisms underlying both celiac disease and liver disease.

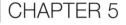

CHAPTER 5

Endoscopy in Celiac Disease

Daniel A. Leffler, MD, MS

José is a 55-year-old man who recently had an immunoglobulin A (IgA) tissue transglutaminase blood test done after his sister was diagnosed with celiac disease. He was quite surprised when the level returned elevated at 88 units (normal is less than 20 units), as he had considered himself quite healthy. Nevertheless, he did have what he considered a "sensitive stomach," with intermittent episodes of diarrhea, especially in times of stress. After reading about how accurate this blood test was for celiac disease, he was willing to begin a gluten-free diet (GFD). But José was dubious when we suggested that, before he starts eating gluten free, he have an endoscopy to biopsy the first portion of his small intestine (the duodenum) to confirm the diagnosis of celiac disease.

What Is an Endoscopy?

An endoscopy of the upper part of the gastrointestinal tract, also known as an esophagogastroduodenoscopy (EGD), is a procedure in which a thin tube (about the width of your little finger) is passed through the mouth into the beginning of the small intestine (Figure 1). Although this procedure is often performed with sedation, many individuals can tolerate this procedure comfortably with only numbing medication sprayed in the back of the throat. The endoscopist will look carefully at your esophagus, stomach, and small intestine for any visual abnormalities. Although changes on the surface can occasionally be seen in celiac disease, looking under a microscope is much more accurate. Once the tube is in the small intestine, the person performing the EGD passes a tiny set of forceps (like tweezers) through the endoscope and takes small pieces of intestinal lining for microscopic examination. The intestine does not have nerves that sense this type of sampling, so you don't feel the biopsies being taken. The entire procedure usually takes only about five minutes, and risks in most individuals are very, very small.

FIGURE 1. Endoscopy

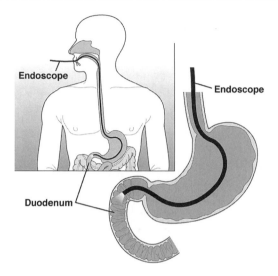

Why Perform an Endoscopy?

Although the current blood tests for celiac disease are very good, they are not perfect. The blood test can be both falsely positive and falsely negative, so deciding what to do with the result depends on the type of symptoms and other risk factors for celiac disease that you have. In other words, someone with significant symptoms associated with celiac disease, such as diarrhea and anemia, should consider an endoscopy even if the blood tests are negative. On the other hand, if you have a positive blood test, you need a biopsy to confirm the diagnosis. The other benefit of having a biopsy for diagnosis is that, regardless of the outcome, it provides a baseline description of the condition of your small intestine. If you have new or continued symptoms, or if other problems occur in the future, your doctor can compare a follow-up biopsy to your initial one to see what changes have occurred (see Chapter 34 on nonresponsive celiac disease). In about a quarter of patients, the endoscopist can see changes consistent with celiac disease right away, while in most, the intestine can look normal at first, but under the microscope there are clear changes related to celiac disease. It is important to have the endoscopy *before* starting a GFD, because once you are on the diet, your intestine will start to heal, which makes diagnosis difficult.[1,2]

When Is an Endoscopy Unnecessary?

Before accurate blood tests were available, we recommended that patients have a routine follow-up biopsy after being on the GFD for some time. This is no longer routinely done as long as your symptoms and blood test results show improvement. If you have a blood test that is positive for celiac disease and a skin biopsy that is consistent with dermatitis herpetiformis, it's not always necessary to have an endoscopic biopsy for diagnosis. We are also studying ways to avoid endoscopy in young children, who tend not to tolerate procedures as well as adults. Although using a biopsy to confirm a diagnosis is still the standard of care for children, some clinicians avoid endoscopy in the very young. For most individuals, diagnosis of celiac disease requires small intestinal biopsy. However, some people, based on their symptoms and blood test results, may, in consultation with their physician, choose not to pursue endoscopy before starting a GFD. In the future, new tests and techniques may take the place of endoscopy for celiac diagnosis in certain populations.

Outcome

We discussed the risks and benefits of undergoing the endoscopy with biopsy with José, and he chose to undergo the procedure in our clinic the next week under standard sedation. In his case, the biopsies showed damage consistent with the diagnosis of celiac disease. He started a GFD and continues to do well.

SELF-MANAGEMENT TIPS

☐ Endoscopy with small intestinal biopsy is currently recommended for confirmation of nearly all cases of suspected celiac disease.[1,2]

☐ Both false negatives and false positives are possible with current celiac blood testing.

☐ Endoscopy is safe and generally very well tolerated.

☐ An initial intestinal biopsy before starting a GFD provides important baseline information for comparison if problems arise in the future.

References

1. Rostom A, Murray JA, Kagnoff MF. American Gastroenterological Association (AGA) Institute technical review on the diagnosis and management of celiac disease. *Gastroenterology* 2006; 131:1981–2002.
2. Green PH, Cellier C. Celiac disease. *N Engl J Med* 2007;357:1731–43.

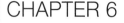

CHAPTER 6

Genetic Testing in Celiac Disease

Michelle Pietzak, MD

Amy will return today to our gastroenterology clinic with her two young children. I first saw Amy, a 28-year-old mother, two years ago with her then 5-year-old son, Brian. At that time, Brian was complaining of abdominal pain daily and having loose bowel movements. His pediatrician had ordered stool studies, which revealed that Brian was infected with a parasite called *Giardia*. Brian was treated several times for this infection and was put on a high-fiber diet for the diarrhea, but nothing made his symptoms better. He was beginning to lose weight, which prompted a referral to a pediatric gastroenterologist.

Amy said that Brian had been toilet trained at age 2½ years but now was having accidents at school. He also seemed more tired than usual and had begun taking naps again after coming home from Kindergarten. On physical exam, Brian was short for his age but of average weight. His mother said that he had been wearing the same sized clothes and shoes for the past year and that he did not seem to be growing. There was a family history of autoimmune diseases. Amy has Grave's disease, a form of hypothyroidism, and required in vitro fertilization to become pregnant with her two children. Amy's niece, Emily, has type 1 diabetes. Amy's mother, Debra, has rheumatoid arthritis for which she takes prednisone, an immune-suppressing steroid medication.

At the first visit, Brian's blood tests showed levels of IgG antigliadin antibody (AGA) greater than 100 units (normal is less than 10 units) but undetectable levels of IgA-AGA, IgA tissue transglutaminase (tTG) antibody, or IgA endomysial antibody (EMA). Further blood tests revealed that this was because his total blood IgA level was very low. He also had iron deficiency anemia and vitamin D deficiency. Brian's liver tests, thyroid studies, and other vitamin levels were normal. He had an upper endoscopy under anesthesia, and his intestinal biopsies confirmed that he had celiac disease.

Brian started a gluten-free diet (GFD) immediately. He also took gluten-free prescription iron and vitamin supplements. Within the first month, Brian's diarrhea and energy level both improved. After about six months, Brian needed larger clothing and shoes. After one year on a GFD, his IgG-AGA had dropped to 7 units, and he no longer had anemia or vitamin D deficiency. I offered antibody testing for celiac disease to Brian's parents, who both stated that they were in good health and did not want to be tested. Brian's father,

Mark, admitted that even if he did have a positive test, that he would "never be able to stick to a GFD because I like beer and pizza too much."

At today's visit, Amy tells me that Brian is doing well and that she has no concerns about him. He is now 7 years old, in 2nd grade, and has regular, daily bowel movements that are formed and not watery. His weight and height are both at the 75th percentile for age. He has an excellent appetite and is active in soccer. However, Amy has concerns both for herself and Brian's new little sister, Olivia. Olivia is now 4 months old, and has been exclusively breastfed since birth. She appears to be growing and gaining weight well and does not have any obvious medical problems. Amy is hesitant to introduce gluten-containing cereals into Olivia's diet, as she does not want her to experience the same medical problems as her brother. Also, during her first trimester of pregnancy, Amy began to experience symptoms of reflux, gas, and bloating. She put herself on a GFD, and her symptoms resolved.

Amy has remained gluten free for the past 10 months. However, she is not sure if she has celiac disease or if her symptoms were because of the pregnancy. She would like to have herself and Olivia tested for celiac disease at today's visit. She is also now advocating that Brian's grandmother eat gluten free to see if it helps her arthritis. What testing options are available to mother Amy and little sister Olivia? Should Grandma Debra and niece Emily be tested? Would genetic testing for celiac disease be helpful in their specific cases?

Which Genes Convey Risk for Celiac Disease?

Like most diseases, celiac disease is caused by both genetic and environmental factors. We believe it occurs only in genetically susceptible individuals who ingest gluten and occurs in about 1% of the U.S. population.[1] We know it runs in families and also that having a family member with another autoimmune disease increases the risk for celiac disease. A twin sibling also has a higher likelihood of having celiac disease if identical, rather than fraternal. This information led researchers to believe that there was a strong genetic component to the condition. However, the question became: which gene or genes? The genetics of celiac disease are complex, as they do not follow a simple dominant or recessive pattern seen with many other diseases thought to be because of genetic components.

The genes thought to play the biggest role in risk for development of celiac disease are the class II human leukocyte antigens (HLA) -DQ2 and -DQ8.[2] HLA are markers found on the white blood cells. The role of class II antigens is to identify "self" versus "nonself" via the immune system. Nonself can be a bacterial or viral infection, a transplanted organ, or even food proteins. In the case of celiac disease, the nonself recognized by the HLA are gluten proteins. When someone with celiac disease ingests wheat, more than 50 large wheat fragments are created during digestion that can be potentially recognized by the immune system as nonself. The enzyme tTG (the same one to which you make the antibody) changes the shape of some gluten fragments into molecules that can then interact with HLA-DQ2 like a key (gluten) in a lock (the HLA) on the immune system's antigen-presenting cell (APC). The APC then presents the gluten-HLA complex as a foreign invader to an army of T lymphocytes (white blood cells that cause inflammation). These T-cells become "activated" and call in the immune army to that site of the small bowel, leading to intestinal damage. They also stimulate

B lymphocytes (white blood cells that produce antibodies) to produce antibodies to gliadin, tTG, and EMA. Without HLA-DQ2, the gluten is not recognized as nonself by the APC and does not stimulate the same vigorous immune response. Thus, without the right HLA, someone can eat as much gluten as they want and not develop celiac disease.

HLA-DQ2 is common in Western Europe, Central Asia, and Northern and Western Africa. Depending on the population studied, HLA-DQ2 occurs in 78–95% of patients with biopsy-proven celiac disease, with HLA-DQ8 or a combination of HLA-DQ2/DQ8 occurring in most of the rest. However, these genes have been found in close to 40% of the population without celiac disease. Because of this, genetic testing is not the best method to diagnose or screen for celiac disease. However, it is very rare for someone to develop celiac disease and not possess HLA-DQ2 and/or HLA-DQ8.

Our research has focused on the HLA genes that put patients at risk for celiac disease. It appears that HLA-DQ2 and HLA-DQ8 in combination with other high-risk genes can increase the risk for celiac disease. We found that, in more than 4,000 people at risk for celiac disease, 28–31% of those who had two copies of the HLA-DQ2 (homozygous for this high-risk gene) were EMA positive.[3] These results were validated in a larger study with samples from more than 10,000 at-risk subjects and held true for both children and adults.[4,5] Therefore, knowing someone's HLA-DQ genotype can be a powerful tool for determining individual risk for celiac disease (Table 1).

Celiac disease is considered to be a complex genetic disorder, with the presence of HLA-DQ2 and DQ8 accounting for about 35 to 40% of the genetic familial load. Researchers have identified eight previously unknown regions in non-HLA genes that contribute significantly toward risk for celiac disease in a Northern European population.[6] These regions harbor genes associated with controlling the immune response, such as IL2–IL21 and IL18RAP (interleukins, signaling molecules from white blood cells, and their receptors), CCR3 (a chemokine/protein receptor), and SH2B3 (a gene that regulates white blood cell

TABLE 1. Genetic Risk for Celiac Disease

HLA-DQ Genotype	EMA Positive	Risk Category
Two copies of DQ2* (DQ2.5 plus either another DQ2.5 or DQ2.2)	28–31%	Extremely high
One copy of DQ2.2 with another high-risk gene	13–16%	Very high
One copy of DQ2 and one copy of DQ8	12–14%	Very high
One copy of DQ2.5	9–10%	High
Two copies of DQ8	8–10%	High
One copy of DQ8	2%	Moderate
One copy of DQ2.2 with another low-risk gene	<1%	Low
Neither DQ2 nor DQ8	<0.1%	Extremely low

*The DQ2 molecule is made up of two chains. The two genes that code for these chains can both be from one parent or one gene can come from each parent. It appears that getting the genes from the same parent is higher risk than getting them from different parents. See references 5 and 10 for further information.

signaling). Some of these reported regions are also of interest in Grave's disease, type 1 diabetes, and rheumatoid arthritis (see Chapter 44 on autoimmune diseases). These eight regions may explain an additional 3–4% of the heritability of celiac disease and why only a minority of people who have the HLA-DQ2/DQ8 genes eventually develop celiac disease. However, testing for these genes is currently just a research tool and not commercially available.

How Is Genetic Testing Done?

HLA testing can be done on any tissue in the body and is commonly performed to find matches for organ or bone marrow transplantation. Testing for the HLA types associated with celiac disease can be done with a blood test, saliva test, or from cells rubbed from the cheek with a cotton swab. Because the test measures the HLA that you were born with and these genes are not changed by diet, HLA testing can be done while on a GFD. This is in contrast to antibody testing, where a prolonged GFD can lead to negative antibody tests.

What If I Test Positive?

Although genetic testing is imperfect, it is safe and easy and can be useful to both patient and physician when deciding on further testing for potential celiac disease under certain circumstances. If someone lacks the HLA-DQ types commonly seen in celiac disease, it makes the diagnosis very unlikely (high negative predictive value). However, most people possessing these genes will not go on to develop celiac disease (low positive predictive value). A small intestinal biopsy documenting the characteristic damage seen in celiac disease is still considered the "gold standard" for diagnosis. It is possible that, in the future, the combination of a person's symptoms, family history, antibody and genetic tests, and response to a GFD may be sufficient for diagnosis. There is a remote possibility that eligibility for employment, health insurance, or life insurance may be adversely affected by knowledge of increased genetic risk for specific diseases. However, current Federal law (Genetic Information Nondiscrimination Act) prohibits the use of genetic testing for employment or health insurance (but not life or disability insurance) purposes.

Outcome of Brian's Family

Relatives of people with biopsy-proven celiac disease have an increased risk for the condition. About 3–6% of people with a first-degree relative (parent, sibling, or child) with celiac disease also have celiac disease themselves; roughly 2–4% of people with a second-degree relative (grandparent, grandchild, uncle, aunt, nephew, niece, or half-sibling) with celiac disease also have celiac disease. Therefore, we offered both blood antibody and genetic tests to the potentially affected members of Brian's family. Table 2 shows the results.

Brian was negative for IgA-tTG and IgA-EMA antibodies because he is IgA deficient. However, his IgG-gliadin antibody was positive. He already had a positive biopsy. The IgA deficiency and celiac disease also put him at risk for recurrent *Giardia* infections. Because

TABLE 2. Celiac Test Results for Brian's Family

Name	Age	Relation	Medical History	IgA-tTG	IgA-EMA	HLA	Risk	Biopsy
Brian	7 yrs		Celiac disease	Neg	Neg	N/D		Pos
Olivia	4 mos	Sister	None	N/D	N/D	DQ2 neg/ DQ8 neg	Very low (<1%)	N/D
Amy	30 yrs	Mother	Thyroid disease	Neg	Neg	Two copies of DQ2.5	High (~30%)	Pending
Mark	32 yrs	Father	None	Neg	Neg	DQ2 neg/ DQ8 neg	Very low (<1%)	N/D
Debra	55 yrs	Grand-mother	Rheumatoid arthritis	Neg	Neg	DQ2.5 pos/ DQ8 pos	High (~13%)	N/D
Emily	12 yrs	Cousin	Type 1 diabetes	Pos	Neg	DQ2.5 pos/ DQ8 neg	High (~10%)	N/D

Neg, negative; pos, positive; N/D, not done.

Brian's diagnosis was already confirmed, genetic testing would not be of direct benefit to Brian. However, knowing his HLA type may make him eligible for future clinical trials for celiac disease therapy. DQ2 has a greater binding affinity for immune-stimulating gluten peptide fragments and is a potential target for drugs and vaccines to either augment or replace the GFD. Knowing Brian's HLA type might also be of benefit to other members of his family and his future children. He continues on a GFD and has IgG-gliadin antibody levels measured at his annual check-up with a pediatric gastroenterologist and registered dietitian who are familiar with the GFD and complications of celiac disease.[7]

Brian's infant sister Olivia, at 4 months of age, had never been exposed to gluten and therefore should not have detectable antibodies in her blood. Also, very young children may not make tTG or EMA. Therefore, instead of antibody testing, genetic testing was done via a cheek swab to assess her future risk of developing celiac disease. She tested negative for both HLA-DQ2 and -DQ8, indicating a very low risk. Amy was advised to breastfeed Olivia for as long as possible, ideally until at least one year of age, which is associated with a decrease in lifelong risk for celiac disease. Amy was told to introduce grains into Olivia's diet at 4 to 6 months of age, per the recommendations of the American Academy of Pediatrics (see Chapter 27 on infant feeding). Olivia does not require further testing or a biopsy for celiac disease.

Brian's mother Amy was negative for IgA-tTG and IgA-EMA. However, this may have been because of her eating gluten free for the preceding 10 months or she may have IgA deficiency. She tested positive for two copies of HLA-DQ2, which, in combination with her symptoms, family history of celiac disease, and coexisting autoimmune thyroid disease, put her at very high risk of having celiac disease. We advised her to undergo a gluten challenge (Chapter 8 on gluten intolerance describes gluten challenge), and she will have a biopsy done in the future to confirm whether or not she has active disease. Being the mother of a child with celiac disease, having Grave's disease, and having a mother with rheumatoid arthritis all increase her risk for celiac disease. Amy's problems with infertility may have been because of undiagnosed celiac disease (see Chapter 50 on fertility).

Brian's father Mark tested negative for tTG, EMA, and HLA-DQ2 and -DQ8. Because of this and Amy's family history of autoimmune disease, the genes for celiac disease were likely coming from Amy's side of the family. Mark does not require further testing or a biopsy for celiac disease.

Brian's grandmother Debra also tested negative for tTG and EMA, but this might have been because of her immune-suppressing medications. She tested positive for both HLA-DQ2 and -DQ8. She is at increased risk for celiac disease not only because she is Brian's grandmother but also because she has rheumatoid arthritis. Like Amy, Debra was advised to have an intestinal biopsy, but she declined due to her poor health. She said she wanted to "try" the GFD and see if it improved her arthritis. Because prednisone is used to treat the intestinal inflammation seen in refractory sprue (see Chapter 43), it is possible that Debra could have a false negative biopsy, even while ingesting gluten.

Brian's cousin Emily, who has type 1 diabetes, tested positive for HLA-DQ2 and had a mildly elevated IgA-tTG. However, she was negative for IgA-EMA. Emily visited a pediatric gastroenterologist and had a normal physical exam, normal growth, controlled diabetes, no gastrointestinal symptoms, and no nutrient deficiencies (such as iron deficiency anemia). Because her IgA-EMA was negative and she had no intestinal symptoms or other symptoms related to celiac disease, we believed that her positive tTG represented latent celiac disease or may have been due to her type 1 diabetes (low positive levels of celiac antibodies may be seen in other chronic and/or autoimmune conditions). HLA-DQ2 is not specific to celiac disease but is also commonly seen in people with type 1 diabetes and other autoimmune diseases.[8,9] Therefore, she did not undergo endoscopy for biopsies. Emily will be monitored closely and offered a biopsy if her health changes.

SELF-MANAGEMENT TIPS

☐ Negative results of genetic testing essentially rule out the possibility of having or developing celiac disease.

☐ The actual risk of having or developing celiac disease depends on which genes you carry. However, even with high-risk genes, most people will never get celiac disease.

- [ ] Consider genetic testing to determine risk of celiac disease for
    - Infants with a family history of celiac disease who have not yet been exposed to gluten in their diet
    - Very young children at risk for celiac disease, or suspected of having celiac disease, who may not make tTG or EMA antibodies
    - People of any age who are suspected of having celiac disease and who are IgA deficient, in whom IgG based testing is inconclusive
    - Patients of any age who are suspected of having celiac disease and who are on immune-suppressing medications, who may not make antibodies
    - Patients with other autoimmune conditions that may produce moderately elevated levels of tTG antibodies, such as type 1 diabetes, autoimmune liver disease, rheumatoid arthritis, and inflammatory bowel disease
    - People of any age who have put themselves on a GFD for several months and have negative antibodies and/or biopsies and are unwilling or unable to undergo gluten challenge
    - People who have inconclusive antibodies and/or biopsies, including those with villous atrophy possibly due to diseases other than celiac disease (see Chapter 7 on diagnostic dilemmas)

References

1. Fasano A, Berti I, Gerarduzzi T, et al. Prevalence of celiac disease in at-risk and not at-risk groups in the United States: a large multicenter study. *Arch Intern Med* 2003;163:286–92.
2. Sollid LM, Thorsby E. HLA susceptibility genes in celiac disease: genetic mapping and role in pathogenesis. *Gastroenterology* 1993;105:910–22.
3. Pietzak M, Schofield T. HLA-DQ2 homozygotes are associated with a 31-fold increased risk of EMA positivity in a large sample of sera (n = 4152) from patients at-risk for celiac disease. *Gastroenterology* 2007;132:2585.
4. Pietzak M, Schofield T, McGinnis M. HLA-DQ2 homozygotes are associated with a 24-fold increased risk of EMA positivity in a large sample of sera (n = 1021) from pediatric patients at-risk for celiac disease in the U.S. *J Pediatr Gastroenterol Nutr* 2007;45(4):539, #124.
5. Pietzak MM, Schofield TC, McGinniss MJ, Nakamura RM. Stratifying risk for celiac disease in a large at-risk United States population by using HLA alleles. *Clin Gastroenterol Hepatol* 2009;7:966–71.
6. Hunt KA, Zhernakova A, Turner G, et al. Newly identified genetic risk variants for celiac disease related to the immune response. *Nat Genet* 2008;40:395–402.
7. Pietzak MM. Follow-up of patients with celiac disease: achieving compliance with treatment. *Gastroenterology* 2005;128(4):S135–41.

8. Bizzaro N, Villalta D, Tonutti E, et al. IgA and IgG tissue transglutaminase antibody prevalence and clinical significance in connective tissue diseases, inflammatory bowel disease, and primary biliary cirrhosis. *Dig Dis Sci* 2003;4:2360–65.

9. Clemente MG, Musu MP, Frau F, et al. Antitissue transglutaminase antibodies outside celiac disease. *J Pediatr Gastroenterol Nutr* 2002;34:31–34.

10. Louka AS, Sollid LM. HLA in coeliac disease: unravelling the complex genetics of a complex disorder. *Tissue Antigens* 2003;61(2):105–17.

Michelle Pietzak, MD, is an Assistant Professor of Pediatrics at the University of Southern California Keck School of Medicine and a pediatric gastroenterologist at Los Angeles County + USC Hospital and Childrens Hospital Los Angeles, caring primarily for children with celiac disease, inflammatory bowel disease, short bowel syndrome, or special nutritional needs requiring either intravenous nutrition or special formulas.

CHAPTER 7

When Celiac Disease Diagnosis Isn't Straightforward

Carlo Catassi, MD

I saw Manuel for a second opinion on suspected celiac disease when he was 15 months old. This baby had a history of delayed growth, poor appetite, and diarrhea starting at 6 months of age. Manuel had been breast fed for 11 months and introduced to gluten-containing cereals at 6 months. He has a second cousin with celiac disease, but there are no other significant gastrointestinal diseases in his immediate family. Manuel had low blood levels of iron and total immunoglobulin (Ig) A (15 mg/dl). His level of IgA tissue transglutaminase (tTG) was within the normal range; however, IgG antigliadin antibodies (AGA) and IgG-tTG antibodies were elevated. Human leukocyte antigen genotyping failed to detect either the HLA-DQ2 or -DQ8 allele.

Although this information suggested that Manuel had celiac disease, I wasn't so sure. Blood tests, particularly IgA-tTG, are sensitive and simple diagnostic tools for celiac disease (see Chapter 4 on blood tests). We also can perform genetic testing (see Chapter 6 on genetic testing). However, these tests have limitations. In particular, if someone has selective IgA deficiency or is already eating gluten free, these tests don't tell the whole story.[1]

IgA Deficiency

Selective IgA deficiency (SIgAD) is a condition that affects about 1 in 500 people of European origin. These individuals do not make or have very low blood levels of IgA antibodies (less than 5 mg/dl) because of a genetically determined failure of B lymphocytes to change into IgA-producing plasma cells. SIgAD may remain clinically silent and not show any symptoms and is usually discovered accidentally when testing for another disorder like celiac disease. However, SIgAD may be associated with an increased risk of infections, allergies, and autoimmune diseases.[2]

Individuals with SIgAD should be screened for celiac disease because an autoimmune reaction to gluten is 10 to 20 times more common in them than in the general population. On the other hand, only around 2% of people with celiac disease also have SIgAD. Because people with SIgAD are usually unable to produce serum IgA celiac antibodies, they should be tested for IgG-tTG antibodies and IgG antiendomysial antibodies (EMA).

The reliability of these tests in those with SIgAD is very high, although not quite as reliable as IgA-based tests in individuals who make sufficient IgA. Therefore, if someone has SIgAD and is positive for IgG anti-tTG antibodies and IgG EMA, he or she still needs to have a small intestine biopsy to confirm the diagnosis of celiac disease.

It's important to determine total blood IgA levels when screening for celiac disease. However, the results of IgA-based celiac tests are valid for infants who have partial IgA deficiency. Partial IgA deficiency is defined as IgA levels lower than is found in 97.5% of a similarly aged population but higher than 5 mg/dl. Unlike SIgAD, which is permanent, partial IgA deficiency is usually transient.

Blood Tests Negative for Celiac Disease Markers

Having normal blood levels of IgA-tTG and IgA-EMA does not necessarily rule out the diagnosis of celiac disease, even in those with normal levels of IgA. It's possible for someone with HLA-DQ2 and/or -DQ8 and typical small intestinal damage (found by biopsy) who is positively responding to the gluten-free diet (GFD) to test negative for celiac disease. This seems to happen more often in adults (10–15% of cases) than in children.

When those with negative blood tests for celiac disease are studied with immunofluorescence, many show deposits of IgA-tTG in the lining of the small intestinal mucosa that disappear after treatment with the GFD. For unknown reasons, autoantibodies such as tTG seem to be stored in the bowel of individuals whose blood tests are negative for celiac disease.[3]

Therefore, it's vital to investigate those whose symptoms strongly suggest celiac disease by small intestinal biopsy, regardless of their blood test results.[4] If biopsy shows the typical damage caused by reaction to gluten, the next step is treating it with the GFD. This diagnosis needs to be confirmed by a second biopsy after 1–2 years of GFD.

However, disorders other than celiac disease can cause intestinal damage very similar to that in celiac disease. Common problems that can mimic celiac disease changes in the intestine include infection with *Giardia*, damage from viral gastroenteritis, immune deficiency states (including HIV and common variable immune deficiency), and other autoimmune diseases. For this reason, further evaluation, such as genetic testing and evaluation of response to gluten withdrawal, is often needed for people who are thought to have celiac disease based on positive biopsy results but negative blood tests.

Eating Gluten Free

Blood markers for celiac disease—tTG and EMA—usually disappear within 6–24 months of treatment with the GFD. If someone is already eating gluten free or is limiting gluten with a "low-gluten diet," blood tests for celiac disease will be falsely negative. If this is the case, the celiac disease diagnosis should be confirmed by gluten challenge, if possible. (Chapter 8 on gluten intolerance describes gluten challenge.) If an individual is unable or does not want to undergo gluten challenge, there is currently no way to diagnose celiac disease. For this reason, patients are strongly encouraged to seek definitive testing before changing their diet. In select cases, such as women planning pregnancy or growing children, it may be reasonable to defer gluten challenge and to continue a strict GFD without being sure of the diagnosis.

What Was Wrong with Manuel

Celiac disease was in Manuel's family, and his blood tests pointed toward him having celiac disease, too; but he did not have HLA-DQ2 or -DQ8 alleles, a result with a strong ability to rule out celiac disease. I concluded that another condition, possibly long-term diarrhea caused by a previously undetected infection, was probably responsible for Manuel's symptoms. The other factor that helped rule out celiac disease was that his level of IgA-tTG antibodies was not elevated. Although Manuel's level of total IgA was lower than normal, it was probably a sign of partial IgA deficiency, which does not significantly affect the accuracy of the IgA-tTG test.

SELF-MANAGEMENT TIPS

☐ If you do not have the HLA-DQ2 or the -DQ8 allele, this excludes you from having celiac disease with 99.9% certainty.

☐ If your blood tests for celiac disease were negative but you were diagnosed with it based on your symptoms and the results of a small intestinal biopsy, you need to have the diagnosis confirmed by another biopsy after 1–2 years of GFD treatment. The second biopsy needs to show clear-cut improvement in the health of your intestinal lining.

☐ If your diagnosis is in doubt, taking a gluten-challenge test or having a small intestinal biopsy are ways to diagnose or rule out celiac disease with more confidence.

References

1. Catassi C, Fasano A. Is this really celiac disease? Pitfalls in diagnosis. *Curr Gastroenterol Rep* 2008;10:466–72.
2. McGowan KE, Lyon ME, Butzner JD. Celiac disease and IgA deficiency: complications of serological testing approaches encountered in the clinic. *Clin Chem* 2008;54:1203–209.
3. Salmi TT, Collin P, Korponay-Szabó IR, Laurila K, Partanen J, Huhtala H, et al. Endomysial antibody-negative coeliac disease: clinical characteristics and intestinal autoantibody deposits. *Gut* 2006;55:1746–53.
4. Abrams JA, Diamond B, Rotterdam H, Green PH. Seronegative celiac disease: increased prevalence with lesser degrees of villous atrophy. *Dig Dis Sci* 2004;49:546–50.

Carlo Catassi, MD, is Co-Director of the Center for Celiac Research, University of Maryland School of Medicine, Baltimore, Maryland, and an Associate Professor at the Department of Pediatrics, Università Politecnica delle Marche, Ancona, Italy.

CHAPTER 8

Gluten Intolerance: You Mean I Don't Have Celiac Disease?

Daniel A. Leffler, MD, MS

Yolanda is a 36-year-old woman who has had chronic gastrointestinal symptoms for many years, including upset stomach, loose stools, and constipation. Soon after a friend was diagnosed with celiac disease, she decided to try the gluten-free diet (GFD) herself. Once she began avoiding gluten products, Yolanda noticed a great improvement in her symptoms, especially the indigestion and loose stools.

About a year later, she asked her primary care physician to test her for celiac disease. Her doctor measured Yolanda's immunoglobulin (Ig) A tissue transglutaminase (tTG) level and total IgA level, both of which turned out to be normal. Yolanda's doctor referred her to our gastro-enterology department to answer her questions regarding her symptoms and the GFD. The most important piece of information we gave Yolanda was that all available tests, including intestinal biopsy, return to normal after people have been on a GFD for a prolonged period. Therefore, the best way to test Yolanda for celiac disease was for her to undergo a gluten challenge test, which would last several weeks.

In the gluten challenge, the subject slowly increases his or her gluten intake for eight to ten weeks, until he or she is eating a normal diet that includes at least two servings of gluten (about four slices of bread) per day. Soon after reintroducing foods with gluten, Yolanda's gastrointestinal symptoms reappeared. However, when we tested her for celiac disease eight weeks later at the end of the gluten challenge, Yolanda's IgA-tTG level was normal; so was her small intestinal biopsy. In a situation like this, it is most likely that Yolanda has gluten intolerance, rather than celiac disease.

What Is Gluten Intolerance?

The terms used in celiac disease and related disorders can be quite confusing. *Celiac disease* refers to an autoimmune reaction that occurs in response to gluten and damages the intestine. *Gluten sensitivity* covers the entire spectrum of gluten-related disorders, including celiac disease, dermatitis herpetiformis (see Chapter 9), gluten-related neurological disorders (see Chapter 51), and gluten intolerance.[1] Gluten intolerance has not been well studied but appears to be quite common, and as many as 25% of

TABLE 1. Gluten Intolerance vs. Celiac Disease

Gluten Intolerance	Celiac Disease
▪ Normal IgA-tTG	▪ Elevated IgA-tTG
▪ Normal duodenal biopsy	▪ Abnormal duodenal biopsy
▪ Baseline risk of autoimmune diseases	▪ Increased risk of autoimmune diseases
▪ Baseline risk of osteopenia/osteoporosis	▪ Increased risk of osteopenia/osteoporosis
▪ Baseline risk of nutritional deficiencies	▪ Nutritional deficiencies common
▪ May have elevated IgA or IgG antigliadin antibodies	▪ Usually have elevated IgA or IgG antigliadin antibodies
▪ Gastrointestinal symptoms common	▪ Gastrointestinal symptoms common

patients with diarrhea-predominant irritable bowel syndrome (IBS) may respond to gluten restriction.[2] When people with gluten intolerance eat a GFD, their symptoms may improve or completely go away. But we see no evidence in the small intestine of the type of damage to the villi that is associated with celiac disease.[3] Also, people with gluten intolerance do not appear to be at increased risk for the common complications of untreated celiac disease, such as nutrient deficiencies or gastrointestinal cancers (Table 1).

Gluten intolerance is generally thought of as a functional disease. That means it affects how your body functions, but no physical reason for the symptoms, such as damage to the intestinal lining, can be detected. We believe that this points to problems with how the nerves control digestion, although subtle changes in the immune system may also play a role. IBS is a common functional disease that affects about 14 million Americans. In general, many people—more than half in some populations—who are diagnosed with IBS appear to respond to dietary changes of some type. But we don't yet know if gluten intolerance is a type of functional disorder, like IBS, or whether some people with gluten intolerance actually have a very mild immune reaction to gluten.

A gluten challenge can help diagnose or rule out celiac disease. The gluten challenge should be undertaken with the guidance of a physician. It is generally done by those on a GFD but who have not been definitively diagnosed with celiac disease and who meet one or more of the following criteria:

- have had no prior duodenal biopsy consistent with celiac disease or skin biopsy consistent with dermatitis herpetiformis
- have had a borderline or inconclusive biopsy with borderline or negative blood tests
- have had poor response to the GFD and prior diagnostic tests appear inconclusive or are not available to review

Treating Gluten Intolerance

There are no specific guidelines or management strategies for living with gluten intolerance. Because the tolerance for gluten can vary so dramatically between individuals, the best advice is to adjust gluten consumption to eliminate symptoms and optimize your quality of life.

TABLE 2. Guidelines for Gluten Challenge

Step 1.	Perform baseline laboratory testing for IgA-tTG and total IgA level.
Step 2.	If tTG is elevated, proceed to step 5.
Step 3.	If tTG is within normal limits and there is a history of severe symptoms with gluten exposure, consider HLA-DQ2 or -DQ8 typing; be cautious with gluten challenge if positive for HLA-DQ2 or-DQ8 (see Chapter 6).
Step 4.	If tTG is within normal limits and there is no history of severe symptoms with gluten exposure, begin gluten challenge with one regular cracker or ¼ slice of regular bread. Double this every 1–3 days until significant symptoms develop or until you are eating the equivalent of 4 slices of bread or 2 cups/servings of pasta per day. Continue a full gluten-containing diet for 2 months. Note: The amount and duration of gluten ingestion can be altered depending on the severity of symptoms.
Step 5.	Perform endoscopy with duodenal biopsies (see Chapter 5) and check IgA-tTG.
Step 6.	If biopsies are negative for celiac disease, continue gluten-containing diet; recheck tTG in 3–6 months or if symptoms develop. Repeat endoscopy with biopsy if tTG is elevated.

Trial and error is the best way to understand what works for you. Remember to keep a list. It is also typical for your sensitivity to fluctuate over time and with stress levels, similar to what happens in IBS.

You need to eat a healthy, balanced diet that includes fruit and vegetables and watch for nutritional deficiencies that may require supplements or changes in eating habits (see Chapter 12 on a balanced gluten-free diet and Chapter 14 on supplements). It's smart to have some counseling sessions with a dietitian, especially if your symptoms bother you a great deal. Also, the diagnosis of gluten intolerance does not mean that you won't develop celiac disease at a later date. If your health and symptoms change, particularly if they are severe or coexist with rashes, burning, or swelling of the lips or inside of your mouth, get retested for celiac disease and for food and environmental allergies. (See Chapter 35 for further discussion of food allergies.)

What Yolanda Did

We counseled Yolanda on the difference between celiac disease and gluten intolerance. Although she initially kept a very strict gluten-free diet, Yolanda gradually added some gluten-containing products back into her diet without triggering her symptoms. She found that she could tolerate the small amounts of gluten that are generally used in sauces, fillers, and medications; however, breads and pastas continued to cause abdominal discomfort, especially if she ate them in large amounts. Because a low-gluten diet typically reduces fiber intake and can contribute to constipation, we also suggested that she use a fiber supplement (see Chapter 16 on constipation and Chapter 13 on whole grains). Yolanda has been healthy on a low-gluten diet with no further issues.

SELF-MANAGEMENT TIPS

☐ Gluten intolerance is a functional disorder that may mimic celiac disease in terms of symptoms and response to lowering the gluten content of meals.

☐ Unlike celiac disease, there is no (or minimal) autoimmune or inflammatory component to gluten intolerance.

☐ Antigliadin antibodies are commonly elevated in gluten intolerance while IgA-tTG levels and duodenal biopsy are normal (unlike celiac disease where all three are usually abnormal).

☐ If having celiac disease has been adequately ruled out, adjust your diet to optimize your health and quality of life.

References

1. Verdu EF, Armstrong D, Murray JA. Between celiac disease and irritable bowel syndrome: the "no man's land" of gluten sensitivity. *Am J Gastroenterol* 2009;104:1587–94.
2. Wahnschaffe U, Schulzke JD, Zeitz M, et al. Predictors of clinical response to gluten-free diet in patients diagnosed with diarrhea-predominant irritable bowel syndrome. *Clin Gastroenterol Hepatol* 2007;5:844–50; quiz 769.
3. Kaukinen K, Turjanmaa K, Maki M, et al. Intolerance to cereals is not specific for coeliac disease. *Scand J Gastroenterol* 2000;35:942–46.

CHAPTER 9

Dermatitis Herpetiformis

John J. Zone, MD

Kristy is a 38-year-old woman who had no skin problems until three years ago, when she began noticing "itchy bumps" on her elbows and knees. She had seen her general physician as well as two dermatologists for this and had been treated with topical steroids with no improvement. When the itching became severe, a dermatologist did a biopsy of a lesion that showed nothing conclusive. Kristy then started a two-week course of oral prednisone, but she had no relief from the itching.

Kristy then visited our dermatology practice. A physical exam showed that she appeared healthy other than abrasions on her elbows, knees, and buttocks from scratching. She said she has had no abdominal pain, diarrhea, or constipation. We took a biopsy of normal-appearing skin next to a lesion and examined it using direct immunofluorescence, which revealed granular deposits of immunoglobulin (Ig) A in the deeper layer of the skin (dermal papillae), a characteristic of dermatitis herpetiformis (DH). Because DH is associated with celiac disease, Kristy had her blood tested. Although other tests were normal, Kristy's IgA tissue transglutaminase (IgA-tTG) was 25 units (normal is less than 20 units), and her IgA epidermal transglutaminase (a blood test related to the celiac tTG test but that measures antibodies that bind to transglutaminase in the skin) was elevated at 30 units (normal is less than 20 units). Kristy was diagnosed with both DH and celiac disease.

What Is Dermatitis Herpetiformis?

DH is an intensely itchy, blistering disease of the skin that is sometimes the only sign of celiac disease. It primarily occurs on the elbows, knees, and buttocks but can also occur on the scalp and around the waist. Lesions start as tiny blisters. The itching can be so severe that patients scratch the individual lesions vigorously, making it difficult to separate from other skin diseases.

Testing for DH

Routine biopsies may show a blister with neutrophils (a type of white blood cell) and suggest that you have DH. However, routine biopsies may not show the characteristic signs because scratching the lesions changes the microscopic findings. The most reliable method of diagnosis is to biopsy normal-appearing (not scratched) skin immediately next to a red bump and then use direct immunofluorescence to identify the grains of IgA in the skin. Direct immunofluorescence should be used even if the routine biopsy shows DH because another disorder (linear IgA disease, which is not related to celiac disease) may have a similar appearance. The two can only be separated by direct immunofluorescence.

All people with DH have celiac disease, but their conditions may vary from severe damage to the intestinal mucosa to only a little inflammation. The severity of DH is independent of the severity of the intestinal disease. Those with DH usually do not have the gastrointestinal symptoms associated with celiac disease, but this skin disease responds to dietary gluten restriction regardless. For these reasons, small intestinal biopsies are not routinely needed for patients with DH who have been identified with direct immunofluorescence.

Most people (70–80%) with DH have higher than normal blood IgA-tTG antibody levels, which can be used to monitor the response of the intestine to gluten restriction. We sometimes also test for IgA epidermal transglutaminase antibodies because these are specific for DH and are deposited in the skin. They are elevated in 70–80% of the people with DH. Consequently, these blood tests can be useful for both diagnosis and monitoring your progress but are not sufficient for either celiac disease or DH.

Treating DH

The treatment of DH centers on a gluten-free diet (GFD) but adding dapsone can provide immediate relief from the itching. It may take several months of complete gluten restriction before you get a response. Virtually all of those with granular IgA deposits in their skin will eventually respond to a strict GFD, allowing them to either decrease or eliminate the need for dapsone. With a prolonged GFD, IgA in the skin decreases and eventually disappears. With the reintroduction of gluten, IgA and skin disease return. Minor fluctuations in the disease are most likely related to oral gluten intake. Eating a large amount of iodide in the form of kelp, cough medicine, or shellfish may also cause DH to flare.

Itching is relieved and new skin lesions cease within 48–72 hours of starting dapsone. The lesions abruptly return within 24–48 hours of stopping this therapy. Dapsone has no effect on the health of your intestine. Initial dosages of dapsone are 25–50 mg in adults with gradual increases as necessary to control symptoms. The daily dose can be regulated on a weekly basis to get the best control. If you are not eating gluten free, you can expect to get one or two new lesions per week, even when taking the optimal dose of dapsone.

Outbreaks of lesions on your face and scalp can occur even when you eating a strict GFD diet and may not respond to dapsone therapy. There is no good method for preventing such

TABLE 1. Side Effect of Dapsone

Anemia
Methemoglobinemia (change in the way your red blood cells carry oxygen)
Leukopenia (low white blood count)
Fatigue
Flu-like syndrome
Neuropathy
Allergic reactions

occurrences, and increases in dapsone dosage seem to have no effect. Breaking the blisters and applying a corticosteroid gel may aid in healing.

Although there are many side effects of dapsone (Table 1), the drug is well tolerated for years in more than 90% of patients. The major side effect is increased destruction of red blood cells (called *hemolysis*). This occurs in nearly everyone on dapsone therapy, because sulfones produce an oxidant stress for aging red blood cells. Increased hemolysis can lead to anemia but is seldom a serious problem as long as your health is monitored as described below. Dapsone is not to be used by nursing mothers, because it is secreted in breast milk and may cause hemolytic anemia in breastfed infants. If you develop persistent severe anemia on dapsone, there may be an underlying cause, such as iron, vitamin B_{12}, or folate deficiencies.

For those with DH, I routinely provide instruction about a GFD and encourage them seek the help of a dietitian and support groups. I use dapsone to control the skin symptoms. As the GFD takes effect, the patient can attempt to decrease the dapsone dose by 12.5 mg (½ of a 25-mg tablet) per week. If there is a flare of more than a few lesions, I increase the dose to a maintenance level, and wait another 2–3 weeks to attempt to lower the dose again. This approach allows you to take the lowest possible dose of dapsone to control your symptoms and minimizes the dapsone complications (Table 1). This approach eventually allows you to stop using dapsone and control the DH with a GFD.

Patients who cannot tolerate dapsone can try sulfapyridine (Jacobus Pharmaceutical is the only known supplier). The initial dose of sulfapyridine is usually 500 mg three times a day, and it can be safely increased to 2 g three times a day. However, some patients may not respond to sulfapyridine at any dose. One side effect is the risk of developing kidney stones, so you will need to drink plenty of water, which decreases this risk by making urine more dilute and less acidic.

Dapsone therapy requires you to have initial and ongoing complete blood counts and liver function tests. Complete blood counts are needed weekly for the first month, monthly for the next five months, and semiannually as long as you remain on dapsone therapy. Liver function tests are repeated after six months on this therapy and annually thereafter. Baseline glucose-6-phosphate dehydrogenase activity should be assessed in African Americans, Asians, and those of southern Mediterranean ancestry. Glucose-6-phosphate dehydrogenase deficiency is a common inherited disorder that makes red blood cells more susceptible to hemolysis.

Sulfapyridine does not produce hemolytic anemia, but the potential for agranulocytosis does exist. Agranulocytosis is a sometimes fatal acute illness characterized by a decrease in granular white blood cells and by lesions of the throat, gastrointestinal tract, and skin. The condition often occurs as a toxic effect of specific drugs. Consequently, similar monitoring is recommended for chronic sulfapyridine therapy.

Some people with DH choose to control their skin lesions with long-term dapsone therapy and continue on a regular diet. This choice means that they will need regular blood testing indefinitely. Also, they are then at risk for the long-term complications of untreated celiac disease, including osteoporosis, anemia, abdominal discomfort, and lymphoma, although these complications are rare.

Outcome

Kristy starting taking 25 mg dapsone daily. Her itching improved within 48 hours, and her lesions healed in two weeks. However, within 48 hours of stopping dapsone, she developed flares of multiple grouped blisters on her elbows. After we discussed the potential risks of untreated celiac disease, Kristy decided to begin a GFD. Strict adherence to the diet allowed her to taper off and finally discontinue dapsone over a 12-month period. Because she stayed on the GFD, Kristy's IgA-tTG and epidermal transglutaminase antibody levels returned to normal.

SELF-MANAGEMENT TIPS

☐ Dermatitis herpetiformis is a condition resulting from celiac disease, in which antibodies deposit in the skin causing a blistering, itchy rash.

☐ DH can be diagnosed through skin biopsy and the standard celiac blood test. IgA-tTG levels are elevated in most of those with DH.

☐ All patients with DH also have celiac disease, although gastrointestinal symptoms are often mild. For this reason, the gluten-free diet is the treatment of choice.

☐ DH usually responds completely to a GFD. However, dapsone can be used to help symptoms of extreme itching resolve faster or to control flares.

☐ Dapsone has significant side effects but can be safely used when you are carefully monitored by a physician.

Further Reading

- Hall RP, 3rd. Dermatitis herpetiformis. *J Invest Dermatol* 1992;99:873–81.
- Jaskowski TD, Hamblin T, Wilson AR, Hill HR, Book LS, Meyer LJ, Zone JJ, Hull CM. IgA anti-epidermal transglutaminase antibodies in dermatitis herpetiformis and pediatric celiac disease. *J Invest Dermatol* 2009;129:2728–30.
- Zone JJ. Skin manifestations of celiac disease. *Gastroenterology* 2005;128:S87–91.
- Zone JJ, Meyer LJ, Petersen MJ. Deposition of granular IgA relative to clinical lesions in dermatitis herpetiformis. *Arch Dermatol* 1996;132:912–18.

John J. Zone, MD, is Professor of Dermatology and Chairman of the Department of Dermatology at the University of Utah School of Medicine, Salt Lake City, Utah.

CHAPTER 10

Who Should Be Tested for Celiac Disease?

Peter H. R. Green, MD

Debra came to the Celiac Center for her annual visit with the gastroenterologist and dietitian. She was doing well after living with celiac disease for more than 20 years. Debra was concerned about her two children and hoped that they could be seen, because she was certain that they both had celiac disease. Several other family members, including her sister and niece, had recently been tested and were diagnosed with celiac disease. Many years ago, Debra asked their pediatrician to perform genetic testing on her children and both were HLA-DQ2 positive, indicating that they could potentially develop celiac disease (see Chapter 6 on genetic testing). Her daughter Allison, now age 28, had been complaining of fatigue and was recently diagnosed with iron deficiency anemia by her primary care physician. Debra's son James, age 20, was reluctant to come for testing. However, a month later, both her daughter and son were seen in the Celiac Center.

Allison had recently graduated from NYU law school and had begun a grueling job with a large New York law firm. Allison doubted that she had made the right decision in her career choice. She had many years of abdominal bloating that would come and go, which she believed was related more to stresses at college and law school than eating. This led to her diagnosis of irritable bowel syndrome (IBS) several years earlier; she still dealt with mild constipation from time to time. She had been taking Zantac for occasional acid reflux and was depressed and very irritable. Her fatigue had caused her to call in sick from work on several occasions. Recently, Allison's primary care physician diagnosed her with hypothyroidism, and she began thyroid hormone replacement, which improved her fatigue somewhat. Subsequently, she was diagnosed with iron deficiency anemia, which was attributed to her heavy periods. Iron pills, however, did not appear to be correcting the anemia.

Allison's blood tests revealed strongly positive tissue transglutaminase and deamidated gliadin peptide antibodies. The endoscopy revealed reduced duodenal folds, and the biopsies confirmed that these changes were consistent with celiac disease. Allison met with the celiac dietitian and readily adopted a gluten-free lifestyle, happy that there was an explanation for her symptoms and hopeful of feeling better. She began to believe that maybe her career choice had been correct after all.

James was reluctant to be tested for celiac disease, to say the least. He claimed to be well. He did not want his mother or sister in the room while he met with me. I asked him about his mother's story that he had not done well at school and had dropped out of college. James said he was currently working as a bartender in an Irish pub. His physical examination was normal, and he reported no gastrointestinal symptoms or other physical complaints. James refused blood testing for celiac disease.

Case Finding vs. Screening

Allison had several conditions, including IBS, fatigue, hypothyroidism, and iron deficiency, that would warrant testing for celiac disease. She met with physicians, asking what was wrong with her and seeking a diagnosis and treatments that might make her feel better. Testing her for celiac disease is known as case finding: She is asking to be tested for celiac disease. She should have been tested earlier because of her symptoms and associated diseases and diagnoses (IBS, reflux, anemia, and hypothyroidism), especially with the family history of celiac disease.

The practice of testing patients with specific symptoms or diseases for celiac disease is called *targeted case finding* and will markedly increase the rate of celiac disease diagnosis.[1] The sooner the disease is diagnosed, the healthier the patients can be. The use of celiac testing by primary care physicians is considered to be responsible for the increased rate of celiac disease diagnosis in Northern Ireland.[2] But there is another advantage to early diagnosis. In a study of those enrolled in an HMO, the diagnosis of celiac disease reduced health care costs.[3] So, the diagnosis of celiac disease has advantages to patients and the health care system.

James does not want to be tested for anything, although he is at high risk for celiac disease. He has a strong family history of celiac disease, is HLA-DQ2 positive, and did not do well academically. A study from Sweden demonstrated that young adults with celiac disease discovered through screening had fewer university degrees and management-level jobs.[4] Reasons for this are unclear but may be related to psychological problems in childhood and adolescence associated with undiagnosed celiac disease. Testing James for celiac disease is screening. In screening an individual, we are testing them for a disease even though they do not come to the doctor with complaints or say "help me, diagnose me."

There is ample evidence that people with celiac disease are better off being diagnosed and treated. However, the evidence for this in silent celiac disease (in which the symptoms are not noticed) is conflicting. On one hand, silent celiac disease was associated with increased risk of death compared with the general population, as shown in a study that tested stored serum samples for celiac disease that had been undiagnosed.[5] Most studies show reduced risk after several years on the gluten-free diet; however, not all studies show this. On the other hand, there are few studies that have shown the benefit of diagnosing those with silent celiac disease.

Celiac disease fulfills World Health Organization criteria for a disease that is appropriate for screening. It is common, there are tests for it, there is a therapy, and there is benefit to diagnosis, at least in those with signs or symptoms of celiac disease. However, screening for the disease in those who do not have symptoms and are not seeking health care is not advised because research does not show a benefit and the therapy is, at least in the United States, difficult.[6] Safe gluten-free restaurant offerings are uncommon, gluten-free food products are more expensive than regular food,[7] and eating gluten free is often socially inconvenient. Therefore, the accepted approach to celiac disease is case finding rather than population-based screening in the United States.

People who should be tested for celiac disease include those with symptoms or diseases attributable to celiac disease, such as IBS, anemia, osteoporosis, deficiency of minerals or vitamins, and neurological symptoms, such as peripheral neuropathy or ataxia. At present, screening may occur in different situations. First, those with health conditions associated with celiac disease, including a variety of autoimmune diseases, such as type 1 diabetes, Sjogren's syndrome, autoimmune thyroid diseases, and autoimmune liver diseases might be screened for celiac disease. However, it's important to realize that there has been no convincing evidence that these people are better off being treated for their celiac disease except for those with liver diseases. The next large group that could be screened are those with genetic disorders, mainly Down syndrome because of the high prevalence of celiac disease in this population. Finally, family members of those with celiac disease could be screened because they are likely to include a large number of undetected celiac disease cases. Some family members have no control over whether they are tested (children) and others are reluctant (James), but the majority appears convinced that it is advantageous to their health to be diagnosed and treated. There is no population-based screening of the general population, as is done for colon cancer.

What James Decided

James was never tested for celiac disease, although his probability of having it is relatively high. Given his family history and poor school performance, James would be better off with his celiac disease diagnosed and treated. Because he may change his way of thinking later in life, I counseled him that if he develops gastrointestinal symptoms or other health issues consistent with celiac disease, he should immediately be tested.

SELF-MANAGEMENT TIPS

☐ Targeted case finding refers to testing people for celiac disease when they present to a clinician with symptoms or issues consistent with celiac disease.

☐ Screening refers to testing people who have not sought care for any related health issues, such as screening colonoscopies or pap smears, which are performed to monitor continued health.

☐ There is a great deal of evidence to support active case finding of celiac disease in those with symptoms or diseases attributable to celiac disease.

☐ On the other hand, we do not know whether testing and treating people with mild or no symptoms of celiac disease significantly improves their health or quality of life (except in those with liver manifestations of celiac disease). For that reason, widespread screening for celiac disease cannot be justified.

References

1. Catassi C, Kryszak D, Louis-Jacques O, et al. Detection of celiac disease in primary care: a multicenter case-finding study in North America. *Am J Gastroenterol* 2007;102(7):1454–60.
2. Dickey W, McMillan SA. Increasing numbers at a specialist coeliac clinic: contribution of serological testing in primary care. *Dig Liver Dis* 2005;37(12):928–33.
3. Green PH, Neugut AI, Naiyer AJ, Edwards ZC, Gabinelle S, Chinburapa V. Economic benefits of increased diagnosis of celiac disease in a national managed care population in the United States. *J Insur Med* 2008;40(3–4):218–28.
4. Verkasalo MA, Raitakari OT, Viikari J, Marniemi J, Savilahti E. Undiagnosed silent coeliac disease: A risk for underachievement? *Scand J Gastroenterol* 2005;40(12):1407–12.
5. Rubio-Tapia A, Kyle RA, Kaplan EL, et al. Increased prevalence and mortality in undiagnosed celiac disease. *Gastroenterology* 2009;137(1):88–93.
6. James SP. National Institutes of Health consensus development conference statement on celiac disease, June 28–30, 2004. *Gastroenterology* 2005;128(4 Pt 2):S1–9.
7. Lee AR, Ng DL, Zivin J, Green PH. Economic burden of a gluten-free diet. *J Hum Nutr Diet* 2007;20(5):423–30.

Peter H. R. Green, MD, is Professor of Clinical Medicine, College of Physicians and Surgeons, Columbia University, and Director of the Celiac Disease Center at Columbia University, New York, New York.

CHAPTER 11

Finding Celiac Disease in Children

Naamah Zitomersky, MD, and Alan M. Leichtner, MD

Cecilia, a 12-month-old toddler of northern European descent, was not gaining weight and had a distended belly and loose, foul-smelling stools, so her mother brought her to the pediatrician. Cecilia had been exclusively breast fed until she was 4 months old, at which point her parents began feeding her pureed solids and multigrain infant cereal. Over several months, her stools had changed from yellow and seedy to loose, watery, and extremely foul smelling and increased to eight times per day. Cecilia was extremely gassy, and her abdomen would intermittently become distended, especially after meals. At her 12-month visit to the pediatrician, Cecilia appeared pale, and blood tests confirmed that she had iron deficiency anemia. Stool tests for infections were negative. Cecilia then began oral iron supplementation, and her parents tried to get her to eat more food.

Despite these interventions, Cecilia's weight gain had not improved by her 18-month visit, and her symptoms persisted. Although her abdomen was large, her arms and legs appeared to be very thin. Cecilia's weight had decreased from the 50th percentile at 6 months to the 15th percentile at 18 months, despite her height remaining at the 50th percentile. At this point, Cecilia was sent to a pediatric gastroenterologist, who tested Cecilia's blood for celiac disease and found that her immunoglobulin A antibody to tissue transglutaminase (IgA-tTG) was greater than 100 units (less than 20 units is normal). The diagnosis of celiac disease was then confirmed with an endoscopy under general anesthesia.

A mother brought her 9-year-old son to his pediatrician because she was concerned that Jack was the smallest child in his third grade class. Jack had a normal appetite and seemed healthy, with no complaints or symptoms. He said he didn't have abdominal pain and had normal bowel movements, although he would occasionally skip a day. Jack's pediatrician referred him to a pediatric endocrinologist, who could identify no hormonal cause for Jack's poor growth. Jack's mother has hypothyroidism, and his 16-year-old sister has type 1 diabetes. Because he has a cousin who was recently diagnosed with celiac disease, Jack's mother requested that he be tested. Jack's pediatrician was surprised when blood testing revealed the IgA-tTG level to be 85 units. A pediatric gastroenterologist confirmed the diagnosis with an endoscopy under sedation, which yielded duodenal biopsies consistent with celiac disease.

Symptoms and Risk Factors

In the first case, Cecilia had classic symptoms of celiac disease in a toddler, with diarrhea, abdominal distension, poor weight gain, and irritability. Before there were specific celiac blood tests, we believed that almost all children who had celiac disease would show these symptoms and that celiac disease was quite uncommon. Over the past 10 years, studies using blood tests have shown celiac disease to be much more common than we thought. Based on a number of studies in Europe and the United States, we know that celiac disease occurs in approximately 1 in 300 to 1 in 80 children between the ages of 2.5 and 15 years.[1]

Physicians are becoming aware of the emergence of new patterns of symptoms of celiac disease in children. Although children are being diagnosed at all ages, from as young as 6 months to the late teenage years, the average age of diagnosis of childhood celiac disease is now 8 years.[2] In addition, we are finding that school-aged children diagnosed with celiac disease are more likely to

- have different gastrointestinal symptoms, for example, constipation rather than diarrhea
- have nongastrointestinal symptoms that are not usually associated with celiac disease, such as short stature and delayed puberty,[3] anemia, behavioral disorders, or dental abnormalities such as enamel defects
- have no symptoms but be a member of a high-risk group who is diagnosed by screening for celiac disease

In one study, 70% of children lacked any gastrointestinal symptoms and about 10% were actually overweight at diagnosis.[2] The differences in symptoms by age at presentation are summarized in Table 1.

Children with a first-degree relative (parent or sibling) or second-degree relative (grandparent, aunt, uncle, or cousin) with celiac disease or with a disease associated with celiac disease are at increased risk of developing celiac disease. These children should be considered for testing, even though they may have no symptoms. Diseases associated with celiac disease are:

- type 1 diabetes
- autoimmune thyroid disease
- Addison's disease

TABLE 1. Celiac Disease Symptoms by Age

Infant, toddler, early school-age children	Gastrointestinal symptoms are more common. Symptoms may include poor weight gain, diarrhea, abdominal pain, abdominal distention, gassiness, vomiting, and irritability.
Older children and adolescents	Atypical symptoms may occur. Symptoms may include delayed puberty, short stature, decreased appetite, abdominal pain, diarrhea, bloating, changes in school performance, headaches, rashes, and fatigue.

- Down syndrome
- Williams syndrome
- Turner syndrome
- IgA deficiency

Blood Testing and Endoscopy

We diagnose celiac disease in children based on a combination of symptoms, positive antibody testing, confirmation with small intestinal biopsies, and improvement on the gluten-free diet (GFD). As in adults, the best blood tests for celiac disease are the IgA-tTG and IgA endomysial (IgA-EMA) antibody tests. Although the IgA gliadin antibody test is not as sensitive or specific as the newer tests, it may be helpful in identifying celiac disease in children younger than 3 years old when there is a strong clinical suspicion for disease and IgA-tTG and IgA-EMA tests are negative. All the IgA-based antibody tests may be negative in children with IgA deficiency. For this reason, levels of total IgA in blood are often tested in conjunction with IgA-tTG and IgA-EMA (see Chapter 4 on serologic testing).

Endoscopy with small intestinal biopsies remains the gold standard for diagnosis of celiac disease in both adults and children. To prevent falsely negative biopsy findings, it is necessary to do the biopsy before the child begins a GFD. Smaller caliber endoscopes are available for small children. Children will be sedated by their gastroenterologist and/or an anesthesiologist with medications to reduce anxiety and discomfort during endoscopy. Younger or very anxious children may require general anesthesia. Because celiac disease can be patchy and not involve the entire intestine, biopsies should be taken at multiple locations within the small intestine, including both the duodenal bulb and other portions of the duodenum (the duodenum is the first portion of the small intestine) (see Chapter 5 on endoscopy).

Protecting against Inadvertent Gluten Exposure

The GFD presents unique challenges for children, not only because they are young and may not be able to take charge of managing their diet, but also because they are more likely to be exposed to gluten in the environment. Because young children often put their hands in their mouths, handling nonfood products containing gluten can sometimes cause symptoms in children with celiac disease. For example, art supplies such as Play-Doh, face paints, and papier maché often contain gluten, so children need to carefully and thoroughly wash their hands after handling these products or avoid using them. Parents need to meet with school nurses and teachers to educate them about the GFD to help create a safe environment in the classroom. Having children bring their own gluten-free products to school events and birthday parties may help your child deal with temptations and peer pressure that can lead to gluten exposure. Anticipating situations, providing safe alternative foods, and even role playing can prepare and empower children and adolescents to advocate for themselves and make good decisions to avoid gluten exposure. Support groups and their Web sites are often a valuable source of information for parents.[4]

Follow-Up Testing

If your child is responding to the GFD, generally symptoms will subside and blood tests will gradually return to normal levels. Repeat endoscopic biopsies to assess intestinal healing are rarely considered necessary in children. IgA-tTG or IgA-EMA levels are often retested six months after diagnosis and, if improved, may only need to be tested annually. An increase in IgA-tTG or IgA-EMA level after an initial decline on a GFD may point to inadvertent gluten exposure. This warrants a careful review of your child's dietary habits and counseling with a dietitian skilled in celiac disease to identify how your child is encountering gluten. Exposure to gluten can result in a return of symptoms but there may be few or no symptoms, especially in older children, despite physical damage to the intestine (see Chapter 18 on cheating).

Testing Siblings

Because first-degree relatives of those with celiac disease are at higher risk of developing celiac disease, parents often ask about testing their other children. Siblings who have either typical or atypical symptoms of celiac disease should be tested immediately. Testing of high-risk children with no symptoms should generally be delayed until age two or three years, provided the child has been on a gluten-containing diet for more than a year.[1] If your child's blood tests are negative, genetic typing with cell surface markers called *HLA markers* can be done to determine his or her potential risk of developing celiac disease. If the genetic typing is negative, then it is very unlikely that your child will develop celiac disease, and follow-up blood testing for celiac disease is not generally needed. If your child has a higher risk HLA genetic group, monitoring with celiac blood testing at 3- to 5-year intervals and being alert to the development of typical or atypical symptoms of celiac disease are necessary (see Chapter 6 on genetic testing).

Preventing Celiac Disease

Parents frequently ask whether celiac disease can be prevented by delaying the introduction of gluten into the diet. There is little scientific evidence on which to base recommendations. One study of infants at high risk of developing celiac disease found that introducing gluten-containing foods was best done between 4 and 6 months of age.[5] The risk of developing celiac disease was higher if gluten was introduced before 3 months of age or after 7 months of age.[5] Introducing gluten while a child is being breastfed may also be protective (see Chapter 27 on infant feeding). Finally, intestinal infections may trigger the onset of celiac disease, and precautions should be taken to prevent spread of viral illnesses, especially rotavirus, a major cause of diarrhea, by using proper hand-washing techniques and vaccination, when appropriate.

What Happened to Cecilia and Jack

Once Cecilia's biopsy confirmed celiac disease, her mother met with a nutritionist and then began feeding Cecilia a GFD. After several weeks, Cecilia had gained weight and again achieved average weight for her age (50th percentile). Her stools became more solid, and she had less bloating and was once again a happy toddler who was able to keep up with her peers. After six months, Cecilia's IgA-tTG level was close to normal.

After three weeks on a GFD, Jack declared that his abdominal pain was gone, noting that he hadn't even realized he had abdominal pain before starting his new diet. Within a year, his IgA-tTG level returned to normal, and Jack was catching up with his peers in height. Jack's sister, who had normal growth and no abdominal symptoms, also tested positive for celiac disease.

SELF-MANAGEMENT TIPS

- ☐ Celiac disease can produce many different kinds of symptoms in infants, children, and teens that may not suggest a gastrointestinal problem.
- ☐ Children at high risk of developing celiac disease include those with a first-degree relative (parent or sibling) with celiac disease and those with a related autoimmune disorder such as type 1 diabetes.
- ☐ Children at high risk of celiac disease should be considered for screening with blood testing, even if they have no symptoms.
- ☐ A GFD is particularly challenging in children, especially in the school environment.
- ☐ A GFD will resolve symptoms, and children usually respond by resuming their expected growth patterns. Repeat blood testing at regular intervals may be useful for monitoring the child's response to the GFD and indicate any inadvertent exposure to gluten.

References

1. Hill et al. Guideline for the diagnosis and treatment of celiac disease in children: recommendations of the North American Society for Pediatric Gastroenterology, Hepatology and Nutrition. *J Pediatr Gastroenterol Nutr* 2005;40(1):1–19. www.naspghan.org/user-assets/Documents/pdf/PositionPapers/celiac_guideline_2004_jpgn.pdf.
2. Telega G, Bennet TR, Werlin S. Emerging new clinical patterns in the presentation of celiac disease. *Arch Pediatr Adolesc Med* 2008;162(2):164–68.
3. Catassi C, Fasano A. Celiac disease as a cause of growth retardation in childhood. *Curr Opin Pediatr* 2004;16(4):445–49.
4. www.childrenshospital.org/celiac.
5. Norris JM, Barriga K, Hoffenberg EJ, et al. Risk of celiac disease autoimmunity and timing of gluten introduction in the diet of infants at increased risk of disease. *JAMA* 2005;293(19):2343–51.

Naamah Zitomersky, MD, is a third-year Fellow in pediatric gastroenterology and nutrition at Children's Hospital Boston, Boston, Massachusetts. **Alan M. Leichtner, MD,** is a pediatric gastroenterologist and Associate Chief of the Division of Gastroenterology and Nutrition and Director of the Center for Celiac Disease, Children's Hospital Boston, and Associate Professor of Pediatrics, Harvard Medical School.

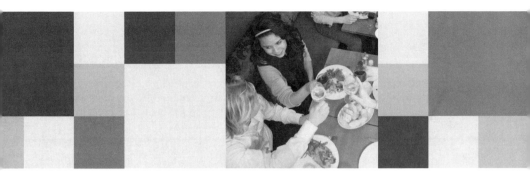

THE GLUTEN-FREE LIFE: SOLUTIONS AND STRATEGIES

The gluten-free diet is the only treatment for celiac disease. Although the gluten-free diet can be well-balanced and healthy, making the dietary and lifestyle changes in a sustainable and optimal way can be tricky. This section addresses some of the most common questions and pitfalls that occur in adopting a gluten-free lifestyle and their solutions.

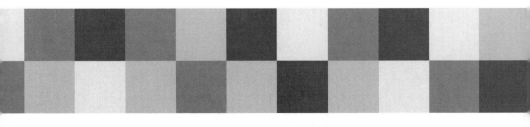

CHAPTER 12

Balanced and Delicious: A *Healthy* Gluten-Free Diet

Nora Decher, MS, RD, CNSC, and Carol Rees Parrish, MS, RD

Emily, a 38-year-old elementary school teacher, was diagnosed with celiac disease one year before coming to our nutrition clinic. Emily enjoys being able to come home and cook a healthy dinner for her two teenage boys and husband. She had researched the gluten-free diet (GFD) on her own, and her celiac blood test (tissue transglutaminase antibody or IgA-tTG) had dropped to 10 units. Emily was successfully avoiding gluten in her diet (Table 1).

Emily was concerned, however, that she would not be able to sustain a varied and healthy diet without gluten. Before her diagnosis, she had always enjoyed sandwiches on whole-grain bread. Emily was now finding it difficult to pack healthy lunches that were gluten free and satisfying. She relied mainly on gluten-free crackers, block cheeses, and plain mixed nuts each day and did not vary her lunch selections because she was com-

TABLE 1. Gluten-Containing Grains, Starches, Flours, and Ingredients

Atta	Hydrolyzed wheat protein
Barley	Kamut
Bulgur	Malt, malt extract, malt syrup, malt flavoring
Couscous	Matzoh, matzoh meal
Dinkel (also known as spelt)	Modified wheat starch
Durum	Oats (unless certified gluten free)
Einkorn	Orzo
Emmer	Rye
Farina	Seitan
Farro or faro (also known as spelt)	Semolina
Fu	Spelt (also known as farro, faro, or dinkel)
Gluten, gluten flour	Triticale
Graham flour	Wheat flour, wheat germ, wheat bran, wheat starch

Adapted with permission from Case S. *Gluten-Free Diet: A Comprehensive Resource Guide*. 4th ed. Case Nutrition Consulting, Inc., 2010, www.glutenfreediet.ca.

forted knowing that these foods were safe. However, she was often hungry after lunch and would snack on a stash of gluten-free snack bars and candies in her classroom for a quick "pick me up." By the time Emily left work, she was usually ravenous and would snack on cheese or treat herself to a bowl of chocolate ice cream when she got home.

Emily's family enjoys eating a wide variety of foods. Emily thought it was unfair to limit her family to eating gluten free, so she found herself spending extra time working in the kitchen to provide both gluten-free meals for herself and gluten-containing choices for the rest of her family. She would frequently prepare additional gluten-free side dishes to ensure that she had something safe to eat. This routine was exhausting.

Balanced Nutrition? I'm Gluten Free! Isn't that Enough?

Although avoiding gluten in the diet takes a little extra effort, it is important not to lose sight of the importance of a healthy, balanced, and wholesome diet. A "balanced" diet is one that includes adequate amounts of the various nutrients required to sustain life, maintain energy, and prevent chronic disease. No one food or food group is superior to any other. What you want is a variety of "nutrient-dense" foods, which are rich in vitamins, minerals, and/or phytonutrients (such as fruits, vegetables, nuts, seeds, dried beans, legumes, whole grains, lean meats, and lean dairy products), and few foods with "empty calories," calories but very little nutrients (such as sodas, baked goods, and alcohol). Table 2 offers guidelines for healthy, balanced eating. Following these basic nutrition guidelines can help you feel great as well as lower your risk for chronic diseases such as diabetes, cardiovascular diseases, and certain cancers. The GFD can be naturally wholesome because so many healthy foods are naturally gluten free.

Scientists have done very little investigating into the adequacy of the GFD. However, surveys conducted in the United States and England suggest that individuals following a GFD may not get enough iron, calcium, fiber, or whole grains.[3,4] Table 3 shows the daily reference intakes and healthy food choices for these nutrients. The U.S. Department of Agriculture's Nutrient Database Web site, www.nal.usda.gov/fnic/foodcomp/search, lists the nutrient content of many more foods.[5]

Although your main source of good nutrition should come from real food like vegetables, fruits, lean meats, gluten-free grains, and healthy fats (rather than food products), your phy-

TABLE 2. Healthy Eating Guidelines

- Balance calorie intake and physical activity to achieve or maintain a healthy weight.
- Consume a diet rich in a variety of vegetables and fruits.
- Choose gluten-free whole-grain, higher-fiber foods.
- Include low-fat or nonfat dairy products.
- Consume 3–4 oz. of omega-3 fatty acids at least twice a week in fish.
- Limit your intake of saturated fat and *trans* fat by cooking at home and including vegetarian dishes.
- Minimize intake of beverages and foods with added sugars.
- If you consume alcohol, do so in moderation.

Adapted from references 1 and 2.

TABLE 3. Nutrients Found to be Low or Deficient in Gluten-Free Diets

Nutrient	Gluten-Free Food Source	Dietary Reference Intake
Iron	▪ Beef, pork, lamb (choose red meats that are lean) ▪ Green leafy vegetables: spinach, asparagus, broccoli, collard greens, mustard greens, kale, turnip greens, parsley, cabbage ▪ Fortified foods: gluten-free oatmeal, rice, corn grits ▪ Salmon, shrimp, tuna, oysters, clams, most kinds of seafood ▪ Most kinds of legumes: lima beans, kidney beans, navy beans, soy beans, chick peas, pinto beans, black-eyed peas ▪ Grains: teff, amaranth, quinoa ▪ Nuts/seeds: almonds, cashews, walnuts, sunflower seeds, sesame seeds or tahini, pumpkin seeds ▪ Dried fruits: apricots, raisins, dates (not rolled in flour), prunes, figs ▪ Turkey, chicken, egg yolks	**8 mg/day** (males >18 yr and females >50 yr) **18 mg/day** (females 19–50 yr)
Calcium	▪ Milk: bottled, canned, evaporated (lactose-free milk if lactose intolerant) ▪ Low-fat or fat-free yogurt ▪ Cheese, ricotta (part skim milk) ▪ Gluten-free chocolate milk ▪ Fortified gluten-free rice, hemp, soy, or nut milk ▪ Collards: frozen, chopped, cooked, boiled, drained, without salt ▪ Rhubarb: frozen, cooked ▪ Anchovies, sardines canned with bone, salmon canned with bone, Atlantic cod, Pacific herring, canned jack mackerel, sunfish, caviar ▪ Shrimp, blue crab ▪ Low-fat gluten-free eggnog	**1000 mg** (males and females 19–50 yr) **1200 mg** (males and females >50 yr)
Fiber	▪ Raspberries, blueberries, strawberries, pear or apple with skin, banana, oranges, dried figs ▪ Split peas, lentils, black beans, lima beans, gluten-free baked beans, sunflower seeds, almonds, pistachios, pecans ▪ Artichokes, peas, broccoli, turnip greens, sweet corn, Brussels sprouts, potatoes with skin, tomato paste, raw carrots ▪ Amaranth, buckwheat, corn, millet, gluten-free oats, quinoa, sorghum, teff, wild rice, brown rice, air-popped popcorn	**38 g** (males <50) **30 g** (males >50) **25 g** (females <50) **21 g** (females >50)

Adapted from references 6 and 7.

sician and nutritionist can advise you about whether you need additional vitamin or mineral supplementation (see Chapter 14 on supplements).

"Recipe" for a Healthy GFD

A healthy GFD contains fruits and vegetables, whole grains and fiber, lean protein, low-fat dairy, calcium and vitamin D sources, and healthy fats.

Fruits and Vegetables

Fruits and vegetables are powerhouse foods because they are important sources of carbohydrates, fiber, vitamin C, folate, potassium, vitamins A and E, and phytonutrients. Phytonutrients (such as carotenoids, flavonoids, phytosterols, and isoflavones) are components of plants that provide health benefits. Deep color is a good rule of thumb to gauge the nutrient density of vegetables and fruits (Table 4). Depending on your calorie needs, 2½ to 6½ servings of vegetables are recommended each day (USDA). The American Cancer Society recommends at least 5 servings of vegetables and fruits (combined) each day to help prevent cancer.

What's a serving size?

- ½ cup fruit
- Medium-sized piece of fruit (the size of a tennis ball)
- ¼ cup dried fruit
- ¾ cup (6 ounces) of 100% fruit or vegetable juice
- 2 cups leafy vegetables (spinach or lettuce leaves)
- 1 cup cooked or raw vegetables

Any plain, fresh, frozen, or canned fruits and vegetables are safe. Dried fruits and vegetables may have gluten added in flavorings, coatings, or sauces, so read the labels (see Chapter 20 on inadvertent gluten exposure and Chapter 22 on food labeling for information on what to look for). Vegetables in sauces or gravies are questionable, and you should give the labels a closer look.

TABLE 4. Nutrient-Dense Fruits and Vegetables

Safe and Nutrient Dense	Safe but Less Nutrient Dense	Questionable	Avoid
Vegetables Carrots, tomatoes, broccoli, kale, spinach, bell peppers, asparagus, sweet potatoes, yams, squash, zucchini, low-sodium gluten-free vegetable juice	Iceberg lettuce, cucumber, corn, potatoes	Dried vegetables or vegetables in sauce or gravy; check labels for added ingredients	Added ingredients, seasonings, or sauces containing gluten
Fruits Berries, apples, cherries, grapes, pomegranates, oranges, peaches, nectarines, plums, melons, bananas		Dried fruit or fruit in sauce; check labels for added ingredients	

Whole Grains and Fiber

Diets rich in whole grains and fiber are associated with better health. Whole grains are an excellent source of soluble fibers, which have been shown to be helpful in decreasing LDL cholesterol (the "bad" cholesterol) levels. Nutrition experts recommend adults consume 21–38 g of fiber per day, along with ample fluid intake.[8]

Some patients complain of constipation after starting a GFD because of a low fiber intake (see Chapter 16 on constipation). Many gluten-free foods are low in fiber. However, fiber-rich gluten-free whole grain sources, such as gluten-free oatmeal, air popped popcorn, and brown rice, are easy to find. There are exotic nutrient-dense gluten-free grains available that add variety, as well as fiber and iron (Table 5). Including gluten-free whole grains significantly increases the quality of your GFD.

In addition to whole grains, fruits and vegetables are excellent sources of fiber. Beans, legumes, nuts, and seeds contain fiber as well as iron and protein. Any grain that does not contain gluten and has not been contaminated by gluten is safe to eat. There is more information on grains and food labeling in Chapters 13 and 22.

The Basics on Protein

Protein is the building block for growth and repair of muscles, red blood cells, skin, and other tissues. Most healthy adults require 0.8–1.0 gram of protein per kilogram of their body weight daily. For example, a healthy 143-pound (65-kg) male should aim for 55–65 grams of protein each day. Special populations, such as endurance athletes, growing children and teenagers, pregnant women, people with malabsorption concerns, people who are on hemodialysis, or those with healing wounds, may have greater protein needs.

It is common for someone with newly diagnosed celiac disease to select high-protein foods such as meat, cheese, and nuts because these foods are typically safe. However, they are also high in fat. Meats, cheese, and nuts are very healthy in moderation but should not be the mainstay of your diet; the calories will add up quickly. Lean gluten-free protein sources are a healthy and easy way to meet the body's protein needs. The lean protein sources below are low in fat, and each provides 8–12 grams of protein per serving:[9]

- 1 cup low-fat yogurt
- ½ cup low-fat cottage cheese
- 1 cup nonfat or low-fat milk or soy milk
- 1.5 oz. grilled or baked chicken, turkey, fish, pork, or lean beef

TABLE 5. Gluten-Free Whole Grains and Legumes

Safe	Questionable	Avoid
Amaranth; flax; millet; ragi (red millet); quinoa; brown rice; wild rice; sorghum; teff; legumes and beans including garbanzo beans, lentils, pinto beans, edamame (soybean), lima beans, black beans, and dried peas	Carob-soy flour, buckwheat pancake mixes, any naturally gluten-free grains that are not labeled "gluten free" on the package	Wheat including bulgur, couscous, durum, farina, graham, kamut, semolina, spelt, triticale, and wheat germ; rye; barley; oats except pure, uncontaminated oats; low-gluten flour

TABLE 6. Gluten-Free Dairy

Safe	Questionable	Avoid
Any plain, unflavored milk or yogurt, buttermilk, cottage cheese, natural and processed cheeses, cream, half and half	Flavored milks or yogurts, cheese spreads or sauces	Malted milk, yogurt with added "crunchies" or toppings

- 3 cooked egg whites
- ½ cup refried beans, kidney beans, chickpeas, soybeans, or black beans

Dairy, Calcium and Vitamin D

Dairy products such as milk, yogurt, and cheeses are important sources of nutrients, and many are reliably gluten free (Table 6). They are a great source of calcium and vitamin D required for bone health; they also provide protein, phosphorus, magnesium, riboflavin, and vitamins A and B_{12}. Lactose intolerance can be a problem for newly diagnosed patients.[10] If this is the case for you, be sure to select from a variety of nondairy sources to get adequate calcium and vitamin D (Tables 7 and 8). Lactose intolerance often subsides with adherence to the GFD after several months (Chapter 37 has information on lactose intolerance and other poorly absorbed carbohydrates).

Although the daily reference intakes (for adults) for calcium and vitamin D are 1000 mg of calcium and 200–400 IU of vitamin D, many nutrition experts recommend at least

TABLE 7. Lean Dairy and Nondairy Calcium Sources

Food	Calcium Content (mg)
1 cup nonfat plain yogurt	452
1.5 oz. romano cheese	452
2 oz. Swiss cheese	438
1 cup low-fat fruit yogurt	345
½ cup part-skim ricotta cheese	335
1 cup nonfat milk	306
1 cup 1% low-fat milk	290
1 cup low-fat buttermilk	284
1 cup fortified gluten-free cereal	varies
1 cup fortified gluten-free soy milk	368
3 oz. sardines, Atlantic, in oil	325
½ cup tofu	253
3 oz. salmon, canned with bone	181
½ cup collards, cooked from frozen	178
1 Tbsp. blackstrap molasses	172
½ cup spinach, cooked from frozen	146

From Reference 7.

TABLE 8. Food Sources of Vitamin D

Food	Vitamin D Content (IU)
1 Tbsp. cod liver oil	1360
3.5 oz. salmon	360
3.5 oz. mackerel	345
3 oz. tuna, canned in oil	200
1.75 oz. sardines, canned in oil	250
1 cup nonfat or low-fat vitamin D–fortified milk	98
1 Tbsp. vitamin D–fortified margarine	60
Cereal, gluten free, vitamin D fortified	varies
Egg, 1 whole (vitamin D found in yolk)	20
3.5 oz. liver, cooked	15
1 oz. Swiss cheese	12

From Reference 7.

1200 mg of calcium, along with 800–2000 IU vitamin D daily, to maintain good health and strong bones. Those who are deficient in vitamin D may require higher doses of vitamin D and should consult with a physician and registered dietitian for specific recommendations (see Chapters 33 on monitoring patients with celiac disease and Chapter 47 on bone disease for more information on monitoring and supplementing calcium and vitamin D).

To avoid piling on extra calories, choose low-fat or nonfat dairy products instead of full-fat choices. Generally, 3–5 servings of calcium-rich foods, such as those listed in Tables 6 and 7, will meet your calcium needs.[7]

Gone Fishing . . . for Healthy Fats
Omega-3 polyunsaturated fatty acids are an important part of a "heart-healthy" diet. The three omega-3 fatty acids are eicosapentaenoic acid (EPA), docosahexaenoic acid (DHA), and alpha-linolenic acid (ALA). The American Heart Association recommends eating a variety of oily fish at least twice per week to obtain the most heart-protective benefit from omega-3 fats and to reduce your risk for cardiovascular diseases.[11]

Table 9 presents the best sources of EPA and DHA. Some farmed fish, such as farmed tilapia and catfish, may contain higher amounts of omega-6 (pro-inflammatory fatty acids) and lower omega-3 than wild-caught fish.[12,13] However, in general, the differences in omega-3 content between farmed and wild-caught fish are negligible, and choosing any source of omega-3 rich fish, such as those listed in Table 8, is beneficial.[14]

Be aware that certain types of fish (tilefish, swordfish, king mackerel, and shark) may contain significant levels of environmental toxins, such as mercury. The FDA recommends that children and women of childbearing age limit their consumption of these types of fish. For up-to-date information regarding the safety of fish and shellfish consumption, refer to the FDA and the Environmental Protection Agency Web sites (www.fda.gov/Food/default. htm and www.epa.gov, respectively).

TABLE 9. Top Sources of Eicosapentaenoic Acid (EPA) and Docosahexaenoic Acid (DHA)

Fish	EPA and DHA Content (g) per 3-oz. Serving	Amount of Fish (oz.) Required to Provide 1 g EPA and DHA
Herring		
Pacific	1.81	1.5
Atlantic	1.71	2.0
Salmon		
Atlantic, farmed	1.09–1.83	1.5–2.5
Atlantic, wild	0.90–1.56	2.0–3.5
Chinook	1.48	2.0
Sockeye	0.68	4.5
Mackerel	0.34–1.57	2.0–8.5
Sardines	0.98–1.70	2.0–3.0
Tuna		
Fresh	0.24–1.28	2.5–12.0
Halibut	0.40–1.00	3.0–7.5
White (canned in water)	0.73	4.0
Flounder/sole	0.42	7.0
Crab	0.35	8.5
Shrimp	0.27	11.0

From Reference 11.

If eating fish is not for you, a capsule containing 1 gram total of EPA and DHA is a reasonable substitute. If you have been diagnosed with a cardiovascular disease or need to lower your triglyceride level, an increased intake of EPA and DHA (in the form of food especially) may be helpful.[15] Consult with a dietitian and physician before using supplements. See Chapter 14 for information on how choose the best fish oil supplement.

Plant sources of omega-3 fats, in the form of ALA, are beneficial for heart health because your body has the ability to convert some ALA to EPA and DHA. EPA and DHA have the strongest effect on heart health. ALA is a good choice for vegetarians or others avoiding fish. Table 10 presents the best sources of ALA.

Any fresh, plain, untreated fish or shellfish, nuts, seeds, or vegetable oils are safe choices for consuming omega-3 fatty acids (see Table 11 for specific sources). Commercially treated, preserved, or marinated fish or shellfish are questionable. Breaded or battered fish should be avoided, unless care was taken to ensure gluten-free preparation such as using gluten-free breading.

It's also important to limit saturated fats to less than 7% of total daily energy intake (calories) and to avoid *trans* fatty acids (trans fats) to reduce your risk for cardiovascular diseases and stroke.[1,15] Saturated fats are typically solid at room temperature (examples include lard, fatty beef, poultry with skin, cream, butter, and cheese). Trans fats are found in oils that have been "hydrogenated" (chemically altered to a more solid form), such as some margarines, baked goods, and snack foods. Simple ways to cut out unhealthy fats include:

TABLE 10. Top Sources of Alpha-Linolenic Acid (ALA)

Food	Serving Size	ALA Content (g) per Serving
Flaxseed oil	1 Tbsp.	8.5
Walnuts, English	1 oz.	2.6
Flaxseeds	1 Tbsp.	2.2
Walnut oil	1 Tbsp.	1.4
Canola oil	1 Tbsp.	1.2
Mustard oil	1 Tbsp.	0.9
Soybean oil	1 Tbsp.	0.8
Walnuts, black	1 Tbsp.	0.6
Olive oil	1 Tbsp.	0.1
Broccoli, raw	1 Tbsp.	0.1

From Reference 11.

- Choosing lean meats and fish instead of full-fat meats
- Substituting beans or legumes for meat in an entrée
- Choosing fat-free and low-fat dairy products
- Reading labels to find and avoid hydrogenated or partially hydrogenated fats
- Choosing foods from the lean protein and lean dairy food lists above

Healthy Snacking

Snacking can be a healthy component of the GFD with numerous benefits. Snacking helps provide calories for those who need to gain weight and energy for physical activity, prevent overeating by staving off hunger, and prevent temptation while on the go. To make a long-lasting, energizing snack, pair a healthy carbohydrate such as whole-grain gluten-free crackers with a protein like cheese, egg, or natural peanut butter. This is healthier than a high-sugar or fat-based snack. Table 12 presents some snack choices.

TABLE 11. Safe Choices for Omega-3 Fats

Safe	Questionable	Avoid
EPA and DHA Any fresh, plain, or untreated fish or shell-fish, such as mackerel, lake trout, herring, sardines, albacore tuna, or salmon canned in brine, gluten-free vegetable broth, or water	Commercially treated, preserved, or marinated fish or shellfish	Breaded or battered fish
ALA Nuts, seeds, and oils, such as walnuts; flaxseeds; soybeans; tofu; canola, soybean, flaxseed, and olive oils	Dry roasted nuts (may be dusted with flour during processing; check with manufacturer)	

TABLE 12. Safe and Healthy Gluten-Free Snack Ideas

- Fresh fruits: peaches, plums, apricots, bananas, melons, oranges, grapefruits, mango, papaya
- Dried fruits (in small servings): cherries, cranberries, apples, pineapple, raisins, peaches, mango, banana chips (check for added ingredients in dried fruit)
- Plain nuts or seeds (in small servings): almonds, walnuts, cashews, soy nuts, pistachio, sunflower seeds, pumpkin seeds
- Gluten-free dry cereals mixed with gluten free yogurt
- Air-popped popcorn
- Trail mix: experiment with a mixture of nuts, dried fruits, gluten-free dry cereal, and gluten-free pretzels, for example
- Tuna and high-fiber gluten-free crackers
- Peanut butter or other nut butters and jelly or honey on whole-grain rice cakes
- Gluten-free granola or energy bars
- Gluten-free crackers or cheese crisps
- Vegetables with hummus, salsa, or other gluten-free dips
- Cottage cheese
- Gluten-free yogurt
- Hard-boiled eggs
- Hard or string cheese

The GFD becomes less healthy when you overindulge in processed gluten-free snack foods. Processed gluten-free cookies, cakes, and other snack products can be enticing because they are labeled as safe. These are sources of empty calories and should be used sparingly. You can save money by making your own snacks.

Expanding Your Palate

A common concern of those with a new diagnosis of celiac disease is that the diet will be restrictive and eliminate many healthy food choices. We find that patients grow to enjoy the taste of a greater variety of foods. With attention to balance and variety, the GFD is a very healthy and enjoyable way to eat.

Emily's Education

We took a good look at Emily's eating plan over a typical week and addressed several nutritional issues, including lack of variety, lack of fruits and vegetables, and high intake of dietary fat, particularly saturated fat from all the cheese. After meeting with a registered dietitian in our nutrition clinic, Emily felt ready to make a few simple changes.

Emily soon began to save time in the kitchen, feel more energized, and enjoy mealtime. She was more satisfied with her diet *and* her life.

Instead of	Emily decided to
Preparing different foods for herself and her family at dinnertime	Try a variety of gluten-free grains, homemade breads (using wheat flour substitutes such as brown rice, amaranth, sorghum, tapioca, and bean flours), and other dishes that they could all enjoy together.
Scrambling to find gluten-free options for lunch	Prepare a little extra and save the leftovers from dinner each night so that she would have a healthy meal for lunch the next day. On weekends, if she had spare time, she also fixed an extra dish or two for the freezer for those nights when she would not feel like cooking.
Snacking on processed gluten-free snacks and candies, which are often high in sugar and fat, low in protein, and costly	Pack healthy snacks such as fresh fruit, gluten-free trail mix, or celery sticks with almond butter.
Feeling alone and defeated with her diagnosis	Attend meetings with her local celiac support group and connect with national support groups on the Internet (see Resources). Emily was able to share recipes and tips with others with celiac disease, as well as build a support network with those experiencing similar issues.

SELF-MANAGEMENT TIPS

- ☐ Following a balanced GFD is an easy way to feel great, improve your overall health, and reduce your risk for chronic diseases such as diabetes, cardiovascular disease, and cancers.
- ☐ A healthy GFD can be achieved through a balance of foods; however, a physician and dietitian can advise you about supplementing specific nutrients, if necessary.
- ☐ Enjoy a variety of foods, including:
  - – Deeply-colored gluten-free fruits and vegetables
  - – Gluten-free whole grains
  - – Nonfat or low-fat dairy products or nondairy calcium-rich foods
  - – Fish or alternative sources of omega-3 fatty acids
- ☐ Planning ahead to prepare gluten-free meals and snacks, especially when you're on the go, will ensure that you always have foods available that are healthy and safe.
- ☐ For more information about building a healthful diet, refer to the *Dietary Guidelines for Americans* at http://www.health.gov/dietaryguidelines/dga2005/document/default.htm and the U.S. Department of Agriculture's food guidance system *My Pyramid* at http://www.mypyramid.gov.

References

1. American Heart Association Nutrition Committee, Lichtenstein AH, Appel LJ, Brands M, et al. Diet and lifestyle recommendations revision 2006: a scientific statement from the American Heart Association Nutrition Committee. *Circulation* 2006;114:82–96.

2. USDA Dietary Guidelines for Americans 2005. http://www.health.gov/DietaryGuidelines. Accessed 8/4/09.

3. Thompson T, Dennis M, Higgins LA, et al. Gluten-free diet survey: are Americans with coeliac disease consuming recommended amounts of fibre, iron, calcium and grain foods? *J Hum Nutr Diet* 2005;18:163–69.

4. Kinsey L, Burden ST, Bannerman E. A dietary survey to determine if patients with coeliac disease are meeting current healthy eating guidelines and how their diet compares to that of the British general population. *Eur J Clin Nutr* 2008;62:1333–42.

5. US Department of Agriculture, Agricultural Research Service. USDA Nutrient Database for Standard Reference, Release 21. Nutrient Data Laboratory Home Page, 2009. http://www.ars.usda.gov/main/site_main.htm?modecode=12354500. Accessed 8/4/09.

6. Food and Nutrition Board, Institute of Medicine, National Academies. Dietary Reference Intakes (DRIs): Recommended Intakes for Individuals, Vitamins and Macronutrients. http://www.iom.edu/Object.File/Master/21/372/0.pdf. Accessed 8/14/09.

7. USDA Dietary Guidelines for Americans 2005. Appendix B. Food Sources of Selected Nutrients. http://www.health.gov/DietaryGuidelines. Accessed 8/14/09.

8. Case S. *Gluten-Free Diet: A Comprehensive Resource Guide.* 4th ed. Case Nutrition Consulting, Inc., 2010, www.glutenfree.diet.ca.

9. Health Canada. *Nutrient Value of Some Common Foods.* Tufts University School of Medicine, Harvard University, and USDA National Nutrient Data Bank, 1999.

10. Barrett JS, et al. Comparison of the prevalence of fructose and lactose malabsorption across chronic intestinal disorders. *Aliment Pharmacol Ther* 2009;30:165–74.

11. Kris-Etherton PM, Harris WS, Appel LJ, American Heart Association Nutrition Committee. Fish consumption, fish oil, omega-3 fatty acids, and cardiovascular disease. *Circulation* 2002;106:2747–57.

12. Weaver KL, Ivester P, Chilton JA, et al. The content of favorable and unfavorable polyunsaturated fatty acids found in commonly eaten fish. *J Am Diet Assoc* 2008;108:1178–85.

13. Hamilton MC, Hites PA, Schwager SJ, et al. Lipid composition and contaminants in farmed and wild salmon. *Enviorn Sci Technol* 2005;39:8622–29.

14. He K, Song Y, Faviglus ML, et al. Accumulated evidence on fish consumption and coronary heart disease mortality: a meta-analysis of cohort studies. *Circulation* 2004;109:2705–11.

15. Van Horn L, McCoin M, Kris-Etherton PM, et al. The evidence for dietary prevention and treatment of cardiovascular disease. *J Am Diet Assoc* 2008;108:287–331.

Further Reading

These resources are from the *Practical Gastroenterology* Celiac Nutrition Series found at the University of Virginia Health System's GI Nutrition Web site: www.healthsystem.virginia.edu/internet/digestive-health/nutrition/celiacsupport.cfm.

- Dennis M. Celiac centers/experts in the U.S. *Pract Gastroenterol* 2006; XXX(9):94.
- Pagano A. Whole grains and the gluten-free diet. *Pract Gastroenterol* 2006;XXX(10):66.
- Cureton P. Dining out gluten free: is it safe? *Pract Gastroenterol* 2006;XXX(11):61.

- Dinga M, Dinga A. Heart health and celiac disease. *Pract Gastroenterol* 2006;XXX(12):70.
- Plogsted S. Medications and celiac disease: tips from a pharmacist. *Pract Gastroenterol* 2007;XXXI(1):58.
- Sharrett MK, Cureton P. Kids and the gluten-free diet. *Pract Gastroenterol* 2007; XXXI(2):49.
- Kupper C, Higgins L. Combining diabetes and gluten-free dietary management guidelines. *Pract Gastroenterol* 2007;XXXI(3):68.
- Cureton P. The gluten-free diet: can your patient afford it? *Pract Gastroenterol* 2007; XXXI(4):75.
- Pagano A. The gluten-free vegetarian. *Pract Gastroenterol* 2007;XXXI(5):94.
- Obrero T. Management of dialysis patients with celiac disease. *Pract Gastroenterol* 2007;XXXI(6):70.

Nora Decher, MS, RD, CNSC, is a Nutrition Support/GI Nutrition Specialist at the University of Virginia Health System (UVAHS), Digestive Health Center of Excellence, Charlottesville, Virginia. She counsels patients with a variety of GI disorders and leads the Celiac Support Group CharlottsVILLI. **Carol Rees Parrish, MS, RD,** is a Nutrition Support Specialist at UVAHS, Digestive Health Center of Excellence, where she began the home nutrition support program, developed the GI Nutrition Clinic, originated the Celiac Support Group, and co-founded both nutrition support traineeship programs.

CHAPTER 13

Whole Grains = Nutritional Gold

Laurie A. Higgins, MS, RD, LDN, CDE

Sara is a 20-year-old college student who was diagnosed with celiac disease over the summer while at home with her parents in Boston. At diagnosis, Sara and her parents met with a dietitian who specializes in celiac disease and who suggested a lot of changes to be sure Sara could eat gluten free. Before she returned to college, Sara and her mother met again with the dietitian to review the gluten-free diet (GFD) and consider some solutions for problems she might encounter while on her own.

Back at school in New York City, Sara is living off campus this year in an apartment with her friends and has found it difficult to balance a busy college life and cook and prepare gluten-free foods. She has been purchasing many ready-to-eat gluten-free foods from the local health food store. Some of her staples include frozen pizza, burritos, canned soups, snack bars, cheese, potato and corn chips, hummus, fresh fruit, and vegetables. Lately, however, Sara has been having increased abdominal pain and constipation.

Before her diagnosis, Sara ate a lot of whole-grain breads, pasta, and crackers. Since transitioning to the GFD, she has found that many of the substitutes are not made with whole grains and don't have much fiber. She suspects this is causing her constipation but is also concerned about the pain. So, while at home for the holidays, Sara met with her dietitian to make sure her diet is gluten free and to get recommendations on how to safely increase dietary fiber in her diet. The dietitian asked her to record a 3-day food diary. Because Sara eats the same foods every day, she did not think that it was necessary to record three days and just wrote down what she eats most days.

Sara's Typical Meal Plan

BREAKFAST: gluten-free rice cereal, low-fat milk, and an orange

MORNING SNACK: gluten-free cookies and low-fat milk or chips

LUNCH: hummus, corn chips, carrots and celery sticks, and a piece of fresh fruit

AFTERNOON SNACK: gluten-free pretzels, rice cakes, or cookies and low-fat milk

DINNER: white rice, chicken, broccoli, and water or juice

EVENING SNACK: gluten-free rice cereal and low-fat milk or ice cream

Sarah reported that she usually cooks a large pot of rice and 3–4 chicken breasts on the weekend and eats that throughout the week in addition to the ready-to-eat food mentioned above.

Sara received praise for her knowledge and understanding of the GFD from the dietitian, who was unable to detect any ways in which gluten could be sneaking into her diet. She suggested that Sara's abdominal pain might be a result of the decrease of fiber in her diet. They talked about the fact that Sara's diet is also low in B vitamins and variety yet high in fat and sodium. The solution was to increase Sara's intake of gluten-free whole grains.

What Are Whole Grains?

Whole grains or foods made with them contain all the parts of the grain: the bran, germ, and endosperm. We have all heard that eating whole grains is good for us because they are high in fiber, low in fat, contain protein, and are rich in B vitamins. These characteristics are because of the bran, the outside wrapping that is mostly fiber plus B vitamins and minerals, and the germ, a rich source of B vitamins. When grains are milled or processed, these healthy nutrients of whole grains are lost and only the starchy endosperm is retained. Milling and processing of grains was originally done to increase the shelf life of the grains. Removing the germ, which contains unsaturated fats that can spoil or go rancid over time when exposed to heat and sunlight, allows the grain to last longer. Many gluten-containing grains that are processed have been fortified with nutrients that don't occur naturally or are enriched with the very nutrients that are lost during milling, although this is not true for the majority of processed gluten-free grains.

The United States Department of Agriculture's (USDA) Dietary Guidelines for Americans[1] and the Whole Grains Council both recommend that at least three 1-oz. servings (48 grams of whole grain; not to be confused with fiber) or half of the grains we consume daily should be whole grains. This recommendation is based on research that suggests that eating whole grains is associated with a reduction in chronic diseases such as coronary heart disease, type 2 diabetes, and obesity.

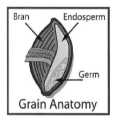

Bran Endosperm

Germ

Grain Anatomy

From Oldways and the Whole Grains Council: www.WholeGrains Council.org.

To help identify foods that have been made with whole grains, the Whole Grain Council launched the "100% Whole Grain" stamp in 2003. This stamp is only placed on foods made with 100% whole grains and that have a minimum of 16 grams of whole grain per serving. For example, Carolina Brown Rice is whole grain with only the outer hull removed but still contains the bran layers and provides 42 grams of whole grain per ¾ cup serving (cooked). The "Basic Whole Grain" stamp signifies that the product has some refined flour, added germ or bran, and at least 8 grams of whole grains per serving. The Whole Grains Council lists products that contain these stamps on their Web site (www.WholeGrainsCouncil.org) to help you locate whole-grain products. Table 1 lists some whole grains and legumes that are gluten free.

What Whole Grains Deliver

There are two reasons why relying heavily on gluten-free food products limits your intake of nutrients. First, many of the gluten-free products on the market are prepared from processed or refined flours and grains, often in an attempt to produce foods that are similar in texture and taste to gluten-containing products. They are missing the fiber, minerals, and vitamins of whole grains. Second, the main source of B vitamins in the American diet—thiamin, riboflavin, niacin, and folate—is enriched flours, breads, crackers, and breakfast cereals. This means that the vitamins removed during refinement are added back. Unfortunately, many gluten-free grains are not enriched and have fewer B vitamins than their gluten-containing counterparts.[2]

By substituting typical gluten-free grains with "alternative" gluten-free whole grains, such as gluten-free oats, high-fiber gluten-free breads, and grains like quinoa, the nutrient content of the diet vastly improves.[3] So, you will reap nutritional benefits if you

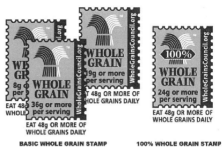

From Oldways and the Whole Grains Council:
www.WholeGrainsCouncil.org

TABLE 1. Gluten-Free Whole Grains and Legumes

Whole Grains	Legumes
Amaranth	Black beans
Buckwheat	Edamame (fresh soybeans in the pod)
Brown rice	Garbanzo beans (chickpeas)
Corn	Lentils
Flax seed	Lima beans
Millet	Peas
Montina Indian rice grass	Pinto beans
Gluten-free oats	Soybeans
Popcorn	Kidney beans
Quinoa	Black-eyed peas
Sorghum	Butter beans
Teff	
Wild rice	

TABLE 2. Gluten-Free Sources of B Vitamins

Thiamine (B₁)
Best: enriched gluten-free grains and flours, pork
Good: gluten-free soy milk, orange juice, legumes (peanuts, beans, and soy), watermelon

Riboflavin (B₂)
Best: enriched gluten-free grains, eggs, meat
Good: liver, mushrooms, spinach and green leafy vegetables, broccoli, asparagus, milk, cottage cheese

Niacin (B₃)
Best: enriched gluten-free grains, beef, chicken, turkey, fish (tuna, halibut, salmon)
Good: peanuts, asparagus

B₆
Best: meat, fish, and poultry
Good: bananas, avocados, potatoes, sunflower seeds

can find and regularly consume gluten-free whole grains (Table 1), enriched foods and gluten-free sources of B vitamins (Table 2). Whole grains also contain other vital minerals, such as iron and calcium, in addition to the fiber and B vitamins (Table 3).

Whole grains also contain two kinds of dietary fiber, soluble and insoluble. Soluble fiber plays a role in lowering cholesterol; it's found in whole grains as well as in many fruits, vegetables, and legumes such as beans, soybeans, and peanuts. Insoluble fiber is

TABLE 3. B Vitamins, Calcium, and Iron Content of Whole Grains (1 cup uncooked)

Flours	Fiber (gm)	Thiamine (B₁) (mg)	Riboflavin (B₂) mg	Niacin (B₃) (mg)	B₆ (mg)	Folate (mcg)	Calcium (mg)	Iron (mg)
Amaranth	12.9	0.22	0.39	1.78	1.14	158	307	14.69
Buckwheat groats	16.9	0.37	0.44	8.42	0.579	69	28	4.05
Millet	17.0	0.84	0.58	9.44	0.77	170	16	6.02
Quinoa	11.9	0.62	0.54	2.58	0.88	313	80	7.77
Sorghum	12.1	0.46	0.27	5.6	1.13	38	54	8.45
Teff	15.4	0.75	0.52	6.49	0.93	—	347	14.73
Wheat flour, whole-grain	14.6	0.54	0.26	7.6	0.41	53	41	4.66
Wheat flour, white enriched	3.4	0.84	0.52	7.3	0.06	245	422	5.84

From USDA National Nutrient Database, http://www.nal.usda.gov/fnic/foodcomp/search/index.html.

TABLE 4. Practical Tips for Using Gluten-Free Whole Grains

Grain	Nutrient Content	Amount of Liquid	Amount of Grain	Cooking Time	Uses
Amaranth	Protein, fiber, iron, magnesium, zinc, calcium, B vitamins	2–3 cups	1 cup	Simmer 7 minutes, let stand covered 10 minutes	Hot or cold cereal, thickener for soups and stews
Buckwheat	Protein, fiber, B₆, niacin, thiamin, iron, zinc	2 cups	1 cup	Simmer 15 minutes	Hot cereal, side dish, soups, stews, casseroles
Quinoa	High-quality protein, fiber, calcium, magnesium, iron, B vitamins	2 cups	1 cup	Simmer 15 minutes	Side dish, cold salad, soups, stews
Teff	Protein, calcium, iron, B vitamins	2 cups	½ cup	Simmer 15–20 minutes	Hot cereal, side dish

Compiled by Anne Roland Lee.

not digested, but it adds bulk to the stool and can be very helpful in treating constipation. Because fiber absorbs a lot of water as it moves through your digestive tract, if you increase the amount of fiber in your diet, it's critical to drink enough fluids. Fiber recommendations for adults range from 21–38 grams daily or 14 grams per 1,000 calories after the age of 1 year.[4]

A 3-day diet analysis of adults on a GFD showed that more than 50% of females did not eat adequate amounts of fiber, iron, or calcium.[5] Sara's typical eating plan provides her with just about 10–12 grams of fiber a day. The dietitian suggested that she increase her fiber intake slowly to a goal of 25–35 grams daily to help her with constipation and abdominal pain. Choosing fresh fruits and vegetables and gluten-free whole-grain foods will enable her to meet this goal. The dietitian reminded her that as she gradually increases her fiber intake, she needs to also increase her fluids so that she is drinking 6–8 glasses of water each day.

Sara had some questions about learning to cook and eat several of the new grains suggested by the dietitian. The advice was to start slowly by choosing one new grain at a time to learn to cook (Table 4), seasoning with salt and butter to taste. The dietitian also urged Sara to consider attending support groups and cooking classes, where she would meet other people with celiac disease to share advice and recipes.

What Sara Decided

After meeting with the dietitian, Sara decided to try to incorporate more gluten-free whole grains into her diet. Here are some of the food ideas that Sara and her dietitian came up with during their session.

Breakfast

- Whole-grain gluten-free waffles: Sara can make a batch and freeze them for the week. Waffles also make great sandwich bread in a pinch.
- Hot gluten-free cereals of buckwheat, amaranth, quinoa, and gluten-free whole rolled oats with sliced almonds, ground flax seed, and dried or fresh fruit
- Baked oatmeal: Mix together 3 cups of gluten-free steel-cut oats or rolled oats, ¾ cup brown sugar, ¼ cup ground flax seed meal, 2 tsp. cinnamon, 2 tsp. gluten-free baking powder, 1 tsp. salt, 1 cup low-fat milk or gluten-free soymilk, 2 eggs or egg substitute equivalent, ½ cup melted butter or canola oil, 2 tsp. vanilla, and ¾ cup dried cranberries or raisins, then pour into 9 × 13-inch baking pan, cover, and place in refrigerator overnight. In the morning, place pan in an oven preheated to 350°F and bake for 40 minutes or until mixture is set in the middle. Serve warm. Stores well in refrigerator and can be reheated in microwave.
- Gluten-free muesli with milk or yogurt: Mix together 4½ cups gluten-free rolled oats, ½ cup ground flax seed, ½ cup rice bran or almond meal, 1 cup raisins, ½ cup chopped walnuts, ¼ cup packed brown sugar, and ¼ cup raw sunflower seeds and store in an air-tight container.
- Whole-grain cold cereals: brown rice, whole sorghum, ground flax seed, and whole grain corn
- Fresh fruit: blueberries, raspberries, or sliced bananas, peaches, apples, or plums

Snacks

- Brown rice or quinoa crackers with nut butter
- Popped corn
- Yogurt with a spoonful of ground flax seed

Lunch and Dinner

- Quinoa salad: cooked quinoa mixed with a variety of chopped vegetables, seeds, nuts, and a mild dressing
- Brown or wild rice with vegetables and meat, poultry, or fish
- Using high-fiber gluten-free breads, make a sandwich in a panini maker (or in a skillet), then wrap it in foil so it will still be soft and moist but not crumbly at lunch time
- Brown rice crackers with hummus and gluten-free tabbouli (made with quinoa or brown rice instead of cracked wheat)
- Buckwheat as a side dish mixed with vegetables
- Enriched gluten-free pasta
- Brown rice and red beans
- Tacos made with 100% corn tortillas, vegetarian refried beans, tomatoes, low-fat cheese, and fresh salsa

There are more gluten-free high-fiber suggestions at www.glutenfreediet.ca/img/WholeGrains.pdf.

In addition to these ideas, the dietitian encouraged Sara to find a celiac support group that meets near her college. Members of the support group will be able to fill her in on foods at local health food stores, specialty shops, and restaurants in the city that are celiac friendly. Because Sara is busy and often eats the same food all the time, the dietitian also suggested that she take a gluten-free multivitamin with minerals. However, Sara is also determined to increase the variety of foods she eats and incorporate some of the ideas about whole grains offered by her dietitian.

SELF-MANAGEMENT TIPS

☐ Look for and purchase mostly whole-grain gluten-free foods.

☐ Choose fortified gluten-free whole-grain products whenever possible.

☐ Add fiber into your diet slowly, accompanied by more fluids, to allow your intestines to adjust to the change in fiber intake.

☐ When you have time to cook, make enough for a few nights, divide it into portions, and freeze it for times when you need a quick meal that you can simply heat up and eat.

☐ Stock your pantry, cabinets, refrigerator, and freezer with canned beans, gluten-free whole grains and flours, fresh and frozen vegetables, and fruit.

☐ Join a support group so you can meet others who can share ideas and recipes that will help you incorporate gluten-free whole grains into your diet.

☐ Meet with a dietitian who is knowledgeable about the GFD to review your typical intake. Almost everyone's GFD can be improved nutritionally.

Laurie A. Higgins, MS, RD, LDN, CDE, is the Coordinator of Pediatric Nutrition Education & Research in the Pediatric, Adolescent and Young Adult Section at Joslin Diabetes Center in Boston, Massachusetts. Her expertise includes nutritional management of diabetes, celiac disease, gastrointestinal diseases, and food allergies. Ms. Higgins was instrumental in the establishment and coordination of the Celiac Support Group at Children's Hospital and is on the boards of the Healthy Villi: The Greater Boston Celiac/DH Support Group, Inc., the Celiac Support Group at Children's Hospital, and the Diabetes Educators Educating Massachusetts.

CHAPTER 14

Supplements 101

Melinda Dennis, MS, RD, LDN, and Christine Doherty, ND

Three months after his diagnosis of celiac disease, Kenny, age 33, visited us for his first nutritional consult. Although he had denied having any of the typical celiac symptoms, Kenny agreed to be screened for celiac disease, along with many family members, after his brother's diagnosis. Kenny is a business man whose work often takes him away from home. He grabs food on the run, eats in hotel restaurants, and to make up for frequent lapses in a relatively healthy diet, occasionally takes one of his wife's multivitamins with iron. His primary complaint at our appointment was of feeling run down.

Kenny provided a detailed food record which showed that he disliked milk and dairy products and that his intake of healthful fatty acids (omega-3) was low. He had recently had blood drawn for testing. Kenny's blood level of vitamin D (25-hydroxyvitamin D) was mildly low at 29 ng/ml. His B_{12} was low normal at 353 pg/ml, and his folate level and iron levels (hemoglobin, hematocrit, and ferritin) were normal. These lab levels indicate that Kenny would likely benefit from additional supplementation.

The Challenge of Good Nutrition in Celiac Disease

Untreated celiac disease causes varying degrees of malabsorption that typically lead to lower than normal levels of important nutrients. Some of the more widely recognized deficiencies include calcium, vitamin D, iron, folate, and B_{12}.[1,2]

After diagnosis, you may find it difficult to restore healthy vitamin, mineral, and essential fatty acid levels with diet alone. Carefully following the gluten-free diet (GFD) is paramount to your health. However, when you eliminate gluten-containing foods, such as wheat bread, pasta, and cereal that are commonly enriched with vitamins, you also eliminate common sources of vitamins, minerals, and essential fatty acids.

Not all GFDs are created equal. Avoiding gluten is the key, but you also have to fill the nutrition gaps with healthy foods (see Chapter 13 on whole grains and Chapter 12 on the balanced diet). Vitamin deficiencies may occur even if you have been carefully following the GFD for several years.[3]

You need to go beyond simply avoiding gluten and choose healthy gluten-free foods to reverse deficiencies. In addition, you will benefit from gluten-free multivitamin, mineral, and essential fatty acid supplements.[4–6] Supplementation can enhance your health and sense of well-being. In this chapter, the term *multivitamin* refers to a multivitamin with minerals, unless otherwise specified.

Using Supplements Wisely

The wide range of supplements available on the market vary in quality, dosage, formula, ability to break apart for absorption, safe levels, and price. Consumer Labs (www.Consumerlabs. com) is a wonderful reference for comparing and evaluating products for quality. Another online resource is www.glutenfreedrugs.com, which lists gluten-free supplements as well as medications. Discuss the best choices for you with your health care provider.

Your supplements, as well as medications, must be gluten free. The inactive ingredients (fillers, excipients, coatings on tablets and capsules) may contain gluten (see Chapter 23 on gluten in medications and supplements). Choose supplements that are labeled gluten free and ideally ones that have been tested to contain less than 20 parts per million gluten.

Given that celiac disease increases your likelihood of having nutritional deficiencies, it is important to work with a physician or dietitian who can direct you to the correct formulas and dosages to meet your needs.

If you choose to use a multivitamin that contains several tablets per serving, split the doses over the course of a day to improve absorption of the full spectrum of nutrients. Multivitamins are better absorbed if taken with food. Some vitamins, especially B_6, can cause nausea if taken on an empty stomach.

Finally, check the label on your supplements for the ingredient polyethelene glycol. This is the drug Miralax, which is used as a "flow agent" to help disperse nutrients equally in tablets and may cause loose stools.

Nutritional Importance of Minerals

Calcium

Calcium deficiency is common in the general population, which puts Americans at greater risk for bone loss and fractures. Individuals with malabsorption disorders such as celiac disease face an even greater risk of calcium deficiency.

Calcium is absorbed in the upper part of the small intestine—the duodenum—which is the part most affected by celiac disease. Damage to the absorption site is the cause of calcium deficiency in those newly diagnosed with celiac disease. Enzymes that digest lactose (the sugar in milk) are also damaged, and this can lead to a condition called *secondary lactose intolerance,* resulting in gas, bloating, and loose stools whenever you ingest dairy products. While this is often temporary and depends on the amount you eat, it can lead you to reduce your intake of milk-based foods, which leads to further calcium depletion and weakening of the skeleton.

The National Osteoporosis Foundation recommends 1200 mg/day of calcium for normal, healthy individuals. Individuals with celiac disease may need more (see Chapter 47 on bone disease). Most patients we see with celiac disease cannot meet their calcium needs using only food. For this reason, we recommend that they take a calcium supplement.

The body absorbs about 500–600 mg of calcium at a time, so you need to split your dose with several hours in between. Most multivitamins, unless taken as several pills over the course of a day, do not contain enough calcium to supply a therapeutic dose. Make sure to understand the serving size of the supplement so that you are actually taking the recommended amount.

In general, there are two types of calcium formulations.

- Calcium carbonate is the form found in many supplements. This is the elemental form and requires healthy stomach acid levels to absorb it efficiently. If you are on acid-blocking medications or have a sensitive stomach, you may do better with a chelated form of calcium.
- Calcium citrate is a chelated form of calcium commonly found in supplements. Chelation is a process used with minerals to enhance their absorption. The process involves attaching or "piggybacking" the mineral onto an amino acid (a protein), taking advantage of the body's more efficient absorption of amino acids. Calcium citrate is a bit more expensive but is the safest for those prone to kidney stones and tends to cause less gas and bloating than the carbonate formula.

Regardless of the formula, if you experience gas, bloating, and constipation, increase your fluid intake and activity level or consider switching formulas. If you have trouble digesting tablets, try gluten-free liquid, gel capsules, or powdered or chewable forms of calcium. You can also crush your calcium supplement to make it easier to swallow.

Your body requires vitamin D and magnesium in order to absorb calcium, so choose a calcium supplement that contains both (unless you are taking a separate magnesium supplement or have high doses in your multivitamin). The ideal calcium-to-magnesium ratio for absorption is 2:1. If you are taking 500 mg of calcium/day, aim to take 250 mg of magnesium/day. If you have issues with chronic constipation, even after you are eating gluten free, you may need a 1:1 ratio of calcium to magnesium, because magnesium's laxative effect balances calcium's constipating effect. See page 102 for the discussion and dosing of vitamin D, which is often combined with calcium in a supplement.

Calcium and iron compete for absorption in the body. If you use a multivitamin with iron or a separate iron supplement, take your calcium several hours before or after you take the iron.

Calcium has a mild relaxing and sedating effect. If you have fatigue or insomnia, taking your doses later in the day may avoid worsening fatigue during the day and will take advantage of the sedating effect at night to improve your sleep.

Speak to your health care provider before starting a calcium supplement, particularly if you take prescription medication or aluminum-containing antacids. If you experience any of the following after starting a calcium supplement, speak to your provider right away: constipation, colitis, diarrhea, nausea, vomiting, stomach or intestinal bleeding, slow or irregular heartbeat, heart problems, kidney disease, poor digestion, headaches, or confusion.

Finally, *do not*

- Take in more than 2500 mg/day of calcium from diet and/or supplementation unless under the supervision of your doctor.
- Take supplements made from bone meal, dolomite, or oyster shell. They may contain toxins.
- Use an aluminum-containing antacid as a calcium supplement.
- Take calcium if you have a high blood calcium level.
- Take calcium if you have sarcoidosis.

Magnesium

Magnesium is an important yet frequently overlooked mineral that is low in the diets of most Americans. Magnesium is required for more than 300 bodily functions, including muscle relaxation, protein and fat synthesis, and energy production. Like vitamin D, it also helps us absorb calcium.

Magnesium is found in large amounts in the germ (central core) of whole grains, an excellent reason to choose gluten-free whole grains such as buckwheat, millet, and brown rice over processed foods that have had their germ removed. Magnesium is also found in nuts, legumes (soybeans, dried beans, lentils), seafood, and green vegetables (kale, spinach, Swiss chard).

Most multivitamins contain only a small percentage of the recommended daily value (DV) of magnesium (450 mg). Some calcium supplements have added magnesium, which is convenient. Calcium is notoriously constipating and magnesium has a laxative effect so, taken in the right doses and preferably taken together, they minimize any intestinal discomfort that may be caused by taking either one alone. While the tolerance level differs widely among individuals, diarrhea can result if more than 600 mg of supplemental magnesium is consumed per day.[7] You can discuss with your doctor or dietitian whether an additional supplement of about 200–300 mg/day of magnesium would benefit you based on your diet and current supplementation. Magnesium citrate and magnesium glycinate are both highly absorbable, chelated forms. Either form is good, although magnesium glycinate tends to have a lesser diarrheal effect. Magnesium oxide, the form found in most supplements, tends to cause more gas and diarrhea than the chelated forms.

Iron

Iron deficiency is very common in people with malabsorptive disorders such as celiac disease as well as menstruating women and vegetarians. Symptoms of iron deficiency include fatigue, pale skin, canker sores, and lack of stamina. Red meat contains heme iron, which is the most easily absorbed food source. Vegetable sources of iron and most supplements contain nonheme iron. Ferrous sulfate is a common supplemental form of iron. As with other minerals, chelated forms such as iron bysglycinate may be better tolerated and absorbed. It is common to experience stomach upset and constipation from iron supplements (see Chapter 49 on anemia). Be aware that iron may limit absorption of replacement thyroid hormone.

Both men and women need to be aware of the individual need for iron. Women who are menstruating experience monthly iron loss and often find it difficult to get enough iron from their diets; for this reason, women's multivitamins generally contain about 18 mg of iron. Otherwise, unless you are anemic or have a low blood ferritin level (low iron stores) and your diet is devoid of iron-rich sources such as red meat and dark meat poultry, it is generally recommended to avoid supplemental iron to prevent iron overload.

Zinc

Although our bodies require relatively little zinc, it is involved in more than 200 enzyme systems in our body, particularly those involving our immune system; sense of taste and smell; growth; health of skin, hair, and nails; and wound healing. Zinc is found in most multivitamins in small amounts. Zinc oxide is the elemental form of zinc, which can cause nausea on an empty stomach.

Low zinc levels are common in celiac disease. If your zinc levels are low, your provider can recommend a zinc supplement. A total dose of 25 mg daily, including what is in a multivitamin, is a safe and effective dose. You can discontinue it after reaching a healthy blood level of zinc.

Selenium

Thyroid disorders and frequent infections can be symptoms of celiac disease. The mineral selenium helps the liver activate thyroid hormone and helps fight infection. Selenium also plays an important role in the production of enzymes and is an antioxidant. Antioxidants are substances that may protect your cells against free radicals, which are molecules that can damage cells and may play a role in heart disease, cancer, and other diseases.

Selenium may be low in some people with celiac disease, and the level can be tested if there is a concern. Not all multivitamins contain this mineral. The ideal or optimal amount of selenium per day is unknown, however, it may be higher than the recommended daily allowance of 55 mcg/day for men and women over age 14 years.[8] The food source with the highest amount of selenium is Brazil nuts.

Iodine

This mineral is found in sea vegetables (seaweed) and iodized table salt and is the central molecule in thyroid hormone. Iodine deficiency can result in a goiter—an enlarged thyroid gland—that in mild cases can cause difficulty swallowing dry foods like breads, crackers, and meat and other symptoms associated with low thyroid function, such as fatigue and weight gain. Be aware that in some cases, a high intake of iodine can exacerbate dermatitis herpetiformis.

Boron

This mineral is often found in bone density formulas because it enhances calcium absorption and protects against calcium loss. It is also commonly found in multivitamins in trace amounts.

Manganese

Lack of this mineral can cause impaired bone development, poor wound healing, and poor carbohydrate metabolism. It is commonly found in trace amounts in a multivitamin.

Copper

Although copper is efficiently absorbed by the body, its absorption competes with that of zinc and calcium. Therefore, if you are taking either one at high doses, make sure that your multivitamin contains copper to avoid copper deficiency. Shellfish and legumes are the richest dietary sources of copper. Deficiency symptoms include anemia, fatigue, bone and joint problems, osteoporosis, and reduced skin coloring.

Fat-Soluble Vitamins

Vitamin D

We cannot say enough about the importance of vitamin D and its multiple benefits for the body. Vitamin D helps prevent cancer and reduce inflammation and influences many hormones in the body. One of its primary roles is to assist in calcium absorption, and vitamin D is needed by the body on a daily basis. Because 10–30% of individuals with celiac disease also have osteoporosis, calcium and vitamin D supplementation is required (see Chapter 47 on bone disease).

Vitamin D is an essential nutrient, which means that the body often cannot produce enough for our needs. People living in southern parts of the United States or near the equator may make adequate vitamin D, when the skin is exposed to sunlight, with just 5 to 15 minutes of sunlight exposure per day. However, there is seasonal variation in sunlight at higher latitudes, which decreases our production of vitamin D in the skin in the winter months. We do not recommend this means of vitamin D supplementation because sun exposure can have deleterious effects on the skin.

Those with darker skin, which prevents ultraviolet radiation from penetrating to the skin layers that make vitamin D, need more sunlight exposure to produce the same amounts of vitamin D as those with lighter skin. Similarly, the use of sunscreen blocks our ability to produce vitamin D. With aging, kidney function declines so there is less conversion of 25-hydroxyvitamin D (the form of vitamin D that circulates in the blood) to the active 1,25-dihydroxyvitamin D. Finally, there are few sources of dietary vitamin D (Table 1), another reason why supplementation is important to you.

The recommended daily dose of vitamin D is 800–1000 international units (IU). People with a known deficiency may require a therapeutic dose of 50,000 IU once or twice a week for six to eight weeks. We monitor vitamin D therapy by checking blood levels of 25-hydroxyvitamin D. There are two forms of supplemental vitamin D: D3 (cholecalciferol) is the natural form of vitamin D and the most useful and absorbable by the body; D2 (ergocalciferol) is not naturally used by the body, and some people do not convert D2 to D3 very well. A quality supplement will contain D3.

Vitamin A

Poor night vision, frequent infections, and small bumps on the skin, often on the backs of the arms, are symptoms of vitamin A deficiency and may occur in some individuals with celiac dis-

TABLE 1. Food Sources of Vitamin D

Food	IUs per serving
Cod liver oil, 1 tablespoon	1,360
Salmon (sockeye), cooked, 3 ounces	794
Mushrooms that have been exposed to ultraviolet light to increase vitamin D, 3 ounces (not yet commonly available)	400
Mackerel, cooked, 3 ounces	388
Tuna, canned in water and drained, 3 ounces	154
Milk, nonfat, reduced fat, and whole, vitamin D–fortified, 1 cup	115–124
Orange juice, vitamin D–fortified, 1 cup (check product labels, amount of added vitamin D varies)	100
Yogurt, fortified with 20% of the DV for vitamin D, 6 ounces (more heavily fortified yogurts provide more of the DV)	80
Margarine, fortified with vitamin D, 1 tablespoon	60
Sardines, canned in oil, drained, 2 sardines	46
Liver, beef, cooked, 3.5 ounces	46
Ready-to-eat cereal, fortified with 10% of the DV for vitamin D, 0.75–1 cup (more heavily fortified cereals might provide more of the DV)	40
Egg, 1 whole (vitamin D is found in yolk)	25
Cheese, Swiss, 1 ounce	6

IUs, international units; DV, daily value.
From National Institutes of Health. Office of Dietary Supplements. Dietary Supplement Fact Sheet: Vitamin D. http://dietary-supplements.info.nih.gov/factsheets/vitamind.asp#h3. Accessed January 22, 2010.

ease. Most multivitamins contain vitamin A. There are two forms of vitamin A: beta carotene, which is water soluble, and retinoids, which are fat soluble. Supplements often contain a mixture of the two forms. Beta carotene needs to be converted in the liver into the fat-soluble form of vitamin A. This conversion process does not always happen efficiently. Therefore, if you are diagnosed with vitamin A deficiency, choose a supplement with the active, retinoid form of vitamin A—retinol, retinal, or retinoic acid—to restore levels and improve symptoms. Vitamin A can be toxic and cause birth defects, so don't take more than 5,000 IU daily without discussing it with your clinician. If you do not have vitamin A deficiency or for general health purposes, use beta carotene or a mixed formula in a multivitamin (recommended amount 3,000–5,000 IU/day). If you have any of the symptoms listed above, talk with your clinician about switching to an active form of vitamin A.

Vitamin K

This vitamin can be made by the beneficial bacteria present in a healthy colon. Vitamin K improves bone health and reduces fractures and may be related to the low bone mineral density common in celiac disease.[9] Vitamin K helps blood to clot, and deficiency symptoms include easy bruising, heavy menstrual periods, and bleeding gums. Individuals taking Coumadin must maintain a consistent dietary and supplement intake of vitamin K to get the most from this medicine. This includes vitamin K from both diet and supplements combined. Most healthy bone supplements contain about 150 mcg of vitamin K, but many multivitamins do not contain vitamin K. Food sources high in vitamin K include dark, leafy greens such as kale, spinach, and turnip greens.

Vitamin E

This vitamin is an antioxidant that protects cells and is occasionally low in individuals with severe malabsorption. Vitamin E deficiency can cause restless leg syndrome and neuropathy (nerve damage that can cause pain, numbness, and tingling). Most multivitamins contain vitamin E; look for the natural form, which is D-alpha tocopherol or mixed tocopherols. Avoid supplements with DL-alpha tocopherol, which is synthetic and not well used by the body. Vitamin E is primarily found in nuts and seeds. Most supplements of vitamin E are derived from soy, but some whole food vitamins use wheat germ oil, which may be unsafe for those with celiac disease because some of the toxic gliadin protein may be left in the oil.

B Vitamins—Better Together

Each of the eight B vitamins is essential to hundreds of critical biochemical processes in our bodies. Because they are water-soluble vitamins and not stored in the body, we need a daily supply from vitamin B–rich foods and supplements. These vitamins are thiamin hydrochloride (B_1), riboflavin (B_2), niacin (B_3), pantothenic acid (B_5), pyridoxine hydrochloride (B_6), folate (B_9), cyanocobalamin (B_{12}), and biotin.

B vitamins are essential to many body functions, such as energy production, digestion, red blood cell production, brain function, and more. Common symptoms of B-vitamin deficiency include fatigue, depression, headaches, and poor memory. Supplements are usually in the form of a mixture of B vitamins (B complex). However, individual uses exist for specific B vitamins, such as using B_2 at high doses to treat migraines.

Researchers examining the GFD emphasize, among other nutrients, the need for an increased intake of B vitamins, particularly folate and vitamin B_{12}.[5,10–12] As is the case with magnesium, food sources of B vitamins are gluten-free whole grains, rather than processed grains and starches such as white rice and potatoes (see Chapter 13 on whole grains and Chapter 12 on a balanced diet). Adequate B-vitamin supplementation is particularly important for gluten-free vegetarians and vegans (see Chapter 15 on vegetarian diet). Folate and B_{12} are commonly checked in individuals with newly diagnosed celiac disease. They play important roles in anemia, a common symptom in untreated celiac disease, as well as in energy, mood, and mental clarity.

Rarely referred to as B_9, folate is commonly known as folic acid in supplement form and folate in food form. The food form is found primarily in dark leafy greens, and the name is derived from the word *foliage*. An inadequate folate level is a risk factor for breast, prostate, and colon cancer, depression, and spinal cord birth defects. For this reason, pregnant women or those who wish to become pregnant should take 800 mcg/day of folic acid in a prenatal supplement in addition to ensuring they get folate in their diet. Most multivitamin formulas contain 400 mcg of folic acid.

Vitamin B_{12} is found mainly in red meat, so vegetarians are at high risk for deficiency. This vitamin plays a vital role in blood formation and cell function, including nervous system function. Intrinsic factor (a substance made in the parietal cells in the stomach) and hydrochloric acid (also produced by the parietal cells) are both needed to aid in the absorption of B_{12}. As we age, less B_{12} is absorbed because we produce less intrinsic factor and hydrochloric acid. Pernicious anemia is a form of anemia related to severe B_{12} deficiency that results from lack of intrinsic factor. Pernicious anemia is common in the elderly and in people who have a family history of pernicious anemia.

Small intestinal bacterial overgrowth often results in B_{12} deficiency because bacteria consume it before it can be absorbed. Symptoms of B_{12} deficiency include muscle weakness and fatigue. Therapeutic doses of B_{12}, when indicated, are available in oral, injectable, and sublingual forms. Sublingual B_{12} tablets dissolve under the tongue and go straight into the bloodstream, which bypasses the need for hydrochloric acid and intrinsic factor. B_{12} is a safe vitamin with no known toxicity.

Multivitamins come with varying amounts of B vitamins included. Choosing one that offers 100% of the DV (the column to the right of the Amount per Serving of each vitamin on a Supplement Facts label) for each of the B vitamins is a safe and reasonable recommendation. B vitamins are generally safe with the exception of niacin (B_3) which can be toxic to the liver in high doses. Also, elevated blood levels of B_6 can cause or exacerbate neuropathy (numbness and tingling in the extremities), a common symptom of celiac disease. Reviewing your blood work and diet history with your doctor or dietitian can help you determine whether you need additional single B vitamins or could benefit from a B complex vitamin.

Vitamin C

Like the B vitamins, vitamin C is water soluble and needs to be replaced each day. It is a powerful antioxidant that travels through the body, neutralizing free radicals (waste products that cause injury to cells). Vitamin C is also critical in the structure of bone, skin, blood vessels, tendons, and ligaments. Symptoms of vitamin C deficiency include fatigue, irritability, loose teeth, easy bruising, nosebleeds, and dry skin and hair. Certain inflammatory diseases, such as celiac disease, diabetes, infections, or stress, can increase the body's need for vitamin C because these conditions result in a greater production of free radicals.

Multivitamins contain varying, but usually minimal, amounts of vitamin C. Fortunately, vitamin C is widely found in the food chain in brightly colored fruits (citrus fruits, strawberries, papaya) and vegetables (green peppers, broccoli, Brussels sprouts), and loading up on them is a great idea. After consulting with your doctor or dietitian, it is reasonable to take 500–1000 mg/day of vitamin C in supplement form spaced throughout the day. If you are taking an iron supplement under the direction of your doctor, you can increase the absorption of iron by taking it at the same time that you are eating food with vitamin C or taking a vitamin C supplement.

Supplemental vitamin C can cause intestinal gas or even diarrhea. Individual tolerance for this vitamin varies widely; if you start a new supplement and experience these symptoms you may be taking too high a dose. Vitamin C is acidic so some people tolerate "buffered" vitamin C better; to buffer the C, a small amount of calcium is added to the formula. Interestingly, humans and guinea pigs are the only mammals that do not make vitamin C in the liver, because we lack a specific enzyme that converts glucose into vitamin C.

Essential Fatty Acids

Celiac disease, like many chronic health conditions, has a strong inflammatory component. Focusing on nutrients that decrease inflammation and protect tissues is important for those with celiac disease. Although there are no data from properly controlled studies on the use of omega-3 fatty acids specifically in celiac disease, we know from studies on other diseases (such as heart disease) that these beneficial essential fatty acids help control inflammation.

One of the most important ways to control inflammation is to pay attention to the ratio of two types of polyunsaturated fats in your diet, omega-6 (linoleic) and omega-3 (alpha linolenic), which are known as essential (because we cannot make them) fatty acids. Omega-6 fatty acids turn on inflammation, and omega-3 fatty acids turn it off. Although the ratio of 4:1 (as in the popular Mediterranean diet) is recommended, the ratio in the typical American diet is closer to 10:1, or worse. Simply put, we eat too much of the wrong kind of fat. Most of us are deficient in the omega-3 fatty acids, found primarily in cold water fish (salmon, mackerel, herring), seeds (including flax seeds), nuts (walnuts), and grains. The easiest way to improve this ratio is to reduce your intake of omega-6–rich food (cooking oils such as sunflower, safflower, corn, soybean, and cottonseed, the primary oils in most processed food) and increase your intake of omega-3–rich foods (see Chapter 12 on the balanced diet).

If you dislike or cannot tolerate eating fish, consider taking a fish oil supplement. Eicosapentanoic acid (EPA) and docosahexanoic acid (DHA) are the specific names of the beneficial omega-3 essential fatty acids. On a supplement label, you will typically see the words "fish oil concentrate" and then a number in milligrams (for example, 1000 mg). Underneath it, you will see the amounts of EPA and DHA in milligrams (example, EPA 300 mg; DHA 250 mg). Add up the EPA and DHA amounts. The difference between the total amount of fish oil concentrate (1000 mg) and the combined amount of EPA and DHA (550 mg) is fish oil that contains no EPA or DHA. Therefore, choose a supplement that has the highest amount of EPA and DHA so that you are getting as much of the omega-3–rich fatty acids as possible. To determine the amount appropriate for your health, speak to your doctor or dietitian.

Here are more tips for getting the most benefit from this supplement.

- Be sure that your supplement contains a small amount of vitamin E to help prevent rancidity of the fish oil in the capsule.

- Choose a supplement that is labeled as having been molecularly distilled to remove the heavy metals, such as mercury, that are found in deep water fish.
- Take your fish oil at night if you are concerned about fish burps. Quality fish oil supplements should not cause burping or have an overpowering smell. Some have a citrus or flavored essence. Refrigerating the capsules may reduce odor and help those who have difficulty swallowing them.
- If you do not like taking capsules, fish oil is also available in liquid, chewable, and paste forms and can be mixed with applesauce or yogurt to disguise the texture and flavor.

Always speak to your doctor or dietitian before beginning a gluten-free fish oil supplement as there may be contraindications. For example, because fish oil supplements have anticoagulant (blood thinning) properties, they are generally discontinued before surgery. For people with ongoing diarrhea, concentrated doses of fats may cause gas or bloating or worsen diarrhea. Sometimes smaller doses taken with food will be better tolerated. If you have an allergy to fish, try a plant-based fatty acid formula.

Vegetarians may choose to take omega-3 in the form of flax seed oil or capsules. Although flax seed oil contains a certain omega-3 fatty acid (alpha linolenic acid, ALA), the conversion of ALA to EPA and DHA is slow and can be inhibited by various conditions. About 15% of ALA converts to EPA, and it is unclear whether it converts to DHA, the form of fat that is particularly important to brain and neurological health. Some forms of algae contain DHA. For this reason, and because the rest of the flax seed is so nutrient dense (containing magnesium, chromium, and lignans that may decrease the risk of breast cancer), it is more beneficial overall to consume ground flax seed versus flax seed oil. When consuming flax seed, be sure to drink plenty of water because it is a significant source of fiber.

What Kenny Decided

We believed that Kenny would benefit from taking a standard gluten-free multivitamin for men that does not contain iron and has at least 100% of the DV of each B vitamin. He also agreed to take a gluten-free B vitamin complex at least a few times each week, particularly if he forgot on occasion to take his multivitamin, to help with energy and mood.

Because Kenny doesn't drink milk (one of the primary sources of calcium in the American diet) and avoids most other sources of dairy, he agreed to start a daily gluten-free 1200 mg calcium citrate supplement that contains vitamin D and magnesium, taking it in divided doses twice a day. His goal was to take in 1,000–2,000 IU of vitamin D per day, 400 IU from his multivitamin and the rest from his calcium supplement and an additional vitamin D3 supplement, if needed. Rather than taking a fish oil supplement to supply his omega-3, he decided to increase his deep-water fish intake to 2–3 servings per week.

Because a healthy GFD is the best protection, Kenny met several times with the dietitian to learn ways to improve his GFD while on the road.

Six months later, Kenny's 25-hydroxyvitamin D level was an acceptable level of 41 ng/ml, and his B_{12} level had risen to 712 pg/ml. Kenny reported that his energy had improved and that he was making more of an effort to eat healthfully on the road. Given these results, he has continued with his multivitamin, calcium, vitamin D, and magnesium supplementation and is taking the B complex supplement several times per week.

Resources

- Balance Point Natural Medicine: www.glutenfreevitamins.com
- Country Life: www.countrylifevitamins.com
- Freeda: www.freedavitamins.com
- Kirkman Labs: www.kirkmanlabs.com
- Nature Made: www.naturemade.com
- Pioneer Nutritionals: www.pioneernutritional.com
- Solgar: www.solgar.com

References

1. Hallert C, Svensson M, Tholstrup J, Hultberg B. Clinical trial: B vitamins improve health in patients with coeliac disease living on a gluten-free diet. *Aliment Pharmacol Ther* 2009;29(8):811–16.

2. Malterre T. Digestive and nutritional considerations in celiac disease: could supplementation help? *Altern Med Rev* 2009;14(3):247–57.

3. Hallert C, Grant C, Grehn S, et al. Evidence of poor vitamin status in celiac patients on a gluten-free diet for 10 yrs. *Aliment Pharmacol Ther* 2002;16:1333–39.

4. American Dietetic Association. Nutrition Care Manual for Dietitians. http://nutritioncare manual.org. Accessed 12/09/09.

5. Thompson T, Dennis M, Higgins LA, Lee AR, Sharrett MK. Gluten free diet survey: are Americans with coeliac disease consuming recommended amounts of fibre, iron, calcium and grain foods? *J Hum Nutr Dietet* 2005;18:163–69.

6. Siguel E, Lerman R. Prevalence of essential fatty acid deficiency in patients with chronic gastro-intestinal disorders. *Metabolism* 1996;45(1):12–23.

7. The Institute for Functional Medicine. *Clinical Nutrition: A Functional Approach.* 2nd ed. Gig Harbor, WA, 2004, p. 165.

8. NIH Office of Dietary Supplements. Dietary Supplement Fact Sheet: Selenium. http://ods.od.nih.gov/factsheets/selenium.asp#h2. Accessed 12/09/09.

9. Weber P. Vitamin K and bone health. *Nutrition* 2001;17(10):880–87.

10. Lee A. Celiac disease: detection and treatment. *Top Clin Nutr* 2005;20(2):139–45.

11. Thompson T. Thiamin, riboflavin, and niacin contents of the gluten-free diet: is there cause for concern? *J Am Diet Assoc* 1999;99:858–62.

12. Thompson T. Folate, iron and dietary fiber contents of the gluten-free diet. *J Am Diet Assoc* 2000;100:1389–96.

Christine Doherty, PhD, has worked primarily with gluten-free patients in private practice at Balance Point Natural Medicine in Milford, New Hampshire. She is a medical advisor and writes the Super Supplements column for *Living Without* magazine. She frequently lectures and writes about celiac disease and gluten-free living and credits the gluten-free diet with saving her life.

CHAPTER 15

The Gluten-Free Vegetarian

Nixie Raymond, MS, RD

Christine was a freshman in college when she decided to give up eating meat, chicken, and fish. Although there were a variety of vegetarian foods offered at every meal in her college dining hall, Christine stuck to the foods she had always eaten and simply dropped most animal products from her diet. Her usual intake consisted of milk, cereal, or pancakes; a peanut butter and jelly sandwich or pizza; fruit and 1–2 servings of vegetables a day; pasta, pizza, or a veggie stir-fry with rice; and chips, pretzels, crackers, cake, cookies, and ice cream for snacks.

By the end of her first semester, Christine began to complain of extreme tiredness and stomach aches. These were initially attributed to the stress of adjusting to college life. Her parents thought it might be because of her vegetarian diet. Worsening stomach cramps and diarrhea led to a doctor's visit, and she was diagnosed with lactose intolerance. Her symptoms subsided some on a lactose-free diet, but she was still exhausted and was found to be anemic. Was Christine's vegetarian diet the cause? No, the source of her poor health was more complex.

Christine was experiencing symptoms of emerging celiac disease. Her diet, which tended to be high in gluten and low in iron, just made matters worse. She was ultimately diagnosed with celiac disease just before the end of her first year at college.

Christine came to me shortly after her diagnosis. She felt strongly that she wanted to continue a vegetarian diet. However, with the added restrictions of the gluten-free diet (GFD), Christine was feeling like there was nothing left for her to eat. Her parents worried that such a limited diet couldn't possibly be adequate. But in fact, with knowledge and planning, a vegetarian GFD can be quite healthful and nutritious as well as varied and tasty. In addition to learning about the GFD, Christine needed to know the key nutrients for vegetarians and their gluten-free sources, as well as how to avoid gluten in specialty vegetarian foods.

Key Nutrients in a Gluten-Free Vegetarian Diet

Protein

Although Christine's diet was not very well balanced, it did provide enough protein to meet requirements. People often think that it is hard to get enough protein in a vegetarian diet. But in fact, protein needs can be easily met on a lacto-ovo (milk- and egg-containing) vegetarian diet as well as a lacto (milk-containing) vegetarian diet. Even those who follow a vegan diet (no animal products whatsoever) can fairly easily meet protein needs if they eat a varied diet. An assortment of plant foods eaten over the course of the day can meet all essential amino acids requirements.[1] Table 1 lists gluten-free vegetarian foods that are high in protein.

Iron

Christine presented with iron deficiency anemia, which is common among those newly diagnosed with celiac disease. In her case, it was most likely because of impaired iron absorption that was made worse by low iron intake. She was prescribed a gluten-free iron supplement to replenish her levels of iron and maintain that status until her gut healed and iron absorption normalized.

In the United States, a significant amount of dietary iron is provided by fortified grains, particularly fortified wheat flour and foods made from it such as breads, cereals, crackers, and pasta. However, gluten-free versions of breads, crackers, cereals, and pasta are not typically fortified with iron, so other sources must be found (Table 2).

The type of iron naturally present in plant foods is called nonheme iron. It is absorbed much less efficiently than the heme iron that is in animal flesh. However, the absorption of iron can be affected by the types of food consumed at the same time. Absorption is enhanced

TABLE 1. High-Protein Gluten-Free Vegetarian Foods

Tofu
Eggs
Milk, gluten-free soy milk
Yogurt, soy yogurt
Cheese
Soybeans, soy nuts, edamame (fresh soybeans)
Quinoa, amaranth, buckwheat, teff, millet, sorghum
Nuts, seeds
Lentils, dried beans, chickpeas
Tempeh*
Vegetarian burgers*
Vegetarian hot dogs*

*Only a few of these products are gluten free; check labels carefully.

TABLE 2. High-Iron Vegetarian Foods

Fortified corn flour (masa) or corn meal
Flour made from soybeans, chickpeas, buckwheat
Quinoa, amaranth, teff
Dark leafy greens: spinach, collard greens, Swiss chard, broccoli
Lentils, chick peas, kidney beans, lima beans
Soybeans, soy nuts, edamame
Blackstrap molasses
Tahini (ground sesame seeds)
Cashew, almonds, sunflower seeds
Gluten-free pasta, cereal, or bread that has been fortified with iron

by the presence of vitamin C, but decreased by calcium and by the tannins that naturally occur in tea and coffee. To increase absorption of iron from a supplement or an iron-rich meal, add a source of vitamin C (such as citrus, red peppers, tomato, broccoli, or kiwi) and wait a few hours before having tea or coffee. Wait two or more hours after taking an iron supplement or eating an iron-rich meal before taking a calcium supplement.

Because the body is less efficient at absorbing iron from plant foods, vegetarians like Christine who rely only on nonheme iron may need to consume almost double the amount of iron than those who regularly eat heme iron.[2] High-iron foods, such as those listed in Table 2, should be included at most meals. Individuals with increased iron needs, such as premenopausal women and children, often need and benefit from taking a multivitamin supplement that contains iron. Those who have difficulty including high-iron foods in their daily diet may also need such a supplement, depending on their age and gender.

Calcium

Because she has lactose intolerance, Christine was avoiding milk and milk products, and consequently, her intake of calcium was quite low. Fortunately, the lactose intolerance that Christine developed was probably because of gluten-induced damage to her intestinal lining and, therefore, likely to be temporary. We recommended she start using 100% lactose-free milk or fortified, gluten-free soy, hemp, nut, or rice milk and limit her intake of cheese to hard, aged cheeses that are naturally low in lactose. Then, as her gut healed over the next few months, she could start trying other types of cheese, plus ice cream and other lactose-containing foods to test her tolerance. Her tolerance to lactose is likely to normalize eventually, allowing her to return to eating all dairy products.

If you follow a diet that is completely free of milk and dairy products, you can obtain calcium from various calcium-containing plant foods, as well as calcium-fortified beverages and foods (Table 3). Use calcium supplements if your needs cannot be met by diet alone. Note that most multivitamins contain only small amounts of calcium, so you'll need a separate calcium supplement (see Chapter 14 on supplements).

TABLE 3. Vegetarian Gluten-Free Calcium Sources

Milk, lactose-reduced or lactose-free milk
Nondairy milks, such as gluten-free soy milk, rice milk, nut milks, and hemp milk fortified with vitamin D and calcium (ideally calcium carbonate rather than tricalcium phosphate for best absorption)[1]
Yogurt, fortified soy yogurt
Cheese, especially hard cheeses (parmesan, edam, romano)
Fruit or vegetable juices fortified with calcium
Tofu made with calcium sulfate
Sesame seeds, almonds
Dried beans
Low-oxalate* greens: bok choy, broccoli, Chinese cabbage, collards, kale

*Oxalate is a compound, naturally present in certain foods, that interferes with calcium absorption. Although vegetables such as spinach and Swiss chard contain calcium, they are high in oxalate and, therefore, are poor sources of usable calcium.[1]

Vitamin D

Vitamin D is a fat-soluble vitamin necessary for bone health and overall well-being. Not surprisingly, Christine's blood levels of vitamin D were low. Because she was avoiding milk, she missed out on a major dietary source of vitamin D. And because of intestinal damage, she likely had poor absorption of what little vitamin D she did take in.

Recent research suggests that many otherwise healthy Americans have less than ideal blood levels of vitamin D.[3] Several health organizations are now recommending increased levels of vitamin D intake: 400 IU (International Units) per day for children, 400–800 IU per day for adults up to age 50, and at least 800–1000 IU for those over age 50. But it is not easy, even on a regular diet, to meet these levels through diet alone. Relatively few foods naturally contain or are fortified with vitamin D. The predominant food sources of vitamin D in the United States are milk, fortified cereals, and oily fish.

In the United States, milk is fortified with 100 IU vitamin D per cup. However, cheese, yogurt, ice cream, and other dairy products are made from milk that has not been fortified, so although they are excellent sources of calcium, they are low in vitamin D. Many breakfast cereals are fortified with vitamin D to provide 40 IU per serving, but only one or two of these are gluten free. Few of the specialized gluten-free cereals are fortified with vitamin D. Another dietary source is egg yolk, but it contains only 20 IU vitamin D per yolk.

Our skin naturally produces vitamin D when exposed to direct sunlight. However, using sunscreen and the amount of daily sunlight in your environment both greatly affect your quality of sun exposure and, therefore, how much vitamin D comes through your skin. For example, in Boston (latitude 42 degrees) where Christine lives, the sun exposure from October to April is not strong enough for skin synthesis of vitamin D.

Given all of these factors, it is difficult to get enough vitamin D through a gluten-free vegetarian diet alone. Supplements are recommended to achieve recommended intake levels. Most multivitamin supplements provide 400 IU of vitamin D. Many calcium supplements also include 200 IU or more of vitamin D. Individuals with the highest requirements (adults over age 50) and/or lowest intake or sun exposure may need additional vitamin D supplements at levels recommended by their health care providers (see Chapter 14 on supplements).

Vitamin B₁₂

Vitamin B_{12}

Vitamin B_{12} is essential for the formation of red blood cells and maintenance of the nervous system. Deficiency can cause anemia, fatigue, confusion, poor memory, and nerve degeneration. Evaluation of Christine's vitamin B_{12} status showed that she was at the low end of the normal range and likely heading toward deficiency because of malabsorption. Once on a GFD, Christine's absorption would improve as her gut heals. However, she would still be at risk for deficiency because of inadequate B_{12} in her diet.

The GFD eliminates most of the fortified grain foods that would be good sources of vitamin B_{12}. Diets without meat or other animal flesh lack the richest dietary sources of the vitamin. Vegan diets, which contain no animal products whatsoever, lack any significant source of vitamin B_{12}, requiring the use of fortified foods and vitamin B_{12}–containing supplements.[4,5] In a gluten-free vegetarian diet, the only reliable sources of vitamin B_{12} are dairy products, eggs, and foods that are fortified with the vitamin. Seaweed, algae, and spirulina may contain some B_{12} but in a form that cannot be used by humans.[6] Although some fermented plant foods, such as tempeh (fermented soybean), miso, and algae, are said to contain B_{12}, the amounts are so small and highly variable that these foods are not considered reliable sources of the vitamin.

Given the limited sources of vitamin B_{12} in a vegetarian gluten-free diet, it is wise to use a gluten-free multivitamin and mineral supplement providing at least 100% of the daily value. However, even with adequate intake, vitamin B_{12} deficiency can develop because of impaired absorption. Stomach acid is necessary to free vitamin B_{12} from food so that it may be absorbed. The production of stomach acid decreases with age, putting those over age 50, as well as those who take medications that decrease stomach acidity, at risk for inadequate vitamin B_{12} absorption. Conditions that damage the stomach lining, such as pernicious anemia, disrupt the sequence of events necessary for B_{12} absorption. In these situations, injections or oral daily supplements of vitamin B_{12} may be necessary to correct deficiencies and maintain adequate stores.

The recommended daily intake of vitamin B_{12} for adults is 2.4 micrograms (mcg). Food sources are listed in Table 4.

Zinc

Zinc

Zinc is a mineral that has a wide range of functions throughout the body. It helps with wound healing and plays an important role in maintaining the immune system. Individuals recently diagnosed with celiac disease may have low zinc levels because of malabsorption. Zinc may also be lost in the stool if persistent diarrhea is present before diagnosis. Zinc is found in a wide variety of foods but the richest sources are meat and other animal flesh. Good sources for vegetarians include dairy products, cooked dried beans and lentils, sea vegetables (seaweed, algae, and spirulina), soy foods, yeast, nuts, seeds, and whole-grain

TABLE 4. Vegetarian Sources of Vitamin B$_{12}$

1 cup milk	=	0.9 mcg
1 cup yogurt	=	1.0–1.4 mcg
1 ounce cheese	=	0.25–0.4 mcg
1 cup cottage cheese	=	1.4 mcg
1 egg	=	0.6 mcg

Foods that may be fortified with vitamin B$_{12}$ (check the labels)
  Breakfast cereals
  Some soy milks
  Some "energy drinks"
  Red Star Nutritional Yeast Vegetarian Support Formula fortified with B$_{12}$ (1 mcg B$_{12}$ in 2 tsp. of flakes)
Note: Most yeast and nutritional yeast supplements, do not naturally contain B$_{12}$.

cereals. However, legumes and unrefined grains contain phytates, a substance that interferes with zinc absorption. Vegetarians whose diets are high in these foods may need somewhat higher intakes of zinc to meet their needs.[1,4] In addition to emphasizing zinc-rich foods in the gluten-free vegetarian diet, you can obtain 100% of the daily allowance of zinc from a multivitamin and mineral supplement.

Avoiding Gluten in Vegetarian Diets

Gluten is present in many commercially produced vegetarian foods (Table 5). In particular, "meat substitutes" often contain wheat gluten as a protein source and/or a binder. Wheat-based soy sauce is also a very common ingredient in these foods. As always, check labels carefully.

TABLE 5. Gluten in Traditional Vegetarian Foods

	Not Gluten Free	Likely Gluten Free
Tofu	Seasoned, flavored, marinated, or baked made with soy sauce; wheat gluten	Plain tofu, packed in water
Seitan	All forms of seitan are made from wheat gluten	None
Vegetarian burgers and hot dogs	Most meat substitutes contain wheat protein and soy sauce	Certain varieties may be gluten free; check individual products
Tempeh (fermented soybeans compacted into a firm cake)	Multigrain tempeh made with wheat and barley; seasoned or flavored tempeh products made with soy sauce	Traditional, plain tempeh, made only with soybeans, rice, and tempeh culture

TABLE 5. Gluten in Traditional Vegetarian Foods (*Continued*)

	Not Gluten Free	Likely Gluten Free
Mycoprotein products (sold as Quorn)	Most Quorn products contain wheat breading or textured wheat protein	A few Quorn products, such as turkey substitute, may be gluten free
Textured vegetable protein (TVP)/soy protein	Almost all flavored TVP products contain hydrolyzed wheat or other gluten-containing ingredients	Plain, unflavored, textured 100% soy protein (can be used to increase the protein content of foods)
Soy, rice, or almond milk	Some brands contain malted wheat and barley extracts	Most are gluten free
Miso (paste made from fermented beans and grains)	Miso made with wheat, barley, or rye	Miso made from rice, millet, amaranth, quinoa, or buckwheat

SELF-MANAGEMENT TIPS

☐ Take a standard, well-balanced gluten-free multivitamin and mineral supplement. Ideally it should include 100% of the daily value for vitamins B_{12} and D, folic acid, and zinc. Avoid taking mega doses of any vitamin without speaking with your health care provider first. If you follow a vegan diet, it is especially important to supplement vitamin B_{12}.

☐ Consider your iron intake. If your iron intake is low and/or you are a premenopausal woman, you will likely need to take a multivitamin that contains iron. Gender and age determine iron requirements, so ask your health care provider how much you need.

☐ Use calcium-rich and -fortified foods. If needed, use calcium supplements to achieve the recommended intake. Remember that vitamin D is necessary for calcium absorption and utilization.

☐ Eat vitamin- and mineral-rich foods frequently, such as dark leafy greens; colorful fruits and vegetables; nuts and seeds; dried beans; and gluten-free flours made from lentils, garbanzo beans, amaranth, and quinoa. These will provide you with folate, fiber, protein, antioxidants, and other valuable nutrients.

☐ Let your physician or gastroenterologist know that you are following a vegetarian GFD, noting any additional diet restrictions. Depending on the degree of diet restriction and your age and medical history, your doctor may want to check your levels of certain nutrients, specifically iron, vitamin D, and vitamin B_{12}. If you have concerns about the quality of your diet, ask for a referral to an experienced dietitian.

References

1. American Dietetic Association. Position of the American Dietetic Association: Vegetarian diets. *J Am Diet Assoc* 2009;109:1266–82.
2. Institute of Medicine, Food and Nutrition Board. *Dietary Reference Intakes for Vitamin A, Vitamin K, Arsenic, Boron, Chromium, Copper, Iodine, Iron, Manganese, Molybdenum, Nickel, Silicon, Vanadium, and Zinc.* Washington, DC: National Academies Press, 2001.
3. Institute of Medicine, Food and Nutrition Board. *Dietary Reference Intakes for Calcium, Phosphorus, Magnesium, Vitamin D, and Fluoride.* Washington, DC: National Academies Press, 1997.
4. Craig WJ. Health effects of vegan diets. *Am J Clin Nutr* 2009;89(5):1627S–33S.
5. Key TJ, Appleby PN, Rosell MS. Health effects of vegetarian and vegan diets. *Proc Nutr Soc* 2006;65(1):35–41.
6. Herbert V. Vitamin B-12: plant sources, requirements, and assay. *Am J Clin Nutr* 1988; 48:852–58.

Nixie Raymond, MS, RD, is a dietitian who is board certified as a Specialist in Pediatric Nutrition. She has been working with children and adults with celiac disease for more than 20 years and is a founding member of the Boston area celiac support group Healthy Villi.

CHAPTER 16

Constipation

Suzanne Simpson, RD

L orenzo, a 65-year-old office worker who belongs to a weekend tennis league, was diagnosed with celiac disease four years before his visit to our clinic. At diagnosis, Lorenzo's symptoms were constipation, abdominal pain, bloating, and gas. He met with a dietitian right after his diagnosis and learned about the gluten-free diet (GFD), which he follows. Lorenzo's celiac antibodies were elevated at diagnosis but returned to normal within eight months of starting the GFD. He takes a gluten-free multivitamin and mineral supplement along with calcium and vitamin D supplements.

Lorenzo came to his recent visit complaining that he had hard stools, hemorrhoids, and bloating. He met with me about his complaints.

What Is Constipation?

Clinically, symptoms of constipation can include infrequent bowel movements (often less than three bowel movements per week), straining, and hard stools.[1] Healthy people can have three bowel movements per day or three per week—and any amount in between. It is not true that you need to have a bowel movement every day to be healthy.

Chronic constipation is a different situation. This is a symptom-based disorder diagnosed by the presence of "unsatisfactory defecation characterized by infrequent stools, difficult stool passage, or both, for at least 3 months."[2] Chronic constipation can lead to other health problems, such as hemorrhoids, fecal impaction (the accumulation of dry, hardened stool in the rectum or colon leading to obstruction), rectal prolapse (weakened muscles in the rectum), anal fissures (tears in the rectal area), and fecal incontinence.[1] Diarrhea may occur when the intestine is blocked with stool (because of constipation) and only the watery stool is able to pass.[1]

Constipation is common in those with celiac disease, both before diagnosis and after starting the GFD. This is true for children and adults.[3-5] For some people, being diagnosed with celiac disease and starting the GFD results in a resolution of the constipation. However, for others, constipation is a new problem that occurs after beginning the GFD.[6,7]

TABLE 1. Adequate Water Intake

Life Stage	Water (liters per day)
Children	
1–3 years	1.3
4–8 years	1.7
Males	
9–13 years	2.4
14–18 years	3.3
≥19 years	3.7
Females	
9–13 years	2.1
14–18 years	2.3
≥19 years	2.7
Pregnant	3.0
Lactating	3.8

Source: National Academy of Sciences, 2004, www.iom.edu/Object.File/Master/21/372/0.pdf.

The most common cause of constipation is believed to be slow colonic transport: Some people move food through their gastrointestinal tract more slowly than others. Other problems that may cause or worsen constipation include inadequate fluid intake (Table 1) or holding in bowel movements. New or worsening constipation can be caused by medications or an indication of another medical disorder, such as thyroid disease, endocrine disorders, neurological disorders, structural abnormalities, or intestinal motility disorders. In those with celiac disease, the most common reason for constipation is not eating enough dietary fiber. Because the typical gluten-free diet tends to be low in fiber,[8] fiber along with adequate fluid is recommended as the initial treatment for constipation.[9]

With these facts in mind, Lorenzo and I went over the kinds of foods he usually chooses for his meals and snacks.

Lorenzo's Typical Meal Plan

BREAKFAST: gluten-free corn flake cereal with 2% milk or a gluten-free bagel with fried eggs

LUNCH: corn tortillas or rice cakes with peanut butter, ham, or tuna; or grilled vegetables and chicken

SNACKS: gluten-free pretzels, cookies, or crackers; chocolate; potato chips; almonds; banana

DINNER: gluten-free pizza, or steak with baked potato, or gluten-free pasta with pesto sauce, or white rice with raw fish (sushi)

BEVERAGES: soda, gluten-free beer, fruit juice

TABLE 2. Fiber Recommendations (Daily Reference Intake)

Age (years)	Gender	Fiber (grams per day)
<1	Both	Not determined
1–3	Both	19
4–8	Both	25
9–13	Male	31
9–18	Female	26
14–50	Male	38
19–50	Female	25
>50	Male	30
>50	Female	21
All ages	Pregnancy	28
All ages	Lactation	29

Source: National Academy of Sciences, 2004, www.iom.edu/Object.File/Master/21/372/0.pdf.

On average, Lorenzo took in 14 grams of fiber and approximately 2,000 calories each day. The usual intake of fiber in the United States is 15 grams per day.[10] However, this is less than half of the amount of fiber *recommended* for someone Lorenzo's age who consumes 2,000 calories per day (Table 2).

Treating Constipation

Increasing dietary fiber is the first and best treatment for constipation and helps many people overcome it.[11] Dietary fiber is found in foods that come from plants and is the indigestible carbohydrates and lignin that give a plant its structure (Table 3). Although we break down fiber from foods into smaller pieces by chewing it and with the chemical and mechanical actions of digestion, we don't actually digest fiber. It moves through our intestines and becomes fecal matter without changing too much.

Dietary fiber comes in two forms: soluble and insoluble fiber. Soluble fiber dissolves in water in the gut to become a smooth, slimy gel that passes slowly through the gastrointestinal tract. Insoluble fiber absorbs water but retains its rough texture, which scrapes old cells off the intestinal lining as it moves through it. Because both types of fiber absorb large amounts of water, you need to drink adequate amounts of water daily for fiber to do its job (Table 1). This helps ensure that the stool, while bulky from the fiber, is soft enough to pass easily out the rectum. Stool softeners are another way to help with constipation but should be considered only when fiber supplementation has not provided sufficient relief.

The amount of fiber necessary to correct constipation varies, but for everyone, it is best to increase the amount of fiber you eat gradually. Eating too much fiber at once or suddenly doubling or tripling your fiber intake can make you very uncomfortable. Because fiber absorbs water, it swells and can make you feel bloated. In addition, helpful bacteria in your

TABLE 3. Fiber in Foods

Food	Portion	Fiber (grams)
Legumes: beans, lentils, chickpeas, etc.	1 cup	8–19
Artichokes (cooked)	1 cup	14
Dates	1 cup	14
Organic fiber bar (Renew Life)	1 bar	14
Buckwheat flour	1 cup	12
Soybeans, mature, cooked	1 cup	10
Pears, Asian, raw	1 pear	9.9
Yellow, whole grain cornmeal	1 cup	8.8
Peas, green, frozen, cooked	1 cup	8.8
Vegetables, mixed, frozen	1cup	8
Raspberries, raw	1 cup	8
Prunes, stewed	1 cup	7.7
Blackberries, raw	1 cup	7.6
Pumpkin, canned	1 cup	7.1
Spinach, frozen, cooked	1 cup	7
Gorge Delights Just Fruit bars	1 bar	3–7
Popcorn, air-popped	5 cups	6
Squash, cooked	1 cup	5.7
Parsnips, cooked	1 cup	5.6
Papaya, raw	1 papaya	5.5
Raisins, seedless	1 cup	5.4
Collards, cooked	1 cup	5.3
Quinoa, cooked	1 cup	5.2
Amaranth, cooked	1 cup	5.2
Broccoli, cooked	1 cup	5.1
Pear, raw	1 pear	5.1
Yoplait Fiber One creamy nonfat yogurt	½ cup	5
Kind Fruit and Nut Bar	1 bar	5
Balance Pure Bar	1 bar	5
Sweet potato, cooked with skin	1 potato	4.8
Carrots, cooked	1 cup	4.7
Buckwheat groats, cooked	1 cup	4.5
Potato, baked with skin	1 potato	4.4
Orange, raw	1 cup	4.3
Yellow beans, cooked	1 cup	4.1
Plantain, raw	1 medium	4.1
Brussel sprouts, cooked	1 cup	4.1

TABLE 3. Fiber in Foods (*Continued*)

Food	Portion	Fiber (grams)
Okra, cooked	1 cup	4
Green beans, cooked	1 cup	4
Oats (gluten free), cooked	1 cup	4
Lara bar	1 bar	4
Mango, raw	1 mango	3.7
Figs, dried	2 figs	3.7
Plantains, cooked	1 cup	3.5
Brown rice, cooked	1 cup	3.5
Water chesnuts	1 cup	3.5
Blueberries, raw	1 cup	3.5
Mushrooms, cooked	1 cup	3.4
Beets, cooked	1 cup	3.4
Strawberries, raw	1 cup	3.3
Apple, raw with skin	1 apple	3.3
Red pepper, raw	1 cup	3.1
Turnip, cooked	1 cup	3.1
Carrot, raw	1 cup	3.1
Banana, raw	1 banana	3.1
Prunes	5 prunes	3
Wild rice, cooked	1 cup	3
Onions, cooked	1 cup	3
Cauliflower, cooked	1 cup	2.9
Cabbage, cooked	1 cup	2.9
Flax seed, whole	1 Tbsp.	2.8
Apples, dried	5 rings	2.8
Applesauce	1 cup	2.7
Kale, cooked	1 cup	2.6
Prune juice	1 cup	2.6
Summer squash, cooked	1 cup	2.5
Cauliflower, raw	1 cup	2.5
Eggplant, cooked	1 cup	2.5
Rice, white, cooked	1 cup	1–2.4
Nectarine, raw	1 nectarine	2.3
Broccoli, raw	1 cup	2.3
Kiwi, raw	1 medium	2.3

(*continued*)

TABLE 3. Fiber in Foods (*Continued*)

Food	Portion	Fiber (grams)
Millet, cooked	1 cup	2.3
Cabbage, raw	1 cup	1.5–2.2
Corn, cooked	1 ear	2.2
Carrot, raw	1 carrot	2
Grapefruit, raw	½ grapefruit	2
Cucumber, peeled, raw	1 large	2
Avocado, raw	1 oz	1.9
Celery, raw	1 cup	1.9
Flax seed, ground	1 Tbsp.	1.9
Kohlrabi, cooked	1 cup	1.8
Endive, raw	1 cup	1.6
Tangerine, raw	1 tangerine	1.5
Tomato, raw	1 tomato	1.5
Peach, raw	1 peach	1.5
Cantaloupe, raw	1 cup	1.4
Grapes, raw	1 cup	1.4
Cherries, raw	1 cup	1.4
Honeydew melon	1 cup	1.4
Peanut butter, chunky	1 Tbsp.	1.4
Asparagus, cooked	4 spears	1.4
Lettuce, romaine	1 cup	1.2
Watermelon, raw	1 wedge	1.1
Leeks, cooked	1 cup	1
Mung beans, cooked	1 cup	1
Peanut butter, smooth	1 Tbsp.	1
Nuts	1 oz	0.9
Seeds	1 Tbsp.	0.9
Hummus	1 Tbsp.	0.8
Olives, canned	5 large	0.7
Pickles	1 pickle	0.7
Apricots, raw	1 apricot	0.7
Mushrooms, raw	1 cup	0.7
Alfalfa seeds, raw	1 cup	0.6
Fruit Juice (e.g., orange, apple)	1 cup	0.5
Rice cakes	1 cake	0.2–0.4

Sources: USDA Nutrient Database, www.nal.usda.gov/fnic/foodcomp/search, www.renewlife.com, www.yoplait.com, www.larabar.com, www.balance.com, www.kindsnacks.com, www.gorgedelights.com.

TABLE 3. Fiber in Foods (*Continued*)

Food	Portion	Fiber (grams)
Coconut flour	1 cup	50
Mesquite	1 cup	46
Green pea flour	1 cup	44
Montina	1 cup	36
Ground flax seed	1 cup	33
Fava bean flour	1 cup	32
White bean flour	1 cup	32
Rice bran	1 cup	24
Garbanzo bean flour	1 cup	20
Black bean flour	1 cup	20
Millet flour	1 cup	16
Teff flour	1 cup	16
Potato flour	1 cup	16
Sweet potato flour	1 cup	16
Almond	1 cup	12
Hazelnut	1 cup	12
Corn flour	1 cup	12
Amaranth flour	1 cup	12
Sorghum flour	1 cup	12
Quinoa flour	1 cup	8
White rice flour, brown rice flour, sweet rice flour	1 cup	4
Tapioca flour	1 cup	0

Sources: www.bobsredmill.com, Casa de Fruta (mesquite), www.amazinggrains.com (montina), www.canadiandryingtechnologies.com (sweet potato flour).

Food	Portion	Fiber (grams)
Flax seed	¼ cup dry	12
Amaranth	¼ cup dry	7
Hulled millet	¼ cup dry	6
Buckwheat groats	¼ cup dry	5
Hulled hemp seed	¼ cup dry	4
Teff	¼ cup dry	4
Steel-cut gluten-free oats	¼ cup dry	4
Quinoa	¼ cup dry	3
Whole-grain oats (gluten free)	¼ cup dry	2

Source: www.bobsredmill.com.

colon digest some of the soluble fiber, producing short-chain fatty acids that are important for your health but also make gas as a by-product. Very severe or persistent gas could signal bacterial overgrowth that needs treatment with antibiotics (see Chapter 40 on small intestinal bacterial overgrowth).

It is best to get your fiber from food.[5] People with celiac disease can meet the recommended daily intake for fiber with fruits, vegetables, legumes, gluten-free whole grains, nuts, and seeds. However, if you can't get all you need from your diet, you can add gluten-free fiber supplements (Table 4). Also, modest physical activity, such as daily

TABLE 4. Fiber Supplements

Product	Gluten free?	Manufacturer/Contact Information
Metamucil		Proctor & Gamble
Capsules	Yes	www.metamucil.com
Powders and singles	Yes	800-983-4237
Wafers	No	
Fibersure		Proctor & Gamble
Powders	Yes	www.fibersure.com
Soft chews	Yes	800-525-2855
Capsules	Yes	
Citrucel		GlaxoSmithKline
Powders	Yes	www.citrucel.com
Caplets	Yes	800-897-6081
FiberChoice		GlaxoSmithKline
All products	Yes	www.fiberchoice.com
		877-553-4237
Konsyl		Konsyl Pharmaceutical, Inc.
Powders	Yes	www.konsyl.com
Caplets	Yes	800-356-6795
FiberCon		Wyeth Consumer Healthcare
No gluten in ingredients but will not guarantee raw ingredients have not been in contact with gluten.	N/A	www.fibercon.com 800-282-8805
Resource Benefiber	Yes	Nestle Nutrition www.nestlenutritionstore.com 888-240-2713
Benefiber		Novartis
All products contain wheat dextrin but test to 10 parts per million of gluten, which is considered gluten free.	Yes	www.benefiber.com 800-452-0051

Adapted from Reference 16, with permission.

walks, may help you overcome mild constipation, although it is not likely to help you improve severe constipation.[12]

If your symptoms persist despite maximizing your intake of dietary fiber and fluid, your doctor can recommend other agents for treatment (Table 5). Psyllium, a bulk-forming agent, has been found to improve stool frequency and consistency.[13] Psyllium comes from the ground seed husk of the isphaghula plant and needs to be taken with plenty of water. You can also ask your dietitian about using ground flax seed or ground hemp seed as a dietary fiber source. Polyethylene glycol laxative (Miralax) is safe and often effective.[14] Other options

TABLE 5. Gluten-Free Agents that Treat Constipation

Type	Generic Name	Dosage	Comments
Bulking laxatives	Psyllium	Up to 30 grams per day in divided doses	Must be taken with plenty of water. May contribute to bloating and gas.
	Methylcellulose	Up to 6 grams per day in divided doses	
Osmotic laxatives	Polycarbophil	Up to 4 grams per day in divided doses	
	Magnesium hydroxide	30–60 ml per day	
	Polyethylene glycol	17 grams per day	
	Lactulose	15–30 ml twice a day	Gas and bloating are common side effects.
Stimulant laxatives			
Anthraquinones	Sennosides	8.6–30 mg twice a day	
Diphenylmethane Derivatives	Bisacodyl	10–15 mg once a day 10 mg rectal suppository daily	
Stool softeners	Docusate sodium Docusate calcium	50–100 mg twice a day 240 mg daily	
Emollients			
	Mineral oil	5–45 ml once a day (before bed)	Long-term use can cause fat-soluble vitamin malabsorption.
Chloride channel activator			
	Lupiprostone	8 mcg twice a day 24 mcg twice a day (chronic constipation)	Nausea is common; administer with food and water.

Reference: www.gastro.org/user-assets/Documents/08_Publications/06_GIHep_Annual_Review/ Articles/ Lembo.pdf.

include lactulose, Senna, Biscodyl, and lubiprostone (Amitiza).[15] Please discuss these options with your doctor.

What Lorenzo Decided

Lorenzo was agreeable to increasing the fiber in his diet gradually with the goal of improving his bowel movements. He was able to implement this recommendation by adding gluten-free cooked buckwheat groats and ground flax seed to his breakfast, quinoa and legumes to his lunch, popcorn and fruits for snacks, and more vegetables to his dinner. He made these changes slowly over a few weeks. He also paid attention to his water intake and made sure he had at least six glasses of plain water throughout the day. Within a month of making these simple changes, Lorenzo was no longer bothered by constipation or hemorrhoids.

SELF-MANAGEMENT TIPS

☐ Increase dietary fiber gradually, as tolerated, until you reach your goal, including drinking 6–8 glasses of water daily and participating in regular physical exercise.

☐ Try gluten-free whole-grain side dishes at meals instead of gluten-free baked goods. Quinoa, amaranth, kasha (buckwheat), gluten-free oats, and whole-grain cornmeal are excellent choices.

☐ Use higher-fiber gluten-free flours in baking, such as buckwheat, bean flours, amaranth flour, gluten-free oat flour, mesquite, montina, and quinoa flour.

☐ Eat the recommended daily amounts of fruits (2 cups/day) and vegetables (2½–3 cups/day), in particular, raw fruits and vegetables.

☐ Eat high-fiber legumes such as peas and beans, nuts, and seeds.

☐ Read labels carefully, choosing higher-fiber gluten-free prepared foods.

☐ Plan portable gluten-free snacks, such as popcorn, fresh fruit, raw vegetables, nuts, and dried fruit.

☐ If your constipation does not resolve with dietary changes, speak to your doctor about starting a fiber supplement or a medicine to treat the constipation.

References

1. Eoff JC, Lembo AJ. Optimal treatment of chronic constipation in managed care: review and roundtable discussion. *J Manag Care Pharm* 2008;14(9, Suppl. S-a):S1–S17.
2. American College of Gastroenterology Chronic Constipation Task Force. An evidence-based approach to the management of chronic constipation in North America. *Am J Gastroenterol* 2005;100(Suppl. I):S1–S4.
3. Rashid M, Cranney A, Zarkadas M, Graham ID, Switzer C, Case S, Molloy M, Warrren RE, Burrows V, Butzner JD. Celiac disease: evaluation of the diagnosis and dietary compliance in Canadian children. *Pediatrics* 2005;116(6):754–59.

4. Cranney A, Zarkadas M, Graham ID, Butzner JD, Rashid M, Warren R, Molloy M, Case S, Burrows R, Switzer C. The Canadian Celiac Health Survey. *Dig Dis Sci* 2007;52:1087–095.

5. Catassi C, Kryszak D, Louis-Jacques O, Durksen D, Hill I, Crowe SE, Brown AR, Procaccini NJ, Wonderly BA, Hartley P, Moreci J, Bennett N, Horvath K, Burk M, Fasano A. Detection of celiac disease in primary care: a multicenter case-finding study in North America. *Am J Gastroenterol* 2007;102:1454–60.

6. Murray JA, Watson T, Clearman B, Mitros F. Effect of a gluten-free diet on gastrointestinal symptoms in celiac disease. *Am J Clin Nutr* 2004;79:669–73.

7. Carroccio A, Ambrosiano G, Di Prima L, Giuseppe P, Iacono G, Florena AD, Porcasi R, Noto D, Fayer F, Soresi M, Geraci G, Sciume C, Di Fede G. Clinical symptoms in celiac patients on a gluten-free diet. *Scand J Gastroenterol* 2008;43:1315–21.

8. Midhagen G, Hallert C. High rate of gastrointestinal symptoms in celiac patients living on a gluten-free diet: controlled study. *Am J Gastroenterol* 2003;98:2023–26.

9. Locke GR, Pemberton JH, Philips SH. American Gastroenterological Association technical review on constipation. *Gastroenterology* 2000;119(6):1766–78.

10. American Dietetic Association. Position of the American Dietetic Association: health implications of dietary fiber. *J Am Diet Assoc* 2008;108:1716–31.

11. Fernandez-Banares F. Nutritional care of the patient with constipation. *Baillieres Best Pract Res Clin Gastroenterol* 2006;20(3):575–87.

12. Meshkinpour H, Selod S, Movahedi H, et al. Effects of regular exercise in management of chronic idiopathic constipation. *Dig Dis Sci* 1998;43:2379–83.

13. Brandt LJ, Prather CM, Quigley EMM, et al. Systematic review on the management of chronic constipation in North America. *Am J Gastroenterol* 2005;100(Suppl. I):S5–S22.

14. Di Palma JA, Cleveland MV, McGowan J, Herrera JL. A randomized, multicenter comparison of polyethylene glycol laxative and tegaserod in treatment of patients with chronic constipation. *Am J Gastroenterol* 2007;102(9):1964–71.

15. Johanson JF, Morton D, Geenen J, Ueno R. Multicenter, 4-week, double-blind, randomized, placebo-controlled trial of linaclotide, a locally-acting type-2 chloride channel activator, in patients with chronic constipation. *Am J Gastroenterol* 2008;103(1):170–77.

16. Gluten-free status of commercial fiber supplements. *Pract Gastroenterol* 2009;XXXIII(1):54.

Suzanne Simpson, RD, is a dietitian-nutritionist in the Celiac Disease Center at Columbia University, New York, New York.

CHAPTER 17

Weight Gain: A Common, and Sometimes Unwelcome, Measure of Healing

Melinda Dennis, MS, RD, LDN

S usan, 54 years old, came to our office frustrated over a weight gain of 20 pounds in the three months following her diagnosis of celiac disease and starting the gluten-free diet (GFD). "I'm not eating more. I'm actually eating less, but I can't stop gaining weight. I've never been this heavy. This is ridiculous."

Susan brought with her a three-day food and beverage record, which is often used in clinic as a snapshot evaluation of nutritional intake and adequacy and, in the case of celiac disease, of adherence to the GFD. One day of Susan's record is below.

Susan's Meal Plan

BREAKFAST: gluten-free English muffin with peanut butter and jelly, coffee, orange juice

LUNCH: corn pasta, meat sauce with vegetables, potato chips, whole milk

SNACK: candy

DINNER: baked potato, grilled chicken, broccoli, gluten-free roll, water

EVENING SNACK: bowl of gluten-free cereal with whole milk

How Absorption Affects Weight and Lipid Levels

The classic clinical symptoms of someone with celiac disease are gas, bloating, diarrhea, and weight loss. In general, unintentional weight loss can be a sign that you are not absorbing nutrients or that there is some other serious medical problem. In celiac disease, weight loss generally means that there has been severe damage to the lining of your small intestine. Although weight loss is a classic symptom of celiac disease, it is becoming less common at the time of diagnosis. Part of the reason for this is that we are getting better at finding celiac disease earlier, before a lot of damage has been done. So these days, weight gain on the GFD is a common report and, in many cases, a common complaint from patients.

Whether you have malabsorption of nutrients depends on the amount and degree of the affected intestine[1] and varies greatly among individuals with celiac disease. Some people will need additional calories and protein to help them with the healing process, whereas others have little or no malabsorption. As the villi and microvilli lining in the intestine heal, your ability to absorb the carbohydrates, protein, fat, vitamins, minerals, fiber, and water in food increases, which can lead to weight gain. This indicates that your body is healing—a good sign. But if the weight gain exceeds an acceptable level, other health concerns arise. Excessive weight gain increases the risk of coronary artery disease, hypertension, type 2 diabetes, osteoporosis, and certain types of cancer.[2]

Another unwelcome sign of intestinal healing is rising total cholesterol and LDL cholesterol levels. Typically, individuals with newly diagnosed celiac disease have low total cholesterol levels and LDL levels, also likely the result of some degree of malabsorption. These will also normalize, and may rise to elevated or high levels, as the intestine heals on the GFD, so you need to pay attention to your lipid levels.

Although most weight gain after going on a GFD results from intestinal healing especially if combined with excess caloric intake, certain medical problems like low thyroid hormone level can also cause weight gain. If your weight gain is unusually severe or resists the lifestyle modifications described below, discuss this issue with your physician.

What's Different about Gluten-Free Foods?

An important contributor to weight gain is the food choices people make on the GFD. It's tempting to search out and use the gluten-free substitutes for the foods you've previously eaten. But they are not all necessarily alike in nutritional quality. For example, a gluten-containing English muffin might have 120 calories, 25 grams of carbohydrates, 1 gram of fat, and 1 gram of fiber; a gluten-free alternative may have 210 calories, 39 grams of carbohydrates, 3.5 grams of fat, and 1 gram of fiber. This is nearly a two-fold increase in calories, and triples the fat content. Gluten-free products commonly have added fat, typically to improve the texture and mouth-feel in the absence of gluten.

In addition, many commercial gluten-free foods are prepared mainly from white rice, corn, potato, and tapioca, which are high in carbohydrates, low in fiber, and tend to have poor nutritional value. A food that is high in carbohydrates and low in fiber breaks down quickly into sugar (glucose) in the body. As a result, you feel unsatisfied and tend to compensate by eating more calories, often of the same type of food. This rise in blood glucose levels triggers a corresponding rise in insulin levels. Although this is particularly unhelpful to those who are managing diabetes, it is not healthy for anyone and is associated with weight gain.

There are healthier choices in gluten-free eating. Consult the food labels to find some of the higher fiber, more nutritious whole-grain gluten-free foods that have made their way into the American marketplace. These grains and starches, namely quinoa, millet, amaranth, sorghum, soy (a legume), teff, buckwheat, wild rice, and brown rice (versus white rice), each have their own nutrient profiles that make them superior to white rice, corn, tapioca, and potatoes (see Chapter 13 on grains).

What Is Healthy Weight Loss?

Calories
The first step is to be aware of "calories in versus calories out." Add up the number of calories you eat in one day and make sure it is less than the total number of calories you use up over the course of a day (see Exercise, below). To lose weight, each day you will need to burn more calories than you ingest. One simple way to do this is to eat 500 fewer calories per day than you usually eat. On paper, this leads to about one pound of body weight loss per week (500 calories × 7 days = 3500 calories = 1 pound of body weight). Several online sites can help you individualize your calorie needs and review calorie counting, such as www.eatright.org and www.fitday.com.

Balance
Next, be aware of which foods you choose and aim for a variety each day, including vegetables, fruits, whole gluten-free grains, lean proteins, and healthy fats. Dietitians refer to this as a *balanced diet*. In fact, meeting with a registered dietitian who has expertise in celiac disease can be extremely helpful. A dietitian can calculate how many calories you need based on your gender, age, height, weight, current physical activity, medical conditions, and weight loss goals so you have an estimated caloric intake per day to use as a goal. You can also review your eating plan with the dietitian to make sure it is realistic as well as nutritionally balanced. Your health depends on getting adequate calcium, vitamin D, B vitamins, iron, and fiber, which are often lacking in the GFD[3] (see Chapter 12 on balanced diet).

Portion Control
The trick is to not overeat. Many dietitians teach how to control portion size using the American plate model. Picture a 10-inch dinner plate that is divided into three sections: 25% of the plate is for your lean protein intake, which includes low-fat dairy foods, poultry, fish, eggs, legumes (dried beans, lentils, soybeans, lima beans, peas), and lean cuts of meat; 25% of the plate is for carbohydrates (starches) such as whole-grain brown rice, wild rice, millet, quinoa, amaranth, buckwheat, and whole-grain corn; and the remaining half of the plate is for nonstarchy vegetables such as dark leafy greens (spinach, kale, Swiss chard), zucchini, broccoli, green beans, romaine lettuce, cucumbers, and tomatoes, to name a few. Keeping in mind that calorie needs are different for each individual, this is a quick and easy way to make sure you are limiting the foods that are higher in calories and fat and maximizing your vegetables. Complete your meal with a side of fresh fruit and a glass of water or low-fat or lactose-free milk (or dairy-free alternative).

Clearing Out Unnecessary Fat
Extra fat is routinely added to many gluten-free foods to improve their taste, so it's wise to read food labels and understand the different types of fat. Saturated fats are solid at room

temperature, such as butter, lard, and some vegetable oils like coconut oil and palm oil. These can raise cholesterol levels and the risk of heart disease. Limit your saturated fat intake to 8–10% of your total daily calories. Unsaturated fats, such as nuts, or vegetable oils, such as olive oil and grapeseed oil, which are liquid at room temperature are a much healthier choice. Trans fats, in which a vegetable oil has been hardened by hydrogenation, occur naturally in beef, pork, lamb, butter, and milk, but their most negative impact can be seen in commercially prepared foods, such as cookies, cakes, pretzels, and other snacks. Avoid trans fats to the best of your ability. Simple changes like reducing your meat intake, increasing your fish intake, and using nonstick cooking oil sprays (from olive oil) instead of pouring oil in a pan can significantly cut your fat intake.

Exercise

Exercise is the "calories out" part of your day and is an essential element of weight loss and a healthy life. Exercise increases your metabolism (the rate at which you burn calories), improves mild-to-moderate depression and anxiety, and reduces the risk of chronic diseases.[3] According to the *2008 Physical Activity Guidelines for Americans,* "most health benefits occur with at least 150 minutes (2 hours and 30 minutes) a week of moderate-intensity physical activity, such as brisk walking."[4] This means that it takes only 30 minutes per day (divided into 10-minute segments if you choose), five days per week to see long-term health benefits of regular physical activity. If weight loss is your goal, you'll see results if you are physically active (moderate-to-vigorous intensity) for about 60 minutes on most days.[4] A few suggestions to consider are walking more, biking to work, joining a gym or group exercise class, hiring a personal trainer, taking vacations that involve more activity, dancing to music, and choosing outside play over TV. Engage your family and friends in fun physical activities. Check with your doctor before starting exercise if you have any health concerns.

What Susan Did

After hearing my suggestions, Susan chose to make a few changes in what she was eating. Here's her more recent one-day food and beverage record.

Susan's Improved Meal Plan

BREAKFAST: bowl of home-cooked hot buckwheat with cinnamon, sliced banana, a few almonds, and low-fat milk

SNACK: gluten-free energy bar

LUNCH: whole-grain brown rice pasta, meat sauce with cooked vegetables, and nonfat milk

DINNER: grilled chicken and broccoli over cooked quinoa, and water

SNACK: piece of fruit or low-fat frozen yogurt

Susan found that when she started eating the whole-grain gluten-free versions of her favorite starches, like English muffins, pasta, rolls, and cereal, she felt satisfied on less food. Because they are high in fiber, which is very filling, gluten-free whole-grain foods are useful when you are trying to lose weight. Remember to slowly increase the amount of fiber you eat and drink extra water so that your gastrointestinal tract can adjust. Doing this helps you minimize or avoid gas and bloating. Chapter 13 has more details on the fiber content and nutritional quality, including vitamin enrichment, of the gluten-free grains. Also, Susan liked experimenting with new grains such as hot buckwheat cereal and quinoa.

She also found that when she chooses a healthy morning snack—one that has equal calories from protein, carbohydrates, and fat—she does not crave sugary candy in the late afternoon. Her strategy of eating small meals and snacking through the day is keeping her blood glucose level more consistent (her blood glucose levels do not rise as much after meals), which helps prevent cravings later in the day.

Changing her evening snack from cereal and whole milk (270 calories) to fruit (~60 calories) saves Susan 210 calories, which is about half of the calories she needs to cut to meet her goal of eating 500 fewer calories per day.

Here are some other dietary suggestions that Susan tried:

- She switched from whole milk to nonfat milk and saved 70 calories per cup.
- She switched to natural peanut butter (no sugar added) and had it only occasionally, substituting whole nuts in 1-ounce servings.
- She bought plates designed with dividers (25%, 25%, 50%) and filled half of her dinner plate each night with nonstarchy vegetables (search for these online using the term *divided plates*).
- She drank hot tea or broth, such as gluten-free chicken broth or a clear, hot Asian soup, as an appetizer about 15 minutes before dinner and found she didn't need to eat as much at dinner. Hot liquids send a message to the brain that you have eaten more than you actually have.
- She had a large breakfast that included more protein, a medium-sized lunch, and a smaller-sized dinner so that she had the whole day to burn off most of her calories. Some people think of this habit as "eating breakfast like a king, lunch like a prince, and dinner like a pauper."
- She set a goal of eating 500 fewer calories less each day than she had been eating. I reminded her that she could also use exercise to burn off calories (rather than just eating fewer calories) to reach her goal.

Susan told me that she saw these changes as lifestyle improvements rather than restrictions and, as a result, felt more motivated to keep making small changes in a healthy direction. She started walking for 45 minutes, at lunch or after dinner, most days of the week, something that fit easily into her schedule. Susan was able to lose about three pounds a month and got back to a weight she was comfortable with after six months.

TABLE 1. Sample 1-Day Gluten-Free Menu

Breakfast	2 slices enriched gluten-free toast* with 1 Tbsp. almond butter
	1 egg
	½ cup strawberries
	8 oz. nonfat milk
Lunch	⅓ of a 9-inch gluten-free pizza
	To prepare the whole pizza, use 1 pizza crust* (homemade or ready-to-eat)
	topped with ½ cup tomato sauce, 3 oz. low-fat cheese, 3 oz. grilled chicken,
	1½ cups fresh vegetables, and
	¾ cup pineapple slices.
	6 oz. water
	1 fresh apple or other medium-sized fruit
Snack	6 oz. low-fat plain yogurt mixed with 2 Tbsp. whole-grain, gluten-free cereal
Evening Meal	1 cup whole-grain or enriched gluten-free pasta topped with
	2 Tbsp. pesto and ⅓ cup chick peas
	2 cups mixed greens salad topped with 4 orange slices and ½ oz. walnuts and
	1 Tbsp. oil and vinegar dressing
	8 oz. seltzer water with lime

*Try to select gluten-free bread and pizza crust with 2 grams or more of fiber per slice that includes at least one gluten-free grain other than rice, corn, or potato. Examples are sorghum, quinoa, buckwheat, millet, teff, and amaranth.
Nutrition Facts: 1802 calories, 64.3 g fat (12.1 g saturated), 71.6 g protein, 234.2 g carbohydrates (27.5 g dietary fiber), 2268.7 g sodium
Source: American Dietetic Association. *Nutrition Care Manual*. (Celiac Disease: Food Recommended) (http://www.nutritioncaremanual.org/index.cfm?Page=Meal_Plans&topic=18174&headingid=18228#18228). Accessed September 22, 2009. Adapted with permission.

Recipe: On the Run Breakfast Smoothie

This drink is nothing special to look at once it's all blended, but it's healthy, high in fiber and protein, low in sugar, and gluten free. If you are on the run, you are maximizing nutrition in a simple, transportable shake. I vary my ingredients depending on what I have available so each week can be different.

1 cup rice milk (gluten free, fortified with vitamins A and D and calcium)
½ banana
1 Tbsp. cashew butter (or peanut or almond butter)
½ cup frozen or fresh fruit (mango, peach, berries, papaya)
2 Tbsp. hemp protein powder

Blend in a blender and drink cold!
Nutrition Facts, per serving (about 8 oz.): 396 calories, 12.6 g fat (2 g saturated, 10.6 unsaturated), 12.4 g protein, 58.4 g carbohydrates (6.4 g dietary fiber)

Options

- Prefer a different liquid? Choose your favorite fruit juice (diluted with water, if you like) instead of rice milk. Or try cow's milk, hemp milk, almond or hazelnut milk, soy milk, or potato milk (I have yet to try it with potato milk). Keep in mind that these vary in protein and vitamin content. Make sure you choose a gluten-free brand.
- Prefer a different gluten-free protein powder? Try soy protein powder (not advised for those who get gassy from soy or have a soy allergy), rice protein powder (low in protein but a reasonable option), pea protein powder, egg white protein powder, or whey protein powder (easily absorbed and high in protein but must be avoided by those with a dairy allergy).
- Want less fiber? Reduce the amount of hemp protein powder. Add only one serving of fruit.
- Want more fiber? Add more hemp protein powder with fiber, ground flax seed, or more fruit.
- Want it to be creamier and higher in fat and calories? Add coconut milk (use sparingly), flax seed oil, avocado, and/or more nut butter.
- Want less fat? Leave out or reduce the nut butter and add applesauce or low-fat yogurt (preferably plain because it contains less sugar).

SELF-MANAGEMENT TIPS

- ☐ Understand that weight gain is a natural healing response of a body that is recovering from some degree of malabsorption.
- ☐ One possible reason for unintentional weight gain is low thyroid; be sure to have your doctor check your thyroid status.
- ☐ Replace at least half of your low-fiber, high-carbohydrate commercially prepared foods with whole-grain gluten-free versions that are more nutritious and filling choices.
- ☐ Eat small meals and snacks at intervals during the day to avoid strong hunger and cravings that may tempt you to eat anything you can find, regardless of its nutritional value.
- ☐ Consult with a registered dietitian to review your eating plan and create one that promotes weight loss and includes fiber and nutrients that can be lacking in the gluten-free diet, such as calcium, vitamin D, iron, zinc, and B vitamins.
- ☐ Engage in regular physical activity that is appropriate for your current fitness level and health goals; seek the advice of your health care provider if you are unsure about your ability to be physically active.

References

1. Farrell RJ, Kelly CP. Celiac sprue. *N Engl J Med* 2002;346:180–88.
2. What is the evidence to support the nutritional adequacy of a gluten free dietary pattern? American Dietetic Association Evidence Analysis Library. www.adaevidencelibrary.com/evidence.cfm?evidence_summary_id=25060. Accessed July 1, 2009.
3. U.S. Department of Health and Human Services. *Dietary Guidelines for Americans 2005*. www.health.gov/dietaryguidelines/dga2005/document/html/chapter4.htm. Accessed July 1, 2009.
4. U.S. Department of Health and Human Services. *2008 Physical Activity Guidelines for Americans*. www.health.gov/paguidelines/guidelines/summary.aspx. Accessed July 1, 2009.

CHAPTER 18

Cheating? Think Again

Dee Sandquist, MS, RD, LD

After a year of dealing with diarrhea, abdominal pain, vomiting, and weight loss, Andy was diagnosed with celiac disease at age 44. He had never heard of it before his diagnosis. His doctor told him that he would need to avoid bread and food with wheat in it for the rest of his life. He gave Andy a list of foods that were now off limits.

Andy did pretty well at making sandwiches without bread using lettuce leaves, saying no to pizza, and switching to wine instead of beer. He started feeling better. But he missed his old life and would occasionally have a bagel with his breakfast eggs. And when he went out with friends, he would have some pretzels or dry-roasted peanuts with his drinks and wasn't choosy about what he decided to order at restaurants. Andy didn't like to make a big deal about his eating requirements. Usually within a day or two of cheating, his diarrhea and discomfort would return. But then he would totally avoid gluten again, and things would settle down.

Who Cheats, and Why?

For some people, following a gluten-free diet (GFD) is a daily challenge. Like Andy, some choose to eat gluten occasionally. In a review of more than 30 studies, the number of people following a completely GFD was between 42% and 91%.[1] People diagnosed with celiac disease in childhood were more likely to cheat, perhaps under the mistaken idea that you can outgrow celiac disease. As far as we know, celiac disease is lifelong, and we can't outgrow it. When someone eliminates gluten from the diet, the intestine has a chance to heal, but once sensitivity to gluten develops, it is there for life. Even after a long period of being gluten free, eating gluten again will trigger an immune response that can reinjure the villi.

Just as symptoms can vary greatly among individuals, the types of questions and problems that arise vary, not just among people, but over time as well. Some adolescents can experience a prolonged remission while off the diet, sometimes called a *honeymoon period*, where they show minimal, if any, symptoms—although it is probable that mucosal damage continues to occur.[2] Many of these individuals will go on to develop symptoms of celiac disease in later life. The gluten-free diet is a lifetime eating plan because it is the only treatment for celiac disease.

It's typical for those newly diagnosed with celiac disease to work at following the GFD because they have not felt well for years and want to feel better. You might have found it difficult to adjust to the taste of gluten-free bread because you're used to the distinctive flavor of wheat. Understandably, there is an adjustment period. Most people adapt and find the benefit of not having symptoms makes following the diet worthwhile. However, it's human nature to sometimes challenge what you know to be good for yourself. Or you may simply tire of advocating for yourself when attending social events or eating out.

Generally, it takes only a few times of eating gluten intentionally for most people to realize the benefit of following the GFD. Others may not have visible symptoms and may indulge occasionally. Still others don't care and choose to eat what they want. If this sounds like you, give some consideration to your self-esteem and self-worth. A professional counselor can assist you in sorting through issues that might be preventing you from keeping yourself healthy.

Excuses, Excuses

"Gluten-free food is expensive." Yes, at first glance, gluten-free foods cost more than their gluten-containing counterparts. However, because following a GFD is the only treatment available for your celiac disease, think of the diet as a prescription because there is no medication. There is no additional medication to purchase. It's not just about the cost of a loaf of bread. Focus on the importance of getting treated for your disease. Not being treated adversely affects your quality of life and health. What is the cost of being too sick to work or to enjoy being with your family and friends?

Solutions
Find a registered dietitian who can help you plan gluten-free meals that meet your budget. Here are a few tips that can help you get the most from your food dollar.

- When you see something on sale, buy extras if you can guarantee that you will use it up within a reasonable time to avoid spoilage. Gluten-free flours can be stored in the freezer to extend their life.
- Buy in season and at farmers' markets. Buy frozen fruits and vegetables. Following a GFD is a great time to increase your intake of fruits and vegetables. Many Americans do not eat the recommended 5–9 servings per day.
- Go in with friends on a mail order and save shipping. Small groups of people find that they can order in quantity and divide the items to reduce shipping costs.
- Call your favorite companies and ask them to send you coupons. As the availability of gluten-free products grows, the competition for customers is also growing. Sign up for Mambo Sprouts (a national coupon booklet that contains many gluten-free products) and Be Free For Me.

- Get into leftovers. If you make a special gluten-free bread, freeze part of it so there's no waste.
- Shop around if you have the time to find less expensive products. Many supermarkets are carrying gluten-free items and may even advertise them in their sales notices.

"It's hard to find gluten-free foods." Gluten-free food is one of the fastest growing retail segments in the food industry. There are areas where your grocery stores may not yet be carrying a range of commercial gluten-free foods. Go to your grocery store customer service counter and ask to speak to the person who is in charge of ordering products. Ask about getting a discount if you buy an entire case. Many gluten-free products come in 6- to 24-pack cases. Most grocery stores are happy to special order products as long as they know they will sell. Consider ordering online. You may need to buy a large quantity of products to keep shipping costs reasonable, so consider whether you can freeze the surplus or split the order with others.

"Gluten-free food doesn't taste as good as regular food." Many flavors are learned by exposure over time. Continue experimenting with new foods and recipes, and you will find ones that you enjoy. Invest in a gluten-free cookbook and follow the recipes. There are a wide variety of gluten-free mixes available. Try several mixes until you find the ones you like. If you don't cook, choose your restaurants carefully and educate the staff.

There's a whole world of ancient grains you can discover when you go gluten free. Experiment with amaranth, millet, teff, quinoa, sorghum, and buckwheat—all are gluten free. For example, use quinoa instead of rice; it's cooked the same way. Experiment with herbs and spices and ethnic foods. Adding herbs and spices is a great way to add a variety of flavors. With so many ready products and mixes on the market, try several until you find one you like. It's out there. The range of products varies from the "white" refined product to the whole-grain product. Have a friend over and do some experimenting in the kitchen. Take a cooking class.

"Why should I follow the diet if I don't have symptoms?" Most people who consume gluten suffer the consequences and try to avoid being sick because they don't want to feel miserable. Some people have no symptoms. But what about consequences over the long run? We don't know enough about the damage that ingesting gluten over time causes. We do know, however, that it doesn't take much gluten ingestion to see inflammation in the small intestine. In fact, 1/50 of a slice of bread is enough to see inflammatory damage in the mucosal layer on biopsy. And persistent inflammation is a bad thing.

Someone who generally follows the GFD but chooses to eat gluten now and then is basically in the same situation as someone who has decided *not* to follow the GFD. We also know that Andy may be at an increased risk of developing another autoimmune disease if he continues to eat gluten.[2] In addition, he may be at a higher risk long-term for developing some cancers, as well as gastrointestinal symptoms, and vitamin and mineral deficiencies leading to such problems as bone disease and osteoporosis. More research needs to be done to see exactly how much damage a little gluten over time does to the body of a person with celiac disease.

Unfortunately, your physician or health care provider may not be an expert in celiac disease and may not stress the need for you to follow a GFD. With the correct amount and kind of education, you will realize the importance of eating gluten free to your health and well-being.

What Andy Decided

Andy asked his doctor for a referral to a dietitian. He was lucky enough to meet with a dietitian who was enthusiastic about cooking gluten free and referred him to a class that met in the evenings once a week to make gluten-free meals. There he learned about all sorts of new food products and tried some tasty grains that he started using as side dishes and in casseroles. He also met a few new friends and heard about some restaurants with specific menu items that were safely gluten free. It took Andy a few months to realize that he had more energy and mental focus when he totally avoided ingesting gluten and committed to being gluten free. After a year of eating gluten free, he felt stronger and healthier than he had in years.

SELF-MANAGEMENT TIPS

☐ Focus on the importance of avoiding gluten to treat your celiac disease.
☐ Think about where and when you cheat and come up with some solutions to keep you from eating gluten.
☐ Visit a dietitian for education on eating gluten free, even if you have to pay out of pocket.
☐ Seek out gluten-free foods. Shop online. Ask your grocery stores to stock your favorite gluten-free items or order them for you.
☐ Find a celiac disease support group that will allow you to meet and learn from others with the same dietary challenges.

References

1. Evidence Analysis Library, American Dietetic Association Aliment Pharmacol Ther 2009L 30 (4): 315–30 30 July, 2009
2. Ventura A, Magazzu G, Greco L, SIGEP Study Group for Autoimmune Disorders in Celiac Disease. Duration of exposure to gluten and risk for autoimmune disorders in patients with celiac disease. *Gastroenterology* 1999;117(2):297–303.

Dee Sandquist, MS, RD, LD, is a dietitian at the Ottumwa North and Mt. Pleasant Hy-Vee food stores in Iowa. Prior to this recent move, she served as the Director of Nutrition, Diabetes, Weight Management, Wellness and Wound Healing at Southwest Washington Medical Center, Vancouver, Washington; Ms. Sandquist and her husband owned and operated a gluten-free grocery store in Vancouver.

CHAPTER 19

Is There a Safe Level of Gluten Ingestion?

Katri Kaukinen, MD, PhD, and Pekka Collin, MD, PhD

Lara, a 52-year-old woman, came to her routine follow-up visit at the gastroenterology outpatient clinic. Lara had been diagnosed with celiac disease five years earlier and began a gluten-free diet (GFD), which resulted in prompt improvement of her abdominal symptoms and normalization of tissue transglutaminase (tTG) antibodies. At her screening colonoscopy, done after she had been on the GFD for one year, she elected to undergo a follow-up biopsy to assess her celiac disease. We saw that the mucosal villi looked normal at that time.

Now, four years later, Lara had no gastrointestinal symptoms, but her tTG antibody level was positive again at 56 units (normal is less than 20 units). Lara also had iron deficiency anemia. So, Lara had a small intestine endoscopy with biopsies, which revealed damage to the villi typical of uncontrolled celiac disease. Lara claimed that she had kept a strict GFD; however, in a detailed interview, she admitted she occasionally consumed foods likely to contain hidden gluten, such as sauces and soups, about two to four times a month while dining out.

Is It Possible to Avoid Gluten Totally?

A lifelong GFD is currently our only treatment for celiac disease. For most of those with celiac disease who follow a strict GFD, their symptoms resolve and the damage to the absorptive cells that line the small intestine (the mucosal villi) heals. Studies have examined people with celiac disease who occasionally consume gluten-containing food, such as normal bread or cake (containing between 500 mg and 2,000 mg [2 g] of gluten) every week or at least once a month. Even though many people do not develop symptoms, the ongoing damage to the mucosa caused by ingesting gluten is clearly visible.[1]

Although most people agree that a GFD should be as gluten free as possible, a diet completely devoid of gluten is probably impossible to maintain. Why? The foods on the market, even naturally gluten-free ones, may contain trace amounts of gluten because of contamination during processing.[2] However, foods containing trace amounts of gluten have been consumed for decades by those with celiac disease in

Northern Europe and the United Kingdom. In both children and adults who use these food products, when adherence to the diet is good, most will have intestinal mucosal recovery and low rates of celiac complications, such as development of cancer.[1] Furthermore, a randomized study comparing wheat starch–based gluten-free products, containing less than 200 parts per million (ppm) gluten, to naturally gluten-free products, such as maize (corn), rice, and buckwheat, showed that the response of both the small intestine lining and symptoms were equally good with either type of food.[3]

In Europe, many of the food products labeled gluten-free are created by purifying wheat starch–based foods to remove the gluten. These industrially purified gluten-free products still contain trace amounts of gluten. The amount of gluten in purified wheat starch products varies greatly, and standards for the definition of "gluten free" varies by country. For this reason, adding wheat starch to a GFD must be carefully considered. Full details on this topic are in Chapter 21.

Finding a Safe Level of Gluten

Because gluten contamination in food is all but impossible to prevent, it's natural to wonder if there is some safe threshold for gluten in gluten-free products. This has recently been under investigation. It is generally accepted that a gluten challenge—feeding specific amounts of gluten to those with celiac disease and measuring the effects—is the gold standard for assessing an individual's level of gluten intolerance (Table 1). However, the fact is that tolerance to trace amounts of gluten is highly variable among individuals with celiac disease. In some with celiac disease, the deterioration of the mucosa starts immediately when the individual eats gluten, but in others, the development of mucosal villous atrophy or appearance of celiac antibodies may take years. Also, it is not well known how much gluten is actually in a typical GFD, which makes assessment of how much is too much quite difficult.

Short-term gluten challenge studies in a small number of subjects may not necessarily give the right answers to the question of whether there is a safe level. But we can conclude that for almost all people with celiac disease daily gluten intake of 200–500 mg (~1/6 of a slice of bread) seems to induce damage to the villi and causes inflammation (Table 1). Recently, a double-blind (neither the subjects nor the researchers knew who ate what) randomized study showed that daily intake of 10 mg gluten (equivalent to a few crumbs of bread) for 90 days was not harmful, whereas eating 50 mg gluten per day resulted in small but significant mucosal damage.[4] To compare, a normal U.S. or Western European diet contains 10–20 g (10,000–20,000 mg) of gluten per day.

The question of tolerable amounts of gluten in celiac disease can also be settled in the context of everyday clinical practice. We know from studies in Europe that both naturally gluten-free and wheat starch–based gluten-free flour contain traces of gluten, ranging from less than 20 to 200 ppm. The median daily consumption of these gluten-free flours in people with celiac disease was 80 g (up to 300 g), and within these limits, the long-term mucosal recovery was good.[2] By setting a safe threshold level for gluten contamination at

TABLE 1. Gluten Challenge Studies

Study	Number of Subjects	Amount of Gluten Consumed	Duration of Gluten Challenge	Abnormal Small Intestine Biopsy?
Ciclitira et al. 1985	10	1.2–2.4 mg gluten/day	6 weeks	No
Ciclitira et al. 1984	1	10 mg gliadin*	4 hours	No
Catassi et al. 2007	13 13	10 mg gluten/day 50 mg gluten/day	90 days 90 days	No Villous shortening, no inflammation
Catassi et al. 1993	10 10	100 mg gliadin/day* 500 mg gliadin/day*	4 weeks 4 weeks	Dose-dependent decrease in villous morphology, increased inflammation
Shrinivasan et al. 1996	2	500 mg gluten/day	6 weeks	Villous shortening
Laurin et al. 2002	1 1 22	200 mg gluten/day 800 mg gluten/day 700 mg–4.3 g/day	39 weeks 5 weeks 5–51 weeks	Increased inflammation No Villous shortening, increased inflammation
Sturgess et al. 1994	4	1 g gliadin*	4 hours	Villous shortening in ¾, increased inflammation in all
Montgomery et al. 1988	8	2.5–5 g gluten/day	6 months	Increased inflammation

*Rough estimate: 1 gram of gliadin = 2 grams of gluten.
Note that 1 gram of gluten is about 1/3 slice of whole wheat bread, and 1 slice of bread contains about 3 grams of gluten.

less than 20 ppm (in the United States) and 100 ppm (in Europe), the daily consumption of even 300 g flour (about the amount in an entire loaf of gluten-free bread) would result in less than 30 mg intake of gluten per day. This amount seems to be safe for most people according to the challenge studies (Table 1).

The Oats Controversy

Despite the evidence that oats are well tolerated by people with celiac disease, making oats a part of a GFD is still a matter for debate. Basically, oats are a grain that is distantly related to wheat, rye, and barley, and its prolamine (a type of protein) content is lower than that of the other cereals. Several studies have shown that in most adults and children with celiac disease and dermatitis herpetiformis, eating oats has no detrimental effect on the health of the small intestine lining or on the symptoms, even in long-term use.[5]

Once they know about oats, most people with celiac disease choose to eat them. Being able to eat oats diversifies a GFD, enhances the quality of the food you are eating, and increases intake of dietary fiber. Although fear of contamination of oat products with other gluten-containing cereals has restricted their use, pure gluten-free oat products with strictly controlled production systems are available (see also Chapter 21 on oats and wheat starch). Yet, some individuals cannot tolerate even pure oats, and some case reports have shown that oat-intolerant celiac patients may have oat-specific inflammatory cells in the small bowel lining.

Outcome

Concerned about excessive gluten exposure, we referred Lara to a celiac dietitian. Lara and her dietitian identified several areas of gluten contamination, among them dining out and consuming oats from a facility not dedicated to gluten-free products. Lara agreed to avoid these items, even if it meant eating out less. At her next follow-up visit, Lara's tTG antibodies were once again negative, and her anemia had resolved.

SELF-MANAGEMENT TIPS

☐ A truly 100% GFD is not possible, but we don't know how much gluten is actually in a typical GFD.

☐ The safe gluten threshold varies from person to person, and it is impossible to reliably assess whether there is ongoing damage in your small intestine. Therefore, it is important to remain as gluten free as possible.

☐ Occasional significant exposure to gluten—accidental or intended—typically causes more damage than ingesting trace amounts of gluten in otherwise gluten-free products daily; this includes both naturally gluten-free and industrially purified wheat starch–based gluten-free products.

☐ Gluten-free oats are safe to eat for most people with celiac disease. If you trace symptoms specifically to eating oats, be sure to follow up with your doctor, because this could be a sign of oat-specific inflammation.

References

1. Hischenhuber C, Crevel R, Jarry B, et al. Safe amounts of gluten for patients with wheat allergy or coeliac disease (review). *Aliment Pharmacol Ther* 2006;23:559–75.
2. Collin P, Thorell L, Kaukinen K, Mäki M. The safe threshold for gluten contamination in gluten-free products: can trace amounts be accepted in the treatment of coeliac disease? *Aliment Pharmacol Ther* 2004;19:1277–83.

3. Peräaho M, Kaukinen K, Paasikivi K, Sievänen H, Lohiniemi S, Mäki M, Collin P. Wheat-starch-based gluten-free products in the treatment of newly detected celiac disease. Prospective and randomised study. *Aliment Pharmacol Ther* 2003;17:587–94.
4. Catassi C, Fabiani E, Iacono G, D'Agate C, Francavilla R, Biagi F, et al. A prospective, double-blind, placebo-controlled trial to establish a safe gluten threshold for patients with celiac disease. *Am J Clin Nutr* 2007;85:160–66.
5. Garsed K, Scott BB. Can oats be taken in a gluten-free diet? A systematic review. *Scand J Gastroenterol* 2007;42:171–78.

Katri Kaukinen, MD, PhD, is a gastroenterologist and **Pekka Collin, MD, PhD,** is Chief Physician in the Department of Gastroenterology and Alimentary Tract Surgery at Tampere University Hospital, Tampere, Finland. Both are also Adjunct Professors at the University of Tampere Medical School and conduct extensive research in celiac disease.

CHAPTER 20

Inadvertent Gluten Exposure

Melinda Dennis, MS, RD, LDN

Stephanie, a 42-year-old woman, came to the clinic three years after her diagnosis of celiac disease. Although in general Stephanie felt well, she noted that about once a month she would have a few days of recurrent symptoms similar to those she experienced before her diagnosis, including fatigue, loose stools, abdominal pain, and gas. She could trace some of these episodes back to possible, accidental gluten exposure, but not all of them. This was troubling to Stephanie, because she was not intentionally eating any gluten-containing foods. She had even tried following a lactose-free diet for several weeks with no improvement.

We noted that her immunoglobulin A tissue transglutaminase (IgA-tTG) level was elevated to 45 units (normal is less than 20 units), and biopsies from a small intestine endoscopy showed mildly active celiac disease. Stephanie appeared to have nonresponsive celiac disease because of inadvertent gluten exposure (see Chapter 34 on nonresponsive celiac disease).

Finding Hidden Gluten

Because gluten exposure is the most common cause for nonresponsive celiac disease,[1] this seemed to be the logical place to begin investigating Stephanie's elevated IgA-tTG and symptoms, so she was advised to meet with the celiac dietitian. Stephanie told the dietitian that she worked hard to avoid gluten. Stephanie and the dietitian carefully reviewed her diet and lifestyle for any of the less obvious ways that she could be exposing herself to gluten and reviewed the commonly overlooked sources of gluten (Table 1). Here are some of the findings.

- Stephanie had confirmed with the pharmaceutical companies that none of her medications contained gluten.
- All of Stephanie's dietary supplements were clearly labeled gluten free on the product packaging or she had checked by calling the manufacturer.
- She did not drink beer, ale, or lager made from gluten-containing ingredients.

TABLE 1. Overlooked Sources of Gluten or Potential Gluten

These foods, beverages, ingredients, and products contain or may contain gluten, depending on their ingredients or how they are derived. This is not a comprehensive list, and the references have more detailed information on these and other foods and products.

Ales
Beer/lagers
Breading
Brewer's yeast
Broth/bouillon
Brown rice syrup
Cake frosting
Candy
Coating mixes
Communion wafers
Condiments
Croutons
Dates (if rolled in oat flour)
Dextrin (in USDA products*)
Drink mixes
Flavored teas and coffees
Flour or cereal products
Gravies
Imitation bacon
Imitation seafood
Licorice
Marinades
Malt, malt flavoring, and malt extract (gluten free if made from corn)
Malt vinegar
Matzo/matzoh meal
Medications (prescription and over the counter)
Modified food starch (in USDA products*)
Oats (see Chapter 21)
Panko
Pasta
Play-Doh[†]
Processed luncheon meats
Rice pilaf
Roux
Salad dressing
Sauces/spreads
Seasonings (or spice blends)

TABLE 1. Overlooked Sources of Gluten or Potential Gluten (*Continued*)

Seasoned chips, nuts, and seeds
Self-basting poultry
Smoke flavoring
Soup stock
Soy sauce (commonly made with both soy and wheat)
Stuffing (for poultry)
Supplements

*See Chapter 22 on food labeling for more details on foods regulated by the United States Department of Agriculture.
†The gluten protein does not pass through the skin. Avoid cross-contamination by washing hands after handling and before eating.
Adapted from the following resources with permission: Horvath K, Cureton P: *Gluten-Free Diet Guide for Families*. Children's Digestive Health and Nutrition Foundation and North American Society for Pediatric Gastroenterology, Hepatology, and Nutrition, 2005. Available at www.naspghan.org/user-assets/Documents/pdf/diseaseInfo/GlutenFreeDietGuide-E.pdf; Case S: *Gluten-Free Diet: A Comprehensive Resource Guide*. 4th ed. Case Nutrition Consulting, Inc., 2010, www.glutenfreediet.ca; and Ref. 2.

Stephanie's habits seemed to support her gluten-free lifestyle. When cooking for her family, she was careful to use separate pots, colanders, and utensils if she was making both gluten-free and gluten-containing pasta or grains. She separated her gluten-free flours from the rest of the family's flours, used her own toaster oven, kept a separate stick of butter to avoid other's crumbs, and had her own condiments labeled "for Mom." Stephanie's husband was supportive in reducing any potential for cross-contamination and even carefully cleaned his mouth if he had eaten gluten before kissing her.

But, some clues emerged from their conversation. At home, she occasionally baked gluten-containing muffins or cookies for her family and occasionally forgot to wash her hands. She acknowledged that her youngest son made his sandwiches on the counter, and she frequently found crumbs lying around. Stephanie realized that the salad dressing she had been using for years had changed its ingredients and now contained malt vinegar. Her favorite chocolate bar now also listed a new ingredient, barley malt powder. When dining out, she generally asked appropriate questions, but on occasion she didn't want to draw attention to herself, so she chose dishes that "seemed safe." She learned that cross-contamination is a common concern when shopping from bulk bins, a habit she had recently begun. She and the dietitian also went over other common questions that arise regarding the gluten-free diet (Table 2).

What Stephanie Did

Although it may seem too small to matter, oral contact with minimal amounts of gluten, such as gluten-containing ingredients (malt vinegar, barley malt powder), occasional exposure to uncertain amounts of gluten when dining out, and small amounts of gluten, such as crumbs, qualifies as exposure. Taken together, these issues can be more than enough to cause

TABLE 2. Commonly Asked Questions about Hidden Gluten

What about natural flavors/natural flavoring?

According to Tricia Thompson, author of *The Gluten Free Nutrition Guide,* "For FDA-regulated foods, if a natural flavoring contains protein derived from wheat, the word *wheat* must be stated on the food label. Natural flavoring could be derived from barley; if so, it will most likely be listed as *malt flavoring* on the food label. Natural flavoring could be derived from rye, but products with rye flavoring are likely to be bread products that a person with celiac disease would not eat. For USDA-regulated foods, if a natural flavor contains wheat, barley, or rye proteins, these ingredients will be stated on the food label by their common or usual names. Therefore, if you don't see the words *wheat, barley, rye* or *malt* on the label of a product containing natural flavor, the natural flavor *most likely* does not contain protein derived from these sources."[3]

What about distilled alcohol?

Also according to Ms. Thompson, "Pure spirits (distilled alcohol from fruit, sugar, or grain) are gluten free. While grain alcohol, such as vodka, gin, and whiskey, may be made from gluten-containing grains, the process of distillation prevents any protein from ending up in the final distillate. Some distilled alcoholic beverages, such as cordials and liqueurs, may have flavorings added after distillation. These flavorings are likely to be gluten free, but if you have concerns, contact the manufacturer."[4]

What about body care products?

The gluten protein can only be absorbed orally. It cannot be absorbed through the skin. In addition, even if a gluten-containing ingredient is used in a body care product, it is likely to contain only a very, very small amount of gluten-containing protein. For this reason, people with celiac disease do not need to worry about products applied to the skin (shaving cream, deodorant, makeup, and perfume) or hair (shampoo and conditioner). For a product such as body lotion or sunscreen that stays on the hands, is not washed off, and could travel to the mouth, it makes practical sense to choose a product that contains no gluten. Because you can spit out toothpaste and mouthwash and rinse your mouth with water, it is unlikely that you will consume much of these products, even if they do contain gluten. If a lipstick contains gluten, the minimal estimated amount is still well under the milligrams of gluten considered safe for those with celiac disease.[5] For most people with celiac disease, body care products are not a source of clinically significant gluten exposure. However, some people are highly sensitive to gluten and will react to it even at extremely low levels. If it concerns you, simply research a lipstick or any other body care product that is guaranteed by the manufacturer to be gluten free.

What about food additives?

The following ingredients are gluten free but often listed on packaged seasonings and mixes.
- Dextrose is glucose, a sugar, and so it is gluten free.
- Maltodextrin is a hydrolyzed (broken down) starch that may be made from cornstarch, potato starch, rice starch, or wheat starch.[6] FDA-regulated foods must list wheat on the food label if the maltodextrin used contains protein from wheat. USDA-regulated foods (meat, poultry, and egg products) may contain maltodextrin with protein derived from wheat but this might not be stated on the food label.[7] Even if a food contains maltodextrin derived from wheat, the amount of gluten will be very low. Therefore, maltodextrin is generally accepted as safe on the gluten-free diet.[8]

TABLE 2. Commonly Asked Questions about Hidden Gluten (*Continued*)

- Most vinegars, including distilled vinegar, cider vinegar, wine vinegar, rice vinegar, and balsamic vinegar, are gluten free. Malt vinegar should be avoided on the gluten-free diet because it is made using barley malt, a fermented product. Some flavored vinegars (such as seasoned rice vinegar) may not be gluten free because other ingredients have been added to the product. According to the FDA, the word *vinegar* on a food label indicates that it is made from the juice of apples, either cider vinegar or apple vinegar.[9]
- Whey is a liquid containing lactose, vitamins, protein, minerals, and traces of fat that separates from milk after curdling. Whey is gluten free. Whey protein is commonly sold as a nutritional supplement because it is an easy-to-digest protein source.

an elevated tTG level and abnormal intestinal biopsy. For this reason, it makes sense to read labels carefully, ask questions when dining out, and to wash hands after exposure to gluten that can stay on your hands and migrate to your mouth.

Stephanie started baking only gluten-free foods for her family. On the rare occasion when she needed to bake with gluten-containing flours, she washed her hands carefully, or asked her husband to bake for her. The family received a quick instruction on "crumb control," and now family members make an effort to clean off countertops. She found a new favorite salad dressing and a gluten-free chocolate and avoids the bulk bins when possible. She also adopted safe strategies for eating outside of the home (see Chapter 26 on dining out) and used them consistently. Three months after making the dietary and lifestyle changes to avoid gluten exposure, her IgA-tTG level was within the normal range. Her intestinal symptoms also resolved.

SELF-MANAGEMENT TIPS

☐ For most people with celiac disease who experience occasional or recurrent symptoms, either accidental or intentional gluten exposure is likely to be the cause (see Chapter 34 on nonresponsive celiac disease).

☐ Minimal amounts of gluten exposure "here and there" can add up to an appreciable rise in IgA-tTG levels and mucosal damage in the intestine. It makes sense to strive to be as gluten free as possible.

☐ A dietitian skilled in celiac disease can perform a thorough diet and lifestyle assessment for the many sources of hidden gluten, including medications and supplements.

☐ Dining out and cross-contamination with gluten in the kitchen are two of the most common reasons for gluten exposure. (See Chapter 26 for ways to dine out gluten free.)

- ☐ You can find information about hidden gluten in over-the-counter and prescription pharmaceuticals at www.glutenfreedrugs.com and www.clanthompson.com.
- ☐ Online subscription services and books that provide impressive databases of gluten-free products include Zeer Select (www.zeer.com), www.clanthompson.com, and www.ceceliasmarketplace.com.
- ☐ Because ingredients in foods, medications, and supplements can change at any time, it is important to read labels each time you purchase a product. When in doubt, avoid it until you can confirm that the product is gluten free by contacting the manufacturer.
- ☐ Small intestinal bacterial overgrowth (see Chapter 40) and refractory celiac disease (see Chapter 43) can falsely elevate the IgA-tTG level; consider these problems along with inadvertent gluten exposure if you experience the return of your typical celiac symptoms.

References

1. Leffler DA, Dennis M, Hyett B, Kelly E, Schuppan D, Kelly CP. Etiologies and predictors of diagnosis in nonresponsive celiac disease. *Clin Gastroenterol Hepatol* 2007;5:445–50.
2. Thompson T. *The Gluten Free Nutrition Guide.* New York: McGraw-Hill, 2008.
3. *Ibid.,* p. 201.
4. *Ibid.,* p. 43.
5. Thompson T. Gluten in personal care products: a need to worry? http://www.diet.com/dietblogs/read_blog.php?title=Gluten+In+Personal+Care+Products%3A+A+Need+To+Worry%3F&blid=16557&page=1. Accessed 09/25/09.
6. Thompson T. In *The Gluten Free Nutrition Guide.* New York: McGraw-Hill, 2008, p. 200.
7. U.S. Food and Drug Administration. Maltodextrin. *Code of Federal Regulations,* Title 21. 1 April 2009. www.accessdata.fda.gov/scripts/cdrh/cfdocs/cfcfr/CFRSearch.cfm?fr=184.1444&SearchTerm=maltodextrin. Accessed 02/10/10.
8. European Food Safety Authority. Opinion of the Scientific Panel on Dietetic Products, Nutrition and Allergies on a request from the Commission related to a notification from AAC on wheat-based maltodextrins pursuant to Article 6, paragraph 11 of Directive 2000/13/EC. (Request N∞ EFSA-Q-2006-163). Adopted on 3 May 2007. *The EFSA Journal* 2007;487:1–7. www.efsa.europa.eu/EFSA/Scientific_Opinion/nda_op_ej487_whear_based_maltodextrins_aac_en.pdf.pdf. Accessed 02/10/10.
9. Vinegar. US Food and Drug Administration. CPG Sec. 525.825 Vinegar Definitions—Adulteration with Vinegar Eels. http://www.fda.gov/ICECI/ComplianceManuals/CompliancePolicyGuidanceManual/ucm074471.htm. Accessed 02/10/10.

CHAPTER 21

Oats and Wheat Starch

Tricia Thompson, MS, RD

Mary is a 63-year-old woman who was diagnosed with celiac disease 20 years ago. She came to the clinic for a routine exam with her gastroenterologist. She follows a gluten-free diet (GFD) and has well-controlled celiac disease but no other health issues. During her exam, Mary brought up the issue of whether it was safe for her to eat oats or wheat starch. When she was diagnosed, she was informed that neither product was recommended for GFDs in the United States. But she had been hearing more and more about gluten-free oats and wondered if it really was okay to eat them. Although she wasn't interested in eating foods containing wheat starch, she was curious why wheat starch might now be allowed in a GFD. Mary was referred to a dietitian well versed in celiac disease and eating gluten free to answer her questions.

Defining "Gluten-Free" Foods

The Food and Drug Administration (FDA) has released a proposed rule for the labeling of food as gluten free.[1] As currently written, food will be able to carry a gluten-free label only if all of the following conditions apply:

- The food does not contain as an ingredient the grains wheat, barley, rye, or a crossbred variety of one of these grains.
- The food does not contain an ingredient that is a derivative of one of these grains that has not been processed to remove the protein gluten. Examples of these ingredients include wheat bran, wheat germ, and barley malt. These ingredients contain protein and under normal processing procedures this protein is not removed.
- The food does not contain an ingredient that is a derivative of one of these grains that has been processed to remove gluten if use of the ingredient results in the final food product containing 20 parts per million (ppm) or more gluten. Examples of ingredients that may be allowed in gluten-free foods, depending on their effect on total gluten content, are wheat starch and ingredients that may be made from wheat starch, such as wheat-based dextrin. These ingredients are not intended to contain protein (although small amounts may remain in the starch).
- The food contains less than 20 ppm gluten.

Although the gluten-free labeling rule has not yet been finalized, many U.S. manufacturers of specially produced gluten-free foods are already testing their products for gluten to make sure they are in compliance with the proposed rule. Gluten-free labeling is voluntary, but once the labeling rule is finalized, manufacturers who choose to label their products gluten free will have to be in compliance.

Gluten-Free Oats

According to the American Dietetic Association's (ADA) *Evidence Based Nutrition Practice Guidelines,* it is generally safe for those on a GFD to eat approximately 50 g of dry oats per day as long as they are not contaminated with wheat, barley, or rye, and having this option improves an individual's ability to stay on the GFD.[2] According to the ADA, the addition of oats to a GFD should be done under the supervision of a physician or dietitian. Under the FDA's proposed rule for gluten-free labeling, oats would be allowed to carry a gluten-free label as long as they contain less than 20 ppm gluten.[1]

If you want to include oats in your GFD, it is exceedingly important that they are labeled gluten free. Most oats that you find on grocery store shelves are contaminated with wheat, barley, and/or rye.[3] Contamination can occur while oats are being harvested because of crop rotation, when they are transported because of the use of railcars that may contain foreign grain from a prior load, or when they are processed because of the use of shared processing equipment.[4]

Currently, there are five major producers of gluten-free oats in North America:

- Bob's Red Mill (www.bobsredmill.com)
- Cream Hill Estates (www.creamhillestates.com)
- Gifts of Nature (www.giftsofnature.net)
- Gluten-Free Oats (www.glutenfreeoats.com)
- Only Oats (www.onlyoats.com)

These companies produce gluten-free oats by very carefully monitoring the growing, harvesting, and processing procedures. Many other manufacturers use gluten-free oats in their processed food products. (For more information, see "Oats and Gluten-Free Labeling," page 164.)

Gluten-Free Wheat Starch and Wheat Starch Products

Some gluten-free foods manufactured in Europe contain wheat starch that has been purified to remove almost all gluten.[5] These products are aptly called *wheat starch–based gluten-free foods.* According to the ADA, people with celiac disease who include wheat starch-based gluten-free foods in their GFD show similar recovery of their symptoms and intestinal health as those who eat only naturally gluten-free foods.[6]

Despite this, there has been a lot of controversy surrounding wheat starch and its use in GFDs. This controversy is less about the actual use of wheat starch and more about the level of gluten it contains. Wheat starch contains small amounts of gluten, with the actual amount varying depending on the quality of wheat starch. We now know that it is possible to make wheat starch–based gluten-free products that contain less than 20 ppm gluten.[4] Once the FDA gluten-free labeling rule becomes law, wheat starch–based gluten-free foods, when sold in the United States, will have to contain less than 20 ppm gluten to be sold as gluten free.[1] If you want to include wheat starch and products that contain wheat starch in your GFD, it is very important to find those that are labeled gluten free.

What Mary Decided

After meeting with the dietitian, Mary decided to try adding gluten-free oats to her diet in the form of oatmeal. She was advised not to eat more than ½ cup dry rolled oats or ¼ cup dry steel-cut oats each day. Mary also was advised that a very small percentage of individuals with celiac disease cannot tolerate oats even if they are labeled gluten free.[2,6,7] Individuals who cannot tolerate oats may have an immune response to a protein in oats called *avenin*. This immune response may cause intestinal damage.

Mary was advised to closely monitor any new gastrointestinal symptoms, such as diarrhea and stomach discomfort, although these could be symptoms related to increasing her fiber intake and not necessarily indicative of an inability to tolerate oats.[2] Mary also agreed to a follow-up appointment with her dietitian in three months to assess how she was doing with the addition of oats to her diet.

Mary thought that she probably would avoid wheat starch and wheat starch–containing products. She had come to enjoy many of the gluten-free whole grains, such as amaranth, buckwheat, quinoa, wild rice, millet, teff, and sorghum, and didn't feel the need to add wheat starch to her diet. Mary's dietitian reminded her that she would be able to avoid products that are labeled gluten free but contain wheat starch by reading the ingredients list or "Contains" statement and looking for the word *wheat*.[8]

Outcome

Three months later, Mary returned to the dietitian and explained that she had successfully added oats to her diet without experiencing any gastrointestinal symptoms. She was thrilled to be able to eat oatmeal again after 20 years.

SELF-MANAGEMENT TIPS

- ☐ It is very important to talk with your physician or dietitian before adding oats to your GFD and have their supervision while adding oats.
- ☐ Only oats and oat products labeled gluten free (or labeled pure and uncontaminated in Canada) are safe. Oats and oat products not labeled gluten free are likely contaminated with wheat, barley, or rye.

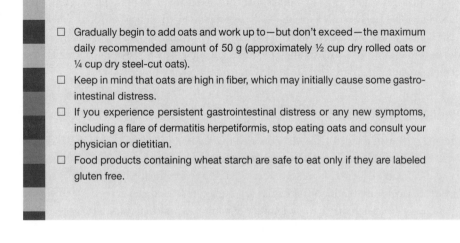

- ☐ Gradually begin to add oats and work up to—but don't exceed—the maximum daily recommended amount of 50 g (approximately ½ cup dry rolled oats or ¼ cup dry steel-cut oats).
- ☐ Keep in mind that oats are high in fiber, which may initially cause some gastrointestinal distress.
- ☐ If you experience persistent gastrointestinal distress or any new symptoms, including a flare of dermatitis herpetiformis, stop eating oats and consult your physician or dietitian.
- ☐ Food products containing wheat starch are safe to eat only if they are labeled gluten free.

References

1. Food and Drug Administration: Gluten-Free Labeling of Foods. Proposed Rule. 21 CFR Part 101, Docket No. 2005N-0279. Federal Register 72(14) (January 23, 2007). http://vm.cfsan.fda.gov/~lrd/fr070123.html.
2. American Dietetic Association. Evidence-based Nutrition Practice Guideline on Celiac Disease. May 2009 http://ada.portalxm.com/eal/topic.cfm?cat=3677&library=EBG.
3. Thompson T. Gluten contamination of commercial oat products in the United States. *N Engl J Med* 2004;351:202–22.
4. Thompson T. *The Gluten-Free Nutrition Guide*. New York: McGraw-Hill, 2008.
5. Codex Alimentarius, www.codexalimentarius.net.
6. American Dietetic Association. Celiac Disease Evidence Analysis Project. http://www.ada evidencelibrary.com/topic.cfm?cat=1403.
7. Arentz-Hansen H, Fleckenstein B, Milberg O, et al. The molecular basis for oat intolerance in patients with celiac disease. *PLoS Med* 2004;1(1):e1.
8. Food and Drug Administration. Food Allergen Labeling and Consumer Protection Act. http://www.fda.gov/Food/LabelingNutrition/FoodAllergensLabeling/GuidanceCompliance RegulatoryInformation/ucm106187.htm.

Tricia Thompson, MS, RD, is an internationally recognized expert on celiac disease and the gluten-free diet (www.glutenfreedietitian.com). She is a consultant, researcher, writer, and author of *The Gluten-Free Nutrition Guide, The Complete Idiot's Guide to Gluten-Free Eating, Celiac Disease Nutrition Guide,* and *American Dietetic Association's Easy Gluten-Free: Expert Advice on Nutrition and More Than 100 Recipes.*

CHAPTER 22

Food Labeling in the United States and Canada

Tricia Thompson, MS, RD, and Shelley Case, RD

aitlin is 23 years old and recently diagnosed with celiac disease. She lives and works in the United States but has extended family in Canada and frequently travels "home" to visit. Caitlin has a lot of questions regarding food labels and whether there are any differences in labeling laws between the two countries that would impact her food choices. She also is concerned about how she will keep all the information straight between the United States and Canada. Her gastroenterologist referred her to a dietitian with expertise in celiac disease. Here is what she learned.

Food Labeling in the United States

All food sold in the United States, regardless of where it is made, including Canada, must comply with current U.S. labeling laws. The information on food labeling in Canada given below applies to products purchased in Canada only.

The FDA regulates all foods with the exception of meat products (such as hot dogs and deli meats), poultry products (such as seasoned chicken breasts), egg products (meaning eggs removed from their shells), and mixed food products that contain more than 3% raw meat or 2% or more cooked meat or poultry. These foods all are regulated by the United States Department of Agriculture (USDA).

Allergen Labeling

The FDA Food Allergen Labeling and Consumer Protection Act (FALCPA) applies to the ingredients in packaged foods, which are defined as conventional foods such as much of the foods in grocery stores; prepackaged foods for sale in retail locations such as delis, restaurants, and supermarkets; medical foods; dietary supplements; and infant formulas. If an ingredient in a packaged food regulated by the FDA contains protein from one of eight major allergens, this must be clearly stated on the food label. Wheat, but not barley or rye, is among these eight allergens (the others are milk, egg, fish, crustacean, shellfish, tree nuts, peanuts, and soybeans). If an ingredient in a food product is wheat or contains protein from wheat, the word "wheat" will be clearly stated in the ingredients list, for instance, "modified food starch (wheat)," or in the "Contains" statement that appears immediately after the ingredients list, for instance, "Contains wheat."

The USDA is considering rulemaking for allergen labeling of USDA-regulated food similar to the FALCPA. Presently, allergen labeling of USDA-regulated food products is voluntary. Nonetheless, the USDA says they have widespread voluntary compliance.

Gluten-Free Labeling

In 2007, the FDA released a proposed rule for the voluntary labeling of food products as gluten free. The rule has not yet been finalized but should be released sometime in 2010, when it will become law. Under the proposed rule, a food may be labeled gluten free only if all of the following apply:

- The food does not contain as an ingredient the grains wheat, barley, rye, or a crossbred variety of one of these grains.
- The food does not contain an ingredient that is a derivative of one of these grains that has not been processed to remove the protein gluten. Examples of these ingredients include wheat bran, wheat germ, and barley malt. These ingredients contain protein and under normal processing procedures this protein is not removed.
- The food does not contain an ingredient that is a derivative of one of these grains that has been processed to remove gluten if use of the ingredient results in the final food product containing 20 parts per million (ppm) or more gluten. Examples of ingredients that may be allowed in gluten-free foods, depending on their effect on total gluten content, are wheat starch and ingredients that may be made from wheat starch, such as wheat-based dextrin. These ingredients are not intended to contain protein (although small amounts may remain in the starch).
- The food contains less than 20 ppm gluten.

The bottom line is that there are certain ingredients that may not be included in a food labeled gluten free. These ingredients include wheat, barley, rye, and crossbred varieties of these grains as well as protein containing derivatives of these grains, such as wheat bran, wheat germ, and barley malt. All of these ingredients contain the protein gluten and are not processed in a way that removes protein. Other ingredients, such as wheat starch, are not intended to contain protein (although they may contain trace amounts) and may be included in a food labeled gluten free as long as the final food product contains less than 20 ppm gluten.

Although the gluten-free labeling rule has not yet been finalized, many (if not most) U.S. manufacturers of specially produced gluten-free foods are already testing their products for gluten to make sure they are in compliance with the proposed rule. Gluten-free labeling is voluntary, but if a manufacturer chooses to label a product as gluten free, it will have to comply with the labeling rule once it is finalized. It is likely that the USDA will adopt the FDA's rule for labeling of food as gluten free once it has been finalized.

Alcohol Labeling

In 2006, the Alcohol and Tobacco Tax Bureau, Treasury (TTB) posted a notice in the Federal Register regarding proposed rulemaking for mandatory allergen labeling of wines, distilled spirits, and malt beverages. The proposed regulation closely follows the FALCPA and states that all major food allergens used in the production of wine, distilled spirits, and malt beverages, including food allergens used as fining agents (used to remove substances that cause cloudiness in wine) or processing agents, must be declared on the label. Included among the major food allergens is wheat but not barley or rye. Because alcohol containers generally do not include an ingredients list, allergens will be declared in a "Contains" statement.

Wine and pure distilled spirits are considered gluten free. Fermented beverages, such as beer, porter, stout, and ale, are not gluten free unless specially processed to be gluten free because they are made using gluten-containing grains.

Reading U.S. Food Labels

FDA-Regulated Foods

When reading the ingredients list and the "Contains" statement to determine whether a food product includes any gluten-containing ingredients, you are looking for the words *wheat*, *barley*, *rye*, *oats* (unless gluten free), *malt*, and *brewer's yeast*.

- Unless otherwise stated on the food label, malt is made from barley.
- Brewer's yeast may be a by-product of the beer brewing process and, as such, may be contaminated with malt and grain.
- Rye and barley may be used as flavoring agents. Rye-based flavoring most likely will be listed as "rye flavoring" on the food label, and barley-based flavoring likely will be listed on the food label as a malt ingredient.

USDA-Regulated Foods

Compared to FDA-regulated foods, reading the ingredients list for USDA-regulated foods is a bit trickier because of the lack of mandatory allergen labeling. For USDA-regulated foods all ingredients must be listed by their "common or usual name." Unfortunately, the common or usual name of an ingredient does not always indicate its source. As with FDA-regulated foods, you are looking for the words *wheat, barley, rye, oats* (unless gluten-free), *malt*, and *brewer's yeast*. In addition, you also are looking for modified food starch and dextrin, both of which may contain wheat protein but not necessarily state this on the food label. It also is important to familiarize yourself with words that mean wheat if used on the label of a USDA-regulated food, including durum flour, enriched flour, farina, graham flour, plain flour, self-rising flour, semolina, and white flour.

In addition to brewer's yeast, you also may come across a few ingredients that occasionally may contain barley protein but don't state this on the food label. These ingredients are brown rice syrup and smoke flavoring. Brown rice syrup may be processed with some form of barley, such as barley enzymes, but it is unclear whether these enzymes sometimes contain residual barley gluten. Some dry smoke flavoring may use malted barley flour as a carrier for the smoke. If this ingredient is in a meat or poultry product (regulated by the USDA), any barley ingredient used in the smoke flavoring will be listed in the ingredients list by its common or usual name. If this ingredient is used in an FDA-regulated food, component ingredients (called *subingredients* of an ingredient) may or may not be included.

Important Points to Remember about U.S. Food Labels
- Allergen labeling of FDA-regulated foods is *mandatory* and applies to *ingredients* only. It does not apply to allergens that may be in a food because of cross-contamination.
- Allergen labeling of USDA-regulated foods is *voluntary.* All ingredients must be listed by their common or usual name, which does not always indicate the source of the ingredient (dextrin, for example, can be made from many starches, including wheat, corn, and rice).
- Allergen advisory statements related to food processing, such as "processed in a facility that also processes wheat" are voluntary and unregulated.
- Gluten-free labeling is voluntary. Once the FDA rule is finalized, it will apply to gluten that may be in a food because of the ingredients and/or because of cross-contamination with a gluten-containing grain. Once final, the rules for gluten-free labeling will likely apply to both FDA- and USDA-regulated food.

Food Labeling in Canada

All food sold in Canada, regardless of where it is made, including the United States, must comply with current Canadian labeling laws. The section above on food labeling in the United States applies only to products sold in the United States.

Health Canada (HC) and the Canadian Food Inspection Agency (CFIA) are responsible for the regulation of all foods including meat, poultry, and egg products. Policies and standards relating to the safety and nutritional quality of foods are established by HC. The CFIA develops regulations and policies related to food labeling and quality and composition standards. In addition, they are also responsible for food inspection, compliance, and enforcement activities.

Allergen Labeling
Canada's *Food and Drug Regulations* (FDR) require a complete list of ingredients on the label of most packaged foods. However, some ingredients used in food products such as seasonings, flavors, hydrolyzed plant/vegetable proteins, starches, and modified food starches do not require a declaration of their components (subingredients) or the source of the specific ingredient. For example, when seasonings are used in a food product, the components of

the seasoning, such as wheat starch or wheat flour, are not required to be listed on the label. Modified food starch or hydrolyzed protein could be derived from wheat but the plant source may not be declared. Also, the name of some ingredients may not be recognized as an allergen or gluten source (such as casein, a type of milk protein, or semolina, which is coarsely ground wheat kernels). These labeling exemptions make it difficult for consumers to identify allergens and gluten sources.

HC recognized these difficulties for consumers with food allergies and celiac disease and proposed changes to the FDR. Until these proposed regulations become law, manufacturers are strongly encouraged by HC and the CFIA to declare on the food label the major food allergens, gluten sources, and sulfites when added as ingredients or subingredients. Many food manufacturers are doing this voluntarily.

The proposed labeling regulations regarding allergens and gluten will apply to food products that *do not* make a gluten-free claim. Therefore, these regulations are different from the gluten-free labeling regulation that has been in effect for more than 24 years (see below). Highlights of the proposed regulations are:

- If an ingredient or component of an ingredient in a food product contains any protein, modified protein, or protein fraction that is derived from the following allergens or gluten sources, it must be declared on the food label.
    - ☐ Food allergens: nuts, peanuts, sesame seeds, wheat, kamut, spelt, triticale, eggs, milk, soybeans, crustaceans, shellfish, fish, or mustard
    - ☐ Gluten: barley, oats, rye, triticale, wheat, kamut, or spelt
- The plant source of a starch, modified food starch, or hydrolyzed protein must be named (for instance, wheat starch, modified wheat starch, or hydrolyzed wheat protein). If wheat flour or wheat starch is used in a seasoning blend in a food product, it must be listed.
- Food allergens and gluten sources in alcoholic beverages (including wine and beer) and vinegars must also be declared.
- The allergen or gluten source can be declared in the list of ingredients or in the "Contains" statement.
- There are some foods where the common or usual name of an ingredient (such as semolina, durum, graham flour, spelt, kamut, or couscous) may not identify the presence of the allergen or gluten source. The new regulation will require the declaration of the allergen or gluten source either in the list of ingredients after the name, such as semolina (wheat), or in the "Contains" statement.

Once the allergen labeling law is passed, there will be some prepackaged products that will continue to be exempt from ingredient declaration. These include:

- Individual portions of foods served by a restaurant or other food-service establishments such as cafeterias and coffee shops

- Individual servings of food sold in vending machines or mobile canteens
- Products packaged from bulk in retail premises, such as small bags of rice flour in a health food store
- Meat, poultry, meat by-products, and poultry by-products that are barbecued, roasted, or broiled in the store, such as rotisserie chicken

Gluten-Free Labeling

The FDR regulations include a specific rule for the labeling and advertising of food products using the term *gluten free* that has been in effect since 1995. These products cannot contain wheat (including spelt and kamut), oats, barley, rye, or triticale or any part thereof.

The CFIA monitors various labeling claims, including the gluten-free claim. If a product making a gluten-free claim is determined to contain gluten or to have been cross-contaminated with gluten, the product may be subject to further investigation. Products found to contain gluten at levels of 20 ppm or higher will undergo a health risk assessment and enforcement actions, including recall, may result.

Oats and Gluten-Free Labeling

Celiac Disease and the Safety of Oats: Health Canada's Position on the Introduction of Oats to the Diet of Individuals Diagnosed with Celiac Disease was published in 2007. They conclude that "the safety/benefit evaluation for the introduction of oats in the gluten-free diet of patients with celiac disease indicates that moderate amounts of pure oats are well tolerated by most individuals with celiac disease and dermatitis herpetiformis. The term *pure oats* is used to indicate oats uncontaminated with gluten from other closely related cereal grains, including wheat, barley, and rye as detected using current test methods. Based on clinical trials in the published literature, the amount of pure oats considered within safe limits is 50–70 grams per day for adults and 20–25 grams per day for children."

Although HC has published this position on the safety of oats, the existing gluten-free regulation includes oats in the list of prohibited grains. Therefore, pure, uncontaminated oats can only be labeled wheat free and not gluten free at this time. To help clarify this issue, and with the approval of HC, some companies also specify on the label that there is no cross-contamination and/or no wheat, barley, or rye has been detected using current testing methods. The gluten-free regulation and the issues of labeling of pure, uncontaminated oats are currently being reviewed by HC.

The Canadian Celiac Association (CCA) has a position statement on oats and supports the use of pure, uncontaminated oats in moderate amounts (same as HC) for individuals with celiac disease once they are stabilized on a gluten-free diet. Because pure, uncontaminated oats cannot be labeled gluten-free at this time, the CCA has developed a trademark called *Pavena* to assist consumers in the identification of these special oats. Manufacturers can apply to the CCA to use the Pavena trademark after meeting specific criteria that includes third party audit to ensure that CCA's standards are met.

Reading Canadian Food Labels

Because the proposed food allergen labeling regulations are not yet mandatory, there are products where gluten is present but may not be declared or obvious. When reading the ingredients list to determine whether a food includes any gluten-containing ingredients, look for any of the following words:

- wheat, bulgur, durum, einkorn, emmer, faro, kamut, semolina, spelt, couscous, graham flour, atta, fu, seitan
- hydrolyzed protein (if it lists only hydrolyzed plant or vegetable protein, call the manufacturer to determine the source)
- modified starch, starch, and dextrin (call the manufacturer to determine the source)
- rye, triticale
- barley, malt, malt vinegar
- beer, ale, lager (these are made from barley); gluten-free beers on the market made from grains not containing gluten, such as sorghum, rice, or buckwheat, are acceptable
- brewer's yeast
- oats (unless pure and uncontaminated and/or Pavena trademark is on the label)

Important Points to Remember about Canadian Food Labels
- The proposed regulations do not apply to allergens and gluten sources that may be present in a food as a result of cross-contamination, which is why a "may contain" or other precautionary statements such as "made in a facility that also processes wheat" can be found on the label of some products. HC is reviewing precautionary statements and developing guidelines for their use.
- The gluten-free regulation was developed more than 25 years ago and prohibits oats in products labeled gluten free. HC is currently reviewing the labeling of pure, uncontaminated oats and the gluten-free regulation. Until changes are made, products with pure, uncontaminated oats can only be labeled as wheat free. In contrast, companies can label these same products sold in the United States as gluten free (see Chapter 21 on oats and wheat starch).
- Gluten-free labeling is voluntary. It applies to gluten that may be in a food because of the ingredients and/or cross-contamination with a gluten-containing grain.

What Caitlin Decided

To help minimize her confusion, Caitlin decided to focus first on learning how to read U.S. food labels with help from her dietitian. She is going to visit family in Canada in three months, so she plans to contact the CCA (www.celiac.ca) for more information about Canadian food regulations one month before she goes home to visit. In addition, she will ask the CCA for practical resources, such as www.celiacguide.org, as well as contact names of local dietitians and celiac group members for further information and local shopping and restaurant options.

Further Reading

- Case S. *Gluten-Free Diet: A Comprehensive Resource Guide.* 4th ed. Case Nutrition Consulting, Inc., 2010, www.glutenfreediet.ca.
- Thompson T. *The Gluten-Free Nutrition Guide.* New York: McGraw-Hill, 2008.
- Canadian Celiac Association. *Pocket Dictionary: Acceptability of Foods & Food Ingredients for the Gluten-Free Diet.* 2009. www.celiacguide.org.
- Food and Drug Administration, Food Allergen Labeling and Consumer Protection Act of 2004 (Title ll of Public Law 108-282). http://www.fda.gov/Food/Labeling Nutrition/FoodAllergensLabeling/GuidanceCompliance RegulatoryInformation/ ucm106187.htm.
- Food and Drug Administration: Gluten-Free Labeling of Foods. Proposed Rule. 21 CFR Part 101, Docket No. 2005N-0279. Federal Register 72(14) (January 23, 2007). http://vm.cfsan.fda.gov/~lrd/fr070123.html.
- United States Department of Agriculture, Food Safety and Inspection Service. Questions and Answers Related to Ingredients of Public Health Concern. http://www.fsis. usda.gov/regulations_&_policihes/FAQs_for_Notice_45-05/index.asp.
- Department of the Treasury. Alcohol and Tobacco Tax, and Trade Bureau. Major Food Allergen Labeling for Wines, Distilled Spirits, and Malt Beverages. 27 CFR Parts 4, 5, and 7. http://edocket.access.gpo.gov/2006/pdf/06-6467.pdf.
- Health Canada's Proposed Amendments "Enhanced Labelling for Food Allergen and Gluten Sources and Added Sulphites." *Canada Gazette.* http://www.gazette.gc.ca/ rp-pr/p1/2008/2008-07-26/html/reg1-eng.html.

- Health Canada Reviews Comments Received on Regulatory Project 1220—Enhanced Labelling for Food Allergens and Gluten Sources and Added Sulphites. http://www.hc-sc.gc.ca/fn-an/label-etiquet/allergen/sum-comm-exa-eng.php.
- Health Canada's Food and Drug Regulations, B.24.018 and B.24.019 Gluten-Free Labeling. http://laws.justice.gc.ca/en/showtdm/cr/C.R.C.-c.870. http://www.hc-sc.gc.ca/fn-an/legislation/acts-lois/index-eng.php.
- Celiac Disease and the Safety of Oats: Health Canada's Position on the Introduction of Oats to the Diet of Individuals Diagnosed with Celiac Disease. http://www.hc-sc.gc.ca/fn-an/securit/allerg/cel-coe/oats_cd-avoine-eng.php.
- Canadian Celiac Association Position Statement and Guidelines for Use of Pure, Uncontaminated Oats and Pavena trademark. http://www.celiac.ca/Articles/PABoats.html. http://www.celiac.ca/Articles/PABoatsguidelines 2007June.html.

Tricia Thompson, MS, RD, is an internationally recognized expert on celiac disease and the gluten-free diet (www.glutenfreedietitian.com). She is a consultant, researcher, writer, and author of the *Gluten-Free Nutrition Guide, The Complete Idiot's Guide to Gluten-Free Eating, Celiac Disease Nutrition Guide,* and *American Dietetic Association's Easy Gluten-Free: Expert Advice on Nutrition and More Than 100 Recipes.* **Shelley Case, RD,** is a leading international expert on celiac disease and the gluten-free diet (http://www.glutenfreediet.ca). She is a member of the Medical Advisory Boards of the Celiac Disease Foundation and Gluten Intolerance Group in the United States and the Professional Advisory Board of the Canadian Celiac Association. A popular speaker, consultant, and writer, Shelley is also author of the best seller *Gluten-Free Diet: A Comprehensive Resource Guide.*

CHAPTER 23

Gluten in Medications and Supplements

Steven Plogsted, RPh, PharmD, BCNSP, and Julie Edmonds, RPh

JoAnne, a 42-year-old marketing director, visited her endocrinologist as part of her usual diabetes follow-up care two years ago. She had begun to experience some mild symptoms typical of celiac disease, such as gastrointestinal upset and bloating, along with unexplained low blood glucose (hypoglycemia). People like JoAnne who have type 1 diabetes are at an increased risk of developing celiac disease, which often occurs years after the diabetes diagnosis. JoAnne's immunoglobulin A tissue transglutaminase (IgA-tTG) antibody level was elevated, and a small intestinal biopsy by endoscopy showed damage to the villi in four separate locations, which confirmed her diagnosis of celiac disease.

JoAnne met with her dietitian to discuss a gluten-free diet (GFD). Joanne was vigilant about following her diabetes care regimen and began the GFD with the same dedication. She has a rigorous work schedule and was determined to stay in the best possible health to meet the demands of her career. As expected, JoAnne's celiac disease symptoms resolved within a number of months, and her IgA-tTG level fell to within normal limits over the course of the first year.

However, JoAnne's celiac disease symptoms returned. She reported that she had frequent bloating and gas pains and felt much more fatigued than normal. Her physician tested her IgA-tTG level again, and it was elevated. Her physician and dietitian wondered whether JoAnne had made changes in her GFD because the blood test indicated that she had ingested gluten. JoAnne assured them that she had not faltered on her diet. She is extremely conscious of product labeling and only eats at restaurants that serve gluten-free choices.

JoAnne had recently been prescribed a medication for high blood pressure. She said she had remembered reading that some drugs may contain gluten and wondered if this could be the cause of her relapse. A pharmacist was consulted to determine the components of her prescription.

How Gluten Gets into Medications

It's possible that the new medication was the source of JoAnne's gluten intake. There is always the potential to have gluten-related components in any medication, whether it's prescription, over-the-counter, or a nutritional supplement.

Oral prescription medications are created using several types of substances. These include the active ingredient and inactive ingredients, which are the excipients, the capsule or tablet shell, and a coating. Excipients are pharmacologically inactive substances that add bulk, control the absorption rate of the active ingredient, and sometimes provide protection from stomach upset. They are also added to give an attractive look to the product. The major concern for people with celiac disease surrounds which excipients are used in the medication. These inactive ingredients can be derived from whole grains, grain flour, and grain starch. Unspecified starch, pregelatinized starch, dusting powder, flour, and gluten may be derived from wheat. Prescription medications containing these items pose the highest risk of containing gluten. Another starch derivative is sodium starch glycolate, which is made from potato predominantly, but may also be made from corn, wheat, or rice.

Even if the word "starch" is not listed in the drug product, there can be hidden sources. Other excipients derived from starch that are used in pharmaceutical manufacturing are dextrins, dextrates, maltodextrin, dextrimaltose, and maltose. Dextrates are obtained by enzymatic hydrolysis of any starch, whereas dextrins are obtained by hydrolysis of corn or potato. Although maltodextrin can be obtained from any starch source, it is usually derived from corn in the United States. Maltose is manufactured similarly to the dextrates and can be obtained from any starch source, and dextrimaltose is a mixture of maltose and dextrin obtained by an enzymatic reaction involving barley malt.

In addition to the inclusion of excipients derived from wheat as a source of contamination, at least one drug company has painted the outside of one of their products with a wheat-based coating.

Some ingredients are processed so that they are free of gluten and, therefore, are safe for people with celiac disease. For example, if an alcohol (a typical drug excipient) is derived from wheat, it can be purified so that no gluten remains. However, additives in medications may become cross-contaminated with gluten during manufacturing even when they contain no gluten to start. This is similar to the concept of oats in a celiac diet. Oats are considered naturally gluten free, yet the growing or milling process allows the oats to be contaminated by wheat or other gluten-containing substances.

The FDA has strict regulations for the *active* ingredient of a preparation. All inactive ingredients (excipients) are reviewed as part of the chemistry review of a medication. The excipients must be FDA approved, but the type and amounts are not regulated. In fact, the drug manufacturer can change the excipients without needing to relabel the product. Generic medications must contain the exact amount of active ingredient, but the excipients can vary. At present, the FDA does not require labeling for gluten content or warnings for celiac disease.

What Gluten Free Really Means

For *food* products, the FDA has proposed that to be labeled gluten free, the product must contain less than 20 parts per million or 20 mg per 2.2 pounds of product. It is an important fact that people with celiac disease show a wide variability in the amount of gluten they can tolerate. This can range from having practically no tolerance (10 mg daily at most) to rare individuals who can tolerate up to 5 g per day. Because the damage to the gastrointestinal tract caused by gluten is cumulative and the long-term effects of repeated gluten exposure are unknown, everyone with celiac disease needs to avoid gluten to the best of his or her ability.

What Drug Manufacturers Can Tell Us

Drug manufacturers were surveyed in 2001 and asked to report on the gluten-containing pharmaceuticals they produce. Only 5 of the 100 survey respondents guaranteed the gluten-free status of their products. Other drug manufacturers *believed* their pharmaceuticals to be gluten free, stating that no wheat, oats, rye, barley, or spelt sources were used. But they were unwilling to guarantee that this was the case because the producers of their raw materials could not confirm that what they supplied was gluten free.

Drug manufacturers are also capable of providing misleading or false information. As explained above, some excipients, even if extracted from a wheat source, can be purified to remove all of the proteins responsible for the gluten reaction. This is the case with the excipients mannitol and xylitol. Both of these excipients are sugar alcohols that can be extracted from many sources, including wheat. At least one manufacturer is telling people that a certain number of their products contain gluten because they use one of these excipients. This would confuse anyone trying to get a clear answer. Ideally, the manufacturer would know the source and purification process for each excipient it uses to help the consumer make the right choice. Unfortunately, this is often not the case because there is no federal mandate to do so.

What JoAnne Did

Because JoAnne's high blood pressure medication clearly could be supplying her with gluten, she consulted the pharmacist. Her pharmacist checked the medication's package insert and then confirmed the fact that the medication had gluten by calling the drug company.

Occasionally, the drug company is not able to answer the question firmly. But because pharmacists know the possible excipients contained in a medication and their typical sources, they can guide you about whether to use it or can name alternative gluten-free formulations. Because her medication contained gluten, JoAnne's pharmacist consulted with her physician, who recommended a different medication. Another option would be to consult with the International Academy of Compounding Pharmacists (www.iacprx.org) to locate a pharmacist who compounds specialty medications. The pharmacy can make medications with the same active ingredient but omit excipients with gluten.

In the future, JoAnne will consult these Web sites about the gluten content of her medications and supplements, in addition to speaking with her pharmacist:

- www.glutenfreedrugs.com
- www.celiacmeds.com
- www.clanthompson.com
- www.stokesrx.com
- http://homepage.mac.com/sholland/celiac/GFmedlist.pdf

SELF-MANAGEMENT TIPS

☐ Any relapse in celiac symptoms should trigger an investigation of all changes in your diet, medications, and supplements. Even if you are not having symptoms from low-level gluten exposure, such as in medications, it is still recommended that you avoid all gluten sources.

☐ Thoroughly evaluate each new medication you are taking. This includes prescriptions, over-the-counter medications, and nutrition products. Start by checking the Web sites listed above for information.

☐ Consult your pharmacist for assistance in evaluating the excipients in your medications. Although a drug company may not state that its products are gluten free, the pharmacist can ascertain if the excipients used are safe.

☐ Medication formulations of inactive ingredients may change. It is important to check your medication's excipient list with each new prescription or refill for changes and possible addition of gluten additives, especially if the shape, size, or color of the product changes.

☐ Regulations that apply to food manufacturing do not necessarily apply to pharmaceutical manufacturing. Drug manufacturers are not required to disclose whether an excipient is obtained from one of the top eight allergens as is required by the food labeling law.

Further Reading

- Plogsted S. Medications and celiac disease: tips from a pharmacist. *Pract Gastroenterol* 2007;XXXI(1):58–64.
- Crowe JP, Filini NP. Gluten in pharmaceutical products. *Am J Health Syst Pharm* 2001; 58(5):396–401.

- King AR. The impact of celiac sprue on patient's medications choices. *Hosp Pharm* 2009;44(2):105–106.
- Gluten-free drugs for celiac disease patients. *The Medical Letter* 2008;50(1281):19–20.
- Colin P, Thorell L, Kaukinen K, et al. The safe threshold for gluten contamination in gluten-free products: can trace amounts be accepted in the treatment of coeliac disease. *Aliment Pharmacol Ther* 2004;19:1277–83.
- Pfizer U.S. Medical Information. June 1, 2009.

Steven Plogsted, RPh, PharmD, BCNSP, is a Clinical Pharmacy Specialist with the Nutrition Support Service at Nationwide Childrens Hospital, Columbus, Ohio. **Julie Edmonds, RPh,** is a doctoral candidate at The Ohio State University College of Pharmacy and Director of Pharmacy, University Optioncare, LLC, Columbus, Ohio.

CHAPTER 24

Combining Diets for Diabetes and Celiac Disease

Cynthia Kupper, RD, CD

Shy and just eight years old, Sarah was diagnosed with type 1 diabetes six months ago. She and her family were instructed on how to use carbohydrate counting to match her insulin needs and were given a carbohydrate meal plan. At that time they were encouraged to include more whole grains and fresh fruits and vegetables to increase the fiber in her diet. The family attended diabetes education classes and learned blood glucose monitoring, insulin injections, and other aspects of diabetes control. Sarah has strong family support from both parents and initially did well controlling her blood glucose level.

Three months ago, Sarah's blood glucose levels became erratic. Although her hemoglobin A_{1C}, a measure of long-term glucose control, was 7.1 mg/dl (normal is 7 mg/dl or less), she began to have frequent low blood glucose reactions (hypoglycemia). She experienced symptoms of failure to thrive, including weight loss, and abdominal pain and diarrhea. She also began restricting her food choices to just a handful of foods. Sarah and her family met with the diabetes care team to review their diabetes care program. Sarah was put on an insulin pump. Sarah was also sent for celiac screening, which revealed a positive result for immunoglobulin A tissue transglutaminase (IgA-tTG). She then had a small intestine biopsy, which confirmed her celiac disease.

I met Sarah and her family a month after her diagnosis of celiac disease to assist with her adjustment to a gluten-free diabetes lifestyle. Sarah had, by her own choice, begun restricting what she ate to 10 foods, avoiding all whole grains, fresh fruits, vegetables, foods with fiber, and many protein foods. Her preferred foods were eggs, juice, milk, gummy worms, cola, peanut butter, Jell-O, yogurt, chicken, and occasionally a hamburger patty. Sarah's parents said she was not normally a picky eater but increasingly over the past year she would not eat many of the foods she used to love, such as pizza, hamburgers, and pasta. Her diet did not meet her needs for vitamins and minerals and was lacking in total calories to sustain normal weight and growth.

What Celiac Disease and Diabetes Have in Common

Celiac disease and type 1 diabetes share common HLA-DQ2 genetic alleles (markers). Associated with the -DQ2 marker is also -DR3, a known genetic marker for type 1 diabetes. Individuals with a genetic predisposition for celiac disease have genetic markers HLA-DQ2 and/or HLA-DQ8. If they carry the -DQ2 marker, they are more susceptible to developing type 1 diabetes. Studies have shown that people with type 1 diabetes have a 5–10% increased incidence of also developing celiac disease.

The two diseases also share symptoms. Uncontrolled celiac disease and diabetes complications both can include bloating, nausea, vomiting, and diarrhea. These symptoms can affect blood glucose control and can mimic uncontrolled diabetes or gastroparesis, a well-known complication of diabetes in which the stomach and bowels are slow to empty. For this reason, some diabetes programs screen those diagnosed with type 1 diabetes for celiac disease.

How Celiac Disease Can Affect Blood Glucose Control

Carbohydrate in food is broken down to become glucose, the body's favorite fuel. During digestion, the glucose moves from the intestines into the bloodstream so it can travel around the body to all the cells. Insulin allows the glucose to get out of the bloodstream and into the cells where it can be used for energy, growth, and repair. People with type 1 diabetes no longer make insulin, so they must adjust the amount of insulin they take to the amount of carbohydrate they eat. They also time the action of the insulin to match the time they expect the food to be digested and the glucose to have entered their bloodstream.

Intestinal damage from celiac disease can lead to problems digesting and absorbing the nutrients from foods. Because of the damage in the upper intestine, foods may be digested more slowly than normal. Conversely, depending on the amount of damage in the intestine and presence of diarrhea, some foods may pass through the intestines without being absorbed, and there are visible food particles in the stool. Clearly, when celiac disease interferes with absorption of foods, so that you are not digesting all of the carbohydrate you eat, and it slows down or speeds up the transit of food through the intestine, it makes correct dosing and timing of insulin very difficult.

Different types of insulin (rapid acting as well as slow acting) are used to help control blood glucose levels. Rapid-acting insulin is given before or after meals and snacks. It aids in the metabolism of glucose, which builds up in the blood as the carbohydrates in food are digested. Slow-acting insulin works over 24 hours to handle the body's small but consistent release of stored carbohydrate in the form of glycogen from the liver. For someone on an insulin pump, like Sarah, which uses only rapid-acting insulin, a small amount of insulin is being released all the time and a larger dose is given for meals. When the intestine is not absorbing foods normally, it is much harder to match the action of insulin to absorption of carbohydrates and release of glucose, which leads to peaks and valleys in blood glucose levels.

Most people with type 1 diabetes use carbohydrate counting to determine the amount of insulin they need to cover meals. The amount of insulin to take can be figured out two ways:

- The person counts the number of carbohydrates he or she plans to eat and then takes the amount of rapid-acting insulin needed to absorb the glucose that will be digested from that carbohydrate. The disadvantage of this method is that if the person does not eat all the food as planned, there will be too much insulin working, which can lead to low blood glucose. If the person wants to eat more food, he or she will need to take additional insulin.
- The person eats first, then counts the carbohydrates ingested and takes the appropriate amount of rapid-acting insulin based on what was actually eaten.

Some carbohydrates, such as breads and grains, contain gluten, which is where celiac disease and diabetes overlap in your food choices. Don't get confused. You must avoid gluten, but you cannot avoid carbohydrates, because they provide your body with its favorite fuel, glucose. When you have these two diseases, you have twice as many reasons to choose your carbohydrates carefully—you want nutrient-rich gluten-free carbohydrates to keep your body well.

Carbohydrate Counting Gluten-Free Foods

Gluten-free carbohydrate foods are made from a combination of gluten-free flours and starches. Often, the gluten-free products that taste the best have a higher ratio of starches to gluten-free flours. The most common gluten-free flours (rice, tapioca, corn, potato, and arrowroot) also have lower ratios of carbohydrates to protein than what is found in wheat products. The more nutritious gluten-free grains and flours have a higher protein-to-carbohydrate ratio and higher fiber content. A protein-to-carbohydrate ratio that is close to 1:2 or one that has a significant source of fiber can slow the overall digestion of the food and thereby slow the release of glucose into the blood. This is important information for managing blood glucose levels, and a good reason to eat the more nutritious grains and flours.

Because fiber is not absorbed, some diabetes dietitians teach patients that they can reduce the total number of carbohydrates counted in a food when the fiber content is high. A typical formula is to subtract the amount of fiber in foods from the total carbohydrates in the food or meal when figuring your insulin needs. For example, if a food has a total carbohydrate content per serving of 25 g of carbohydrates and 5 g of fiber, the patient would administer insulin to cover 20 g of carbohydrates, not 25 g. Table 1 shows the fiber content of gluten-free grains and starches.

I find that patients with celiac disease and diabetes have an easier time controlling blood glucose when their diet includes gluten-free carbohydrates that are high in total fiber and have a higher protein-to-carbohydrate ratio (as close to 1:1 as you can get). In other words, when the ratio of protein to carbohydrate is as close as possible, the food converts more slowly to glucose. Also, if a food contains a lot of fiber, the food digests more slowly. For example, soy flour has a higher ratio of protein to carbohydrates than arrowroot and also more fiber, making it a better choice of flour or grain for helping to control diabetes (Table 2).

TABLE 1. Fiber in Gluten-Free Grains and Starches

Serving Size (1 cup)	Fiber (g)
Soy flour, defatted	18
Corn flour, masa, enriched, yellow	16
Wheat flour, whole grain (for comparison)	15
Amaranth flour	13
Buckwheat flour, whole groat	12
Chickpea flour (besan)	10
Potato flour	9
Rice flour, brown	7
Quinoa, cooked	5
Buckwheat groats, roasted, cooked	5
Rice, brown, long grain, cooked	4
Rice flour, white	4
Arrowroot flour	4
Wheat flour, white, all purpose, enriched, bleached (for comparison)	3
Corn flour, degermed, unenriched, yellow	2
Cornstarch	1
Rice, white, long grain, regular, cooked	0.6

From www.nal.usda.gov/fnic/foodcomp/search.

Not All Gluten-Free Products Are Created Equal

Many gluten-free foods are higher in total carbohydrates than wheat-based foods for the same portion size. Similar gluten-free products can have very different carbohydrate counts, as well, so Sarah and her family need to read food labels to count carbohydrates. Table 3 provides some sample carbohydrate counts for gluten-free foods. When reading labels, it is important to look at the manufacturer's serving size as well as the carbohydrate count. If your actual serving is twice the size of that listed on the label, then you are eating twice as much carbohydrate as is listed on the label.

The Plan for Sarah

I taught Sarah and her family about the gluten-free diet and offered suggestions of foods to try. We reviewed the foods that Sarah would be eating and talked about ways to make the family's favorite foods gluten free. I gave Sarah's parents guidelines for how to substitute gluten-free products in her meals and how to read labels for carbohydrate counts. I recommended that Sarah take a daily gluten-free children's vitamin and min-

TABLE 2. Protein-to-Carbohydrate Ratios of Gluten-Free Grains and Starches

Serving Size (1 cup)	Protein (g)	Carb (g)	Fiber (g)	Ratio
Soy flour, defatted	49	40	18	1:1
Chickpea flour (besan)	21	53	10	1:2
Quinoa, cooked	8	39	5	1:5
Amaranth flour	26	126	13	1:5
Wheat flour, whole-grain (ref. comparison)	16	87	15	1:5
Buckwheat groats, roasted, cooked	6	34	5	1:6
Buckwheat flour, whole-groat	15	85	12	1:6
Wheat flour, white, all-purpose, enriched, bleached (ref. comparison)	13	95	3	1:7
Corn flour, masa, enriched, yellow	11	87	n/a	1:8
Nuts, acorn flour, full fat (100 gm)	9	64	n/a	1:8
Rice, brown, long-grain, cooked	5	45	4	1:9
Rice flour, brown	11	120	7	1:11
Rice, white, long-grain, regular, cooked	4	45	0.6	1:11
Potato flour	11	133	9	1:12
Rice flour, white	9	127	4	1:14
Corn flour, degermed, unenriched, yellow	7	104	2	1:15
Arrowroot flour	0.4	113	4	1:282
Cornstarch	0.3	117	1	1:390

From www.nal.usda.gov/fnic/foodcomp/search.

eral supplement. Because Sarah's intake at each meal is unpredictable, I asked them to consider administering insulin after meals so that the insulin amount would more closely match her actual carbohydrate intake.

We discussed my concern about Sarah's limited food intake. Sarah insisted that she didn't want to try gluten-free versions of the foods that she had previously eliminated by choice. I felt that Sarah's food restrictions might in part be because of her symptoms after eating wheat-based products and a natural desire to avoid these symptoms. I assured her that once she's on a gluten-free diet, these symptoms would lessen over time. The family agreed to begin slowly introducing gluten-free carbohydrate choices into Sarah's diet. Although gluten-free food products are expensive, I suggested that Sarah's parents enjoy some gluten-free foods with her to encourage her in trying new foods. Another way to do this is for Sarah and her family to attend local support group meetings and events, where Sarah could try foods to see which products she likes and to meet other children with celiac disease.

TABLE 3. Sample Carbohydrate Counts for Gluten-Free Foods

	Company	CHO (g)/ Suggested Serving	Suggested Serving Size
Breads			
Light brown rice loaf	Ener-G Foods, Inc.	7	1 slice
Light tapioca loaf	Ener-G Foods, Inc.	7	1 slice
White rice flax loaf	Ener-G Foods, Inc.	14	1 slice
Hi-fiber loaf	Ener-G Foods, Inc.	18	1 slice
White rice bread	Ener-G Foods, Inc.	19	1 slice
Bread mix homestyle	Authentic Foods	23	¼ cup mix
Four flour bread	Ener-G Foods, Inc.	48	1 slice
Tapioca hamburger buns	Ener-G Foods, Inc.	21	1 bun
Seattle Brown hamburger buns	Ener-G Foods, Inc.	43	1 bun
Tapioca hot dog buns	Ener-G Foods, Inc.	21	1 bun
Seattle Brown hot dog buns	Ener-G Foods, Inc.	43	1 bun
Rice pizza shells (6 inch)	Ener-G Foods, Inc.	7	¼ crust
Pizza crust mix	Authentic Foods	27	1 serving (36 g)
Pancake and baking mix	Authentic Foods	24	¼ cup
English muffins with tofu	Ener-G Foods, Inc.	43	1 muffin
Crackers and Snacks			
Crackers	Glutino	15	4 each
Gourmet crackers	Ener-G Foods, Inc.	23	3 crackers
Original crackers	Mary's Gone Crackers	21	13 crackers
Wylde sesame pretzels	Ener-G Foods, Inc.	24	40 pieces
Crisp pretzels	Ener-G Foods, Inc.	25	25 pieces
Pasta			
White rice macaroni	Ener-G Foods, Inc.	43	2 oz.
Rice and corn pasta, gluten-free	Orgran Foods	57	2 oz.
Rice, potato, and soy pasta	BioNaturae	57	2 oz.
Quinoa pasta	Andean Dreams	42	2 oz.
Cereals			
Crispy brown rice cereal	Erewhon	25	1 cup
Perky O's original	Enjoy Life Natural Brands	33	¾ cup
Mighty Tasty GF hot cereal	Bob's Red Mill, USA	42	¼ cup dry
Oats, rolled (certified gluten free)	Gifts of Nature	40	½ cup dry
Desserts			
Ginger cookies	Ener-G Foods, Inc.	9	1 cookie
Plain doughnuts	Ener-G Foods, Inc.	14	1 doughnut
Chocolate cake mix	Authentic Foods	23	1 slice (28 g)
Vanilla cake mix	Authentic Foods	24	1 slice (28 g)
Biscotti	Ener-G Foods, Inc.	24	1 cookie
Carmel apple snack bar	Enjoy Life Natural Brands	28	1 bar

What Sarah Decided

At a follow-up meeting a few months later, Sarah's family reported that Sarah was now eating several new foods and had gained five pounds in the past month. She was still a finicky eater but getting better. Her parents reported Sarah's meals and snacks for a typical day. In addition, Sarah was taking a daily gluten-free multivitamin.

Sarah's Typical Eating Plan

	Carbs
Breakfast	
Gluten-free oatmeal with cinnamon (½ cup dry, cooked)	40 grams
Low-fat milk (1 cup)	12 grams
Raisins (2 Tbsp.)	15 grams
Total	67 grams
Lunch	
Half of a 6-inch gluten-free pizza with sauce, sausage, and cheese	15 grams
Carrot and celery sticks with ranch dip	5 grams
Small apple	15 grams
Milk (1 cup)	12 grams
Total	47 grams
Afternoon Snack	
Caramel apple snack bar	28 grams
Dinner	
Barbecued chicken (gluten free)	
Small baked potato with sour cream and chives	25 grams
Green tossed salad with Italian dressing	
Milk (1 cup)	12 grams
Gluten-free chocolate cake (1 slice)	23 grams
Total	60 grams
Bedtime Snack	
Cheese stick	
Gluten-free pretzels	25 grams

Sarah seemed happy and outgoing and willing to try a new gluten-free product that I offered her. Sarah's parents reported that her blood glucose levels were more stable once they began giving rapid insulin after she ate. She had had only one hypoglycemia reaction in the last month, which they thought was because of her forgetting to eat a snack after school while playing soccer. Sarah is complaining less of stomachaches, and her parents said that she no longer has loose stools.

The family had recently attended a gluten-free food fair and found a few new products that Sarah will eat. They now carry snacks for her that will quickly raise her blood glucose level. They have met with Sarah's teacher to explain her needs while at school. Sarah's parents feel confident in their ability to manage Sarah's diabetes and celiac disease. They will continue to follow up regularly with her diabetes care team, and I encouraged them to follow-up with me as needed.

SELF-MANAGEMENT TIPS

☐ Check your blood glucose level frequently, for example, first thing in the morning, right before and two hours after meals, and at bedtime. Write the numbers in a notebook. Also write down the amount of carbohydrates that you ate that day and when you ate them. Soon you will have solid information about yourself and be able to see patterns in your blood glucose levels so you can begin to understand what affects them. It also helps to make a note of any high stress events or significant physical activity, because these affect blood glucose levels, too. A flare of celiac gastrointestinal symptoms will also affect blood glucose levels.

☐ Include in your daily meals gluten-free carbohydrates that are high in total fiber and have a higher protein-to-carbohydrate ratio (closer to 1:1), such as foods made with soy, chickpea, or amaranth flours or cooked quinoa or gluten-free oatmeal. These carbohydrates are absorbed slowly, which helps you maintain normal blood glucose levels.

☐ You can adjust the total number of carbohydrates in a food when the fiber content is high. Subtract the amount of fiber from the total carbohydrates in the food or meal before figuring your insulin needs.

☐ Choose the healthiest habits for you and your family: Eat high-fiber foods (especially fruits and vegetables), limit sugar intake, be physically active daily, drink water, and get enough rest. Children like Sarah will not exercise in a gym or on machines the way adults do—they prefer to play outdoors with you and others.

☐ If you are not sure how much you (or your child) will eat at meals, count the carbohydrates after you finish eating and give the proper amount of insulin then. This will help you better manage blood glucose levels.

☐ Check the ingredients list on the food label for sources of gluten (see Chapter 22 on reading food labels) and carbohydrate. Look at the Nutrition Facts on the food label to find the amount of carbohydrate and fiber in one serving. Check the serving size. Do not assume that similar foods, such as gluten-free breads or cereals, have the same carbohydrate count or the same amount of fiber. Keep checking the labels, because manufacturers change ingredients from time to time, too.

☐ Eat more vegetables, gluten-free whole grains (see Chapter 13 on whole grains), fruits, and cooked dried beans. These are high in fiber and other nutrients, lower in carbohydrates than processed foods, and are gluten free.

☐ As you add fiber to your diet, be sure to drink more water.

☐ Eat more single-ingredient foods, such as apples, walnuts, red bell peppers, roasted squash, eggs, or meat. These foods are nutrient rich and have not been processed by a food manufacturer. None of them have a food label, but you can easily learn the amount of carbohydrate and fiber in the vegetables and fruit.

- ☐ Your child may need a gluten-free multivitamin and mineral supplement, especially in the period of adjusting to eating gluten-free foods and carbohydrate counting.
- ☐ As you become accustomed to counting carbohydrates and eating a gluten-free diet, it is important to keep a daily log of your blood glucose readings and to consult with your health care team if your blood glucose levels are not doing what you expect them to do.

Resources

- Thompson T, Simpson S. *Counting Gluten-Free Carbohydrates*. 2009. www.glutenfree dietitian.com/gluten_free_books.php.
- Case S. *Gluten-Free Diet: A Comprehensive Resource Guide*. 4th ed. Case Nutrition Consulting, Inc., 2010, www.glutenfreediet.ca.
- Gluten Intolerance Group. *Adding Fiber to Your Diet.* http://gluten.net/downloads/print/Adding%20fiber.pdf.

Recommended Reading

- Kupper C, Higgins LA. Combining diabetes and gluten-free dietary management guidelines. *Pract Gastroenterol* 2007;XXXI(3):68–83.
- Kupper C. *Gluten Intolerance and GI Disorders*. 2nd ed.
- Araujo J, da Silva GA, de Melo FM. Serum prevalence of celiac disease in children and adolescents with type 1 diabetes mellitus. *J Pediatr (Rio J)* 2006;82(3):210–14.
- Schuppan D, Hahn EG. Celiac disease and its link to type 1 diabetes mellitus. *J Pediatr Endocrinol Meta,* 2001;14(Suppl. 1):5973–605.
- Zbikowski-Bojko M, Szaflarska-Poplawska A, Pilecki O, et al. Selected aspects of the epidemiological analysis of celiac disease and diabetes mellitus type 1 coexistence in children and youth. *Pol Merkur Lekarski* 2006;20(117):322–25.

Cynthia Kupper, RD, CD, is the Executive Director of the Gluten Intolerance Group of North America, a national nonprofit organization supporting individuals with celiac disease and other forms of gluten intolerance. A clinical dietitian, she speaks on celiac disease and the gluten-free diet at government and regulatory agency meetings and to the food and hospitality industries, health care professionals, and patient organizations.

CHAPTER 25

Celiac Disease and Religious Practices

Nancy Patin Falini, MA, RD, LDN

Depending on your religion, celiac disease may pose a unique challenge to the way you practice your faith. Some religions, such as Judaism and Roman Catholicism, require gluten-containing grains for worship. Fortunately, special considerations have been established that can help with this requirement. Other religions, including the Catholic Eastern, Eastern Orthodox, and Ancient Eastern Churches, don't have formal written standards, so it is best to seek individual guidance for managing communion from your own clergy. Protestantism and nondenominational Christianity do not require a particular grain or grains for communion and may, depending on the pastor, use a gluten-free cracker or piece of bread for communion. Alternatively, you might prefer to use a gluten-free rice- and potato-based communion wafer (www.ener-g.com). The Muslim religion, as well as Hinduism and Buddhism, have no obligations for eating any type of gluten-containing substance.

Judaism

My initial contact with Rachel, 72 years old, was in late February, when she was newly diagnosed with celiac disease. Reluctantly, she made an appointment for medical nutrition therapy, disheartened by the constraints the gluten-free diet would inflict on Jewish dietary laws, particularly during the upcoming Pesach holiday (Passover). Because she believed herself to be asymptomatic, she was even less interested in changing her eating habits, especially those mandated by Jewish tradition.

Rachel's medical history included 30 years of iron deficiency anemia with periods of intravenous iron infusions. She also had osteopenia. The biopsy showed that her intestinal mucosa was so damaged that the villi were flat, and her immunoglobulin A tissue transglutaminase (IgA-tTG) was more than 100 units (normal is less than 5 units for this lab). Iron studies confirmed her anemia, including serum ferritin of 2 ng/ml, iron saturation of 6%, hemoglobin of 9.8 g/dl, hematocrit of 31.7%, mean corpuscular volume of 68.1 fl, and mean corpuscular hemoglobin of 20.8 pg. All of these parameters were well below normal levels. Her liver enzymes were slightly elevated.

I assured Rachel and her husband at the beginning of our session that there are gluten-free options to her religious dietary practices and we would address them in detail. Although she seemed to believe that eating gluten had no deleterious impact, we reviewed her health, especially the condition of her blood, bones, and liver, which were obviously affected. When she acknowledged the healing potential that the gluten-free lifestyle would have on these aspects of her health, she found a strong motivation for eliminating gluten.

Which Foods Typically Used for Jewish Religious Observance Contain Gluten?

Matzoh, the holy mark of freedom from Egyptian bondage and the sole form of bread during Pesach, and its derivatives contain wheat. Matzoh meal, cake meal, and matzoh farfel all contain wheat. Matzoh replaces bread during the eight days of Pesach, during which all leavened products, such as yeast, quick breads, muffins, and biscuits, are forbidden foods. On the first two nights, dinner is the traditional Pesach seder during which participants perform the special mitzvah (religious act) of eating matzoh. On the first two and last two days, there is an obligation to eat two meals that include matzoh. Foods commonly eaten during Pesach, like matzoh balls and gefilte fish, are customarily made with matzoh meal.

Shabbat (the Sabbath) and other Jewish holidays also include the obligation of eating beautiful and special meals and saying prayers and blessings and singing songs to fulfill the mitzvot (religious acts). Only matzoh or challah bread is consumed with these meals. Challah represents the manna sent from God to nourish the Israelites during their journey from Egypt back to their promised land. According to the Shulchan Aruch (Code of Jewish Law), only five special grains may be used to make the breads intended for satisfying these mitzvot: wheat, spelt, rye, barley, and oats. Matzoh used for Pesach must be made under strict rabbinical supervision and, therefore, cannot be homemade. Matzoh used for Shabbat and other Jewish holidays must be made in compliance with Jewish law and be baked in a special oven, making it impractical to make at home. Only gluten-free oats are safe for people with celiac disease. However, the use of gluten-free oat matzoh and oats should be postponed until adequate healing of the small intestine has been determined by your health care provider (see Chapter 21 on oats and wheat starch). If it's too soon to have gluten-free oats, there are no other alternatives to matzoh. You must consult a local rabbi to determine the waiving of this requirement.

Incorporating Gluten-Free Modifications into Religious Dietary Practices

Because Passover dietary laws require the elimination of grains such as wheat, spelt, rye, barley, and oats with the exception of matzoh, many foods used to observe this lengthy religious holiday are gluten free. As long as a food is marked "kosher for Passover" and is free of any form of matzoh, which would be clearly stated in the ingredients list, the product is gluten free. To eliminate the fear of possible leavening, some very observant Jews avoid matzoh as an ingredient when mixed with liquids during Passover. The interchangeable terms that may be used to distinguish the absence of matzoh are *non-gebrokts, non-gebroktz,* and *non-gebroks.* When any such term is on the label of a kosher-for-Passover product, it is easily identified as wheat free, which in this case indicates gluten free. A variety of companies, such as Manischewitz, Gefen,

Lieber's Kosher Products, and Paskez, sell kosher-for-Passover ingredients and foods that are also free of derivatives of matzoh and, therefore, gluten free. These include Passover noodles, kugel mixes, and mixes ideal for making matzoh balls and replacing matzoh meal.[1,2] Pancake mixes made from potato starch make a good replacement for matzoh meal. Kosher-for-Passover foods begin to appear on grocery store shelves and in kosher stores and bakeries as early as one month or more before Passover, so it is wise to stock up on all of your favorites while they are available. A variety of cookbooks provide gluten-free recipes for Pesach as does the Internet.

When your doctor deems it safe to introduce gluten-free oats, you may eat a total of 50 grams or less a day. Gluten-free oat matzoh is available from Rabbi E. Kestenbaum in England (http://mdkwi.com/OatMatza.html) and Lakewood Matzoh (www.Lakewoodmatzoh.com). Both contain less than 20 parts per million (ppm), the proposed FDA gluten-free standard. Both handmade and machine-made gluten-free oat matzoh are available from these sources, and the former also supplies gluten-free oat matzoh meal until supplies are depleted.

The seder mitzvah during Pesach requires a minimal amount of matzoh. For those with medical conditions, the requirement is less and well below the 50-gram or 1¾-oz. daily limit of gluten-free oats, which allows you to have matzoh for other meals, too. When referring to portion sizes, take into account that gluten-free oat matzohs, both hand and machine made, can vary in size and weight. Table 1 provides general guidelines for portions.[3] Moreover, oat matzoh has been described as absorbing much more water compared with wheat matzoh. However, because the exact water content is unknown, the exact weight of the actual oats is also not known. For this reason it is wise to be conservative and weigh out no more than a total of 50 grams of oat matzoh for an entire day. For a rough comparison, 1¼ pieces of gluten-free oat machine-made matzoh weighs 50 grams or 1¾ oz. This is based on 1 whole piece of matzoh measuring 7 inches by 6¼ inches (43.75 square inches). Consider purchasing a food scale that measures both in grams and ounces, which can be found in stores selling kitchen items. Finally, it is important to determine the amount of matzoh you will need for the year so that you purchase enough.

The mitzvot on Shabbat and other holidays also require a minimum amount of matzoh or challah. For each of the three special meals for Shabbat (one Friday night and two on Saturday) as well as the two meals on other holidays, one golf ball–sized piece of matzoh or challah is recommended for those with medical conditions. For matzoh, the golf ball exemplifies approximately a 36-gram or 1.3-oz. portion. In order to fulfill the mitzvot, this portion is expected to be consumed a maximum of two times in one day. Because these

TABLE 1. Minimum Matzoh Requirements for the Pesach Seder for Those with Health Conditions

Oat Matzoh Type	Amount Required	Square Inches
Handmade matzoh	⅛th of a piece	13.75
Machine-made matzoh	¼th of a piece	10.75

Note: These measurements are based on wheat matzoh from Tzelem Pupa Bakery; only gluten-free oat matzoh should be considered for consumption.

breads may only be made from the same five grains required for Pesach, gluten-free oats are the only option. Two golf ball–sized portions of gluten-free oat matzoh weigh 72 grams, thus exceeding the general recommendation to limit oat consumption to 50-grams per day. However, many experts now believe that consumption of significantly greater amounts of gluten-free oats is safe for most individuals; discuss your needs with your health care provider. Additionally, challah is not currently made from gluten-free oats, so you may need to consult a local rabbi.

As always, care should be taken at a seder to prevent contact or cross-contamination of gluten-free and gluten-containing foods. Be sure to keep wheat matzoh separate from gluten-free oat matzoh and items made with wheat matzoh, such as gefilte fish, separate from matzoh-free foods. Explain your gluten-free requirements to the host or cook your own food in advance when celebrating in the homes of others or outside your home.

To aid in the use of kosher-for-Passover nonfood items, specifically medications and supplements, the annually updated *Passover Guide to Cosmetics and Medications* is a very informative resource available from Kollel Los Angeles. This guide is also incorporated into the *Star-K Passover Directory* by Kosher Certification (www.star-k.org) that is sold in Jewish bookstores one month before Pesach. Note: Continue to take any life-sustaining medications even though they do not meet kosher-for-Passover requirements; consult your rabbi and physician regarding this issue.

What Rachel Decided

Once Rachel better understood celiac disease, realized the healing benefits of the gluten-free lifestyle, and learned about the options that enabled her to follow her faith, she was relieved. Because it was too early to introduce gluten-free oat matzoh into her diet, she consulted with her rabbi, who excused her. Despite the exclusion of matzoh and challah for the holiday and Shabbat meals, she was going to partake in the wine. However, because previous tests had revealed her slightly elevated liver enzymes, Rachel consulted first with her gastroenterologist, who determined that the liver inflammation was a result of active celiac disease with no other underlying cause. The doctor approved wine for religious purposes.

In anticipation of introducing gluten-free oats, particularly gluten-free oat matzoh, in the coming year, Rachel planned ahead and ordered some to have on hand. Because this matzoh is made only of oat flour and water, it has a very long shelf life (well over 1 year). Rachel stored them in a cool, dry place. If necessary to maintain crispness, she planned to warm them in an oven for a few minutes, being careful not to burn them. She found that her local grocery stores had a wide variety of kosher-for-Passover gluten-free foods and stocked up on these for the following year. She found a recipe for Mock Matzoh Balls in *The Gluten-Free Gourmet Cooks Fast and Healthy* by Bette Hagman. Following Pesach, she took advantage of the clearance sales on these specialty foods. She also referred to the *Passover Guide to Cosmetics and Medications* to guide her in using only kosher-for-Passover medications and supplements, which under the circumstances would also be wheat free because a matzoh derivative would not be used in these types of products.

Outcome

In a follow-up phone conversation, it was evident that Rachel was responding favorably, both physically and spiritually, to living gluten free. Within three months, her IgA-tTG dropped from greater than 100 to 43 units (not negative, but improved), indicating that she was doing well at reducing her gluten exposure and that intestinal healing was occurring. Although Rachel was very outgoing, her long history of iron deficiency anemia had accustomed her to having little energy. Much to her surprise, she began to feel a sense of rejuvenation as a result of living gluten free. Because Jewish mitzvot and prayer are so interactive, despite her need to omit matzoh (initially) and challah, she did not feel excluded. She participated in seders in the home of dear friends, as well as at her synagogue, which required her to plan ahead and tell others about her medical nutritional needs. She explained her need to avoid matzoh and its derivatives and showed how to prevent cross-contamination to those she assisted in preparing the foods. Rachel understands that she requires ongoing monitoring of her IgA-tTG until the level is normal and remains that way.

Catholicism

Mary, a 60-year-old director of religious education, saw me shortly after her diagnosis of celiac disease. Mary's job allowed her to receive Holy Communion (or Eucharist) daily. As she pondered the implications of celiac disease on expressions of her faith, she experienced denial and was overcome with frustration and confusion. She questioned why she could no longer receive the sacrament of Holy Communion (an outward sign of God's love and grace) that is central to her faith.

Mary's symptoms of celiac disease were abdominal pain and diarrhea, and rising liver enzymes prior to her diagnosis indicated liver involvement. Despite supplementation of 4500 IUs of vitamin D daily, her serum 25-hydroxyvitamin D (the form of vitamin D that circulates in the blood) remained low. Her IgA-tTG was greater than 100 units (normal is less than 5 units for this lab), and biopsy of her small intestine revealed serious intestinal damage, specifically severe and diffuse villous atrophy.

During our nutrition counseling session, I explained how gluten causes damage to the intestine, the daily maximum level of gluten that is believed to be safe if ingested inadvertently, and safe options for the host used in Holy Communion. Mary feared the harm in receiving the regular wheat host but questioned even the minute amount of gluten in the wheat starch–based low-gluten communion host.

Church Doctrine Defining Catholic Communion

Canon Law Number 924 reveals the manner in which communion may occur. Section 1 states, "The Most Sacred Eucharistic Sacrifice must be celebrated with bread and wine, with which a small quantity of water is to be mixed." Section 2 states, "The bread must be made from wheat alone and recently made so that there is no danger of corruption." Section 3 states, "The wine must be natural wine of the grape and not corrupt." Canon Number 925 reveals that "Holy Communion is to be given under the form of bread alone or under both kinds in accord with the norm of the liturgical laws or even under the form of wine alone in case of necessity."

During the time of Jesus, barley was the grain used in common bread. However, the use of wheat for the communion host dates from the early days of the church, a practice probably related to Scriptures that imply wheat to be the finest among the various grains, including Psalms 81:1 6, 147:14 and Revelation 6:6. The church believes that no one has authority to change a tradition that is universal and immemorial regarding this requirement for the Holy Eucharist. His Holiness Pope Pius XII further justifies this principle by stating, "To the Church there is no competency given over the 'substance of the Sacraments,' that is, over those elements which Christ the Lord himself, as witnessed by the sources of divine revelation, established to be observed as the sacramental sign."[4]

A Special Provision for Eucharist for Celiac Disease

As described in the Congregation of the Doctrine of Faith, specific considerations for Holy Communion are granted for those who are gluten intolerant, similar to those for people who are alcohol intolerant.[5] No longer is medical certification a requirement. Under canon 137.1, the ordinary (bishop who has jurisdiction over a diocese) may delegate to the local clergy the authority to permit the use of the low-gluten hosts. The communicant needs only to ask his or her local clergy once for permission to receive the low-gluten host or wine only, either of which conveys the whole presence of Christ according to the church.

Although the church grants permission for people who are gluten intolerant to have the option of taking a small amount of the regular wheat host, this is not safe for those with celiac disease. Most wheat flour contains 11–14% total protein, and generally 75% of that protein is gluten. The regular wheat host contains about 22 milligrams of gluten. The Benedictine Sisters of Perpetual Adoration provide low-gluten altar breads (www.benedictine sisters.org/bread) inspired by the requirements of church teaching for those with celiac disease. They developed a low-gluten communion wafer from wheat starch and pregelatinized wheat starch. The particular wheat starch used results in a low-gluten host that is free of most protein (and thus free of most gluten), resulting in 0.01% or 100 parts per million (ppm) gluten. These hosts are produced in a dedicated area and are packaged and shipped separately from wheat hosts. The low-gluten hosts have a characteristic golden color that distinguishes them from regular wheat hosts.

The proposed FDA standard for a food to be considered gluten free is less than 20 ppm gluten (read more in Chapter 19 on safe level of gluten ingestion). Because ppm is a percentage based on a standard quantity, 1 ppm is 1 milligram of any given substance in 1 kilogram of a food product. A kilogram is equal to 2.2 pounds (35 oz.). Therefore, the FDA proposes that a product that contains a maximum of 19 milligrams gluten in 1 kilogram of the product can be considered gluten free. The amount of gluten necessary to cause damage varies from individual to individual; however, studies suggest that most people can tolerate 10 mg per day, while 50 mg or more per day causes intestinal changes in most people.[6] The low-gluten hosts contain 100 ppm gluten, or 100 milligrams of gluten in 1 kilogram of the host. That sounds like too much gluten, but a typical host weighs a mere 0.0005 kilograms. The average gluten content in one low-gluten host is just 37 micrograms[7] (1000 micrograms equal 1 milligram). This amount of gluten is just 0.4% of the 10 milligram gluten threshold. It would take 270 low-gluten hosts to equal 10 milligrams gluten. Therefore, low-gluten hosts are safe, even on a daily basis. Even a priest who might consume 2–3 low-gluten hosts in a day would consume well under the amount of gluten considered to be the limit. However, as noted above, tolerance for gluten intake varies from person to person, so whenever you add a new potential gluten source into your diet, watch for symptoms and plan on rechecking your blood for celiac antibodies after three months (or sooner if symptoms develop).

In a situation in which there are no low-gluten hosts, the communicant may choose to receive wine alone, regardless of whether it is made available to the rest of the faithful. It's vital that this wine be offered from a chalice that has not come into contact with a regular wheat host. If you are traveling or attending Mass where you cannot make prior arrangements for a modified communion, it is possible to partake in a spiritual communion. Seek the advice of your pastor about this.

What Mary Decided

After being educated on the gluten content of regular wheat hosts and the safe amount of gluten contained in one low-gluten host, Mary was relieved. She found herself highly motivated and felt empowered to request that she receive the low-gluten host daily at her workplace as well as in her own parish on the weekend. She consulted with the pastors at the church where she worked and at her home parish to explore procedures for receiving the low-gluten host. Because there is no one method for keeping low-gluten hosts separate from the regular hosts and accommodating the way in which Holy Communion is distributed to those with celiac disease, they devised a system that incorporated the dynamics of each parish and its communicants.

Monday through Friday, Mary receives communion at her workplace through the use of a pyx (container specifically for the hosts). Before Monday morning Mass, the sacristan stocks a clean pyx designated for only low-gluten hosts and it is labeled as such, with enough hosts for each day of that given week. The pyx is then placed on the altar to be consecrated (thus becoming the presence of Christ) along with the wheat hosts. From the front pew, Mary lines up first to receive Holy Communion. Following communion, the priest returns the pyx to the Tabernacle for the next day.

Mary and her priest worked out two methods for communion at her home parish. Generally, she attends the 10:30 a.m. Mass, where the sacristan places a low-gluten host alone on a separate paten (Communion plate) on the altar. At the sign of peace, when the extraordinary ministers of Holy Communion assemble near the altar, Mary lines up alongside them to receive communion from the priest and then returns to her pew. In the event she chooses to attend a different Mass, she informs the church in advance to forgo the preparation of the low-gluten host. Instead, Mary supplies her own low-gluten host, which she purchases and keeps frozen at home for up to 4 to 6 months. Prior to Mass, she places a host in a pyx given her by the church and arrives at church several minutes early to place the pyx on the altar with the other hosts to be consecrated. The reception of Holy Communion is conducted in the same manner as it is for the 10:30 Mass, except that the priest returns the pyx to her immediately after she receives the host.

Outcome

In addition to avoiding gluten in her food, supplements, and medications, Mary has exchanged the use of regular wheat communion hosts for the low-gluten ones. She is also taking various nutrient supplements to compensate for malabsorption, inadequate dietary intake, and deficiencies. With time, Mary has regained a sense of well-being as her abdominal pain and diarrhea have resolved. Her energy level has improved, and the elevated liver enzymes continue to decline as does her IgA-tTG, all suggesting that she has been eliminating gluten successfully and healing. Mary and her health care providers will continue to monitor her IgA-tTG level to ensure that it falls to and remains in the normal range.

SELF-MANAGEMENT TIPS

☐ Holy Communion may be received with a low-gluten host or by taking wine alone. Together with your priest, establish a method for receiving communion.

☐ You only need to seek permission once from your local priest to obtain special accommodations for receiving Holy Communion, but discuss what to do if you have a new or visiting priest.

☐ Some priests may not be aware of the special accommodations discussed in this chapter. Be patient as you explain your need and educate these individuals.

☐ Consider purchasing and supplying your own low-gluten hosts for Mass.

☐ Special care should be taken to keep the low-gluten host and wine separate from any regular wheat hosts. This means the use of a separate paten or pyx for the low-gluten hosts and a separate chalice of wine for you, if used. It is wise to inform others of the characteristic golden color of the low-gluten hosts to help distinguish them from regular wheat hosts.

References

1. Mandl L. Passover provides unique opportunities for the gluten-free diet: a Passover reminder. www.glutenfreebay.com. Celiac Support Group, Children's Hospital, Boston. Feb. 2008.
2. Ratner A. Passover paradise. www.glutenfreeliving.com. July 2009.
3. *2009 Passover Directory.* Pesach Guide for those with Diabetes. Nechama Cohen/Jewish Diabetes Assoc. Star-K Certification, Inc. http://www.star-k.org/cons-pesach-flash.htm.
4. Apostolic Constitution Sacramentum Ordinis, 30 November 1947: AAS 40 (1948) 5.
5. Congregation for Doctrine of the Faith. July 24, 2003 Prot. 89/78-174 98. Statement by the National Conference of Catholic bishops on the use of low gluten hosts at Mass.

6. Catassi C, Fabiani E, Iacono G, et al. A prospective, double-blind, placebo-controlled trial to establish a safe gluten threshold of patients with celiac disease. *Am J Clin Nutr* 2007;85:160–66.
7. Crowe JP. Catholic celiacs can now receive communion. *Gluten-Free Living Magazine.* 2004; 9(1):3,6,8.

Acknowledgments

Special gratitude goes to Rabbi Dovid Heber, a Kushrus Administrator at Star-K Kosher Certification, for his generous expert insights and Marcy Glazman Levy, RD, LDN, and Keith J. Laskin, MD, for their gracious review of the information on Judaism.

For the information on Catholicism, special gratitude goes to Sr. Jeanne Patricia Crowe, IHM, PharmD, RPh, for her kind, invaluable contribution to weighing and calculating the regular wheat hosts and Monsignor Michael Magee, SSL, STD, for his generous time, guidance, and wisdom in interpreting and translating documents.

Nancy Patin Falini, MA, RD, LDN, is in private practice specializing in celiac disease. She is a consultant to the Celiac Center at Paoli Hospital in Pennsylvania, author of *Gluten-Free Friends: An Activity Book for Kids,* and is on the Dietetic Advisory Board of Gluten-Free Living and the Scientific/Medical Advisory Board of the National Foundation for Celiac Awareness.

CHAPTER 26

Dining Out Gluten Free—Locally and While Traveling

Pam Cureton, RD, LDN, and Mary C. McKenna, PhD, LDN, CNS

Jenny, a 16-year-old newly diagnosed with celiac disease, came to the clinic for her six-month follow-up visit. Jenny was doing well with no complaints. However, her mother was concerned that a recent episode in which Jenny was exposed to gluten would cause a setback in her healing.

Jenny had dined out with a group of friends at a local restaurant. Being a typical teenager, she did not want to call attention to herself and quietly ordered what she thought was a safe, gluten-free meal. Later that day, she complained to her mother of stomach pain. When Jenny's mother asked her what she had eaten at the restaurant, she replied, "I only had the roast beef, mashed potatoes, and gravy." "Gravy!" shouted Mom. "Gravy has wheat flour in it!" To which, Jenny replied, "But Mom, I have gravy at home all the time."

How Celiac Disease Affects Eating Away from Home

Jenny is like the other 130 million individuals who eat out on any given day in the United States. In fact, the average American eats out 4.2 meals per week.[1] Jenny, however, often faces difficult decisions when dining out because of her celiac disease. Dining out and travel are at the top of the list of quality-of-life concerns faced by people with celiac disease.

A large survey that included individuals with celiac disease and hospitality and food service professionals that cater to special dietary needs was conducted by AllergyFree Passport and GlutenFree Passport. Among the survey's key findings was that most people with celiac disease eat out less after their diagnoses. This is because they fear that lack of knowledge on the part of food service staff will allow them to be exposed to gluten and possible side effects.[2] Another large survey of those with celiac disease found that, even though most respondents followed a strict gluten-free diet (GFD), more than 80% acknowledged some level of dietary indiscretion when eating in a restaurant.[3] A survey of Canadian Celiac Association members found that 54% of respondents avoid dining out altogether and 15% avoid traveling.[4]

SELF-MANAGEMENT TIPS FOR SAFE DINING OUT

Dining out need not be a thing of the past. Armed with knowledge of the GFD, a little prep time, and a positive attitude, safe gluten-free dining is possible. Follow these 10 steps to gluten-free dining, and bon appétit!

1. **Know the GFD.** Before venturing out to a restaurant, arm yourself with knowledge about the GFD (see Chapter 12 on the balanced diet and Chapter 20 on inadvertent gluten exposure). Knowing where gluten normally is or can be hiding will help you avoid it. As you learn the different places that gluten is found, for example, wheat in soy sauce, barley in beer, and malt in malted vinegar, you will be able to easily identify potential problem dishes. Some less obvious places to find gluten include broths, artificial bacon bits, marinades, and imitation crab meat. Basic knowledge of the GFD would have saved the day if Jenny had known that gravy is traditionally thickened with flour. Parents need to instruct their children with celiac disease about the dishes and recipes they alter to make them gluten free. Reading recipes can also provide clues as to when wheat is used, such as in a roux (to flavor or thicken gravy), au gratin, or batter for tempura, fried, or "encrusted" foods.

2. **Know the restaurant.** Some restaurants make better, safer choices than others. A pizza place that only serves pizza cannot provide as many choices as a place with a varied menu. If you are just starting to eat out after a celiac disease diagnosis, you may want to start with a restaurant that has a gluten-free section listed in its menu (Table 1).

TABLE 1. Sample of Chain Restaurants that Offer a Gluten-Free Menu

Biaggi's Ristorante Italiano	Fleming's Steakhouse
Bonefish Grill	Kona Grill
Carrabba's Italian Grill	Legal Seafoods
Cheeseburger in Paradise	Mitchell's Fish Market
Denny's	Outback Steakhouse
First Watch	Pei Wei Asian Diner
P. F. Chang's China Bistro	Roy's Restaurants
Z' Tejas	

3. **Identify yourself to the wait staff.** If Jenny had followed this rule, an alert server might have saved her the discomfort of her mistake. If you are also shy, try calling ahead to ask questions. The best time to call a restaurant and speak to a chef is before the lunch or dinner rush gets underway. You still need to identify yourself when you arrive at the restaurant, but most of your questions will have been answered ahead of time. Also, Triumph Dining sells a set of laminated, portable cards specially designed to help you communicate your dietary requirement in 10 different languages and for several types of cuisine (Table 2).

TABLE 2. Resources for Gluten-Free Dining Out

Materials	
Triumph Dining The Essential Restaurant Guide Dining Cards (10 languages)	www.triumphdining.com
Gluten Free Passport Let's Eat Out series	www.glutenfreepassport.com
Waiter, Is There Wheat in My Soup? The Official Guide to Dining Out, Shopping, and Traveling Gluten-Free	www.whatnowheat.com
Celiac Resource Guide Helping to Navigate LifeDetour	www.CeliacResourceGuide.webs.com
Internet Sites	
Gluten Intolerance Group Gluten Free Restaurant Awareness Program	www.glutenfreerestaurants.org
Bob and Ruth's Gluten-Free Dining & Travel Club	www.bobandruths.com
Gluten Free Passport iPhone/iPod Touch Applications iEatOut Gluten & Allergen Free iCanEat On The Go	www.glutenfreeonthego.com www.glutenfreepassport.com
Urban Spoon	www.urbanspoon.com
Clan Thompson	http://www.clanthompson.com/ life_travel_whereeat_us.php3
Specialgourmets: Global guide of restaurants for celiacs	www.specialgourmets.com
International Travel	
TheCeliacScene: Guides for the gluten free in Canada	http://www.theceliacscene.com
A.I.C. (Italian Celiac Association) Eating Out Project	www.celiachia.it/ristoratori/default_ eng.asp
Dining info service from Coeliac UK	www.gluten-free-onthego.com
Celiac Travel: Restaurant cards and travel tips	www.celiactravel.com

4. **Ask specific questions.** Politely and respectfully win over your server so he or she can help champion your cause to the kitchen staff. Pick specific menu items and ingredients about which to inquire. For example, ask whether the steak or seafood is marinated in soy sauce, the short ribs are dredged in flour before cooking, the French fries are cooked in the same oil as the onion rings, or the vegetables are steamed over pots of boiling pasta water. Even if you are ordering from a restaurant's gluten-free menu, be sure that your server delivers your message to the kitchen.

5. **Ask again.** Explain your need to avoid contamination and emphasize that, for instance, removing croutons from the top of the salad won't work. Ask for your order to be cooked on a clean grill with fresh utensils so your food will not come in contact with gluten-containing foods.

6. **When in doubt, go simple.** Most restaurants can provide salads without croutons, plain grilled fish or meat, baked potatoes, and steamed vegetables. You may not get the most exciting meal, but it will be a safe meal.

7. **Do not accept mistakes.** If the hamburger comes on a bun, do not just remove the bun and eat the hamburger anyway. Remember that you identified yourself as someone who would get sick if you eat wheat, so politely remind your server and ask for a new hamburger. (You may want to cut the meat to identify it so they won't be tempted to send you back the same one.)

8. **Do your homework before you go.** Let today's technology work for you in your search for gluten-free dining. Check the restaurant's Web site beforehand. Many list the wheat/gluten ingredients and will indicate that they have a gluten-free menu (Table 1), or are willing to fax you a copy of their menu. Jenny, for example, could have benefitted from new technology from GlutenFree Passport (Table 2) or an application for iPhones and the iPod Touch that offers instant information about gluten-free dining while at the restaurant. Jenny could have used this application to learn that wheat is used in gravy, but her friends would assume she is just texting or checking her iPod. Another useful application from www.urbanspoon.com lists restaurants by location, cost, and type of food served, with gluten-free being one of the choices. Chain fast-food restaurants list the allergen/nutritional information on their sites. Download the information of your favorite places to eat out and keep it in a notebook in your purse or car for quick reference when away from home.

9. **Try to go early or go late.** Eating out at peak times increases the likelihood that busy servers and cooks may not give your meal proper attention. Try to eat out before the rush hour or dine fashionably late.

10. **Say thank you.** Say thank you to your server, not only with a generous tip but by taking the time to talk to the manager about the wonderful experience you had in his or her restaurant. Being a repeat customer also shows your appreciation. Share your experiences with others who might benefit, such as your support group or health care providers. Not feeling the love from the restaurant staff? Be prepared to leave and try again at another restaurant looking for your business!

How Restaurants Are Reacting

More than ever, restaurants are seeing the need for, and the financial benefit of, safely serving people with celiac disease by offering gluten-free menu options. When surveyed in October 2008, the National Restaurant Association membership indicated in the category of "culinary themes" that gluten free and allergy conscious were the top two trends.[5] It's good business to address special diet requests where possible.

Some restaurants offer a few choices, and others offer entirely gluten-free menus, but the need for gluten-free dining has had an impact on the bottom line of many eateries. For example, P. F. Chang's, a Chinese restaurant chain, has worked to meet the needs of gluten-free customers since 2003 and can attest to the growth in its popularity. At first, the chain would have one order from their gluten-free menu every one to two weeks. In 2009, the restaurant served about 38 gluten-free orders per unit per day, or about 56,000 per week.[5]

What Jenny Learned

Fortunately for Jenny, symptoms caused by her exposure to wheat in the gravy were short-lived, and repeat testing showed that she had normal celiac antibody levels. Because Jenny still wants to eat out with her friends, she has researched their favorite restaurants and found a few options to order at each one that are safe for her. She has promised her mother that she still will mention her need to eat gluten free when ordering. Jenny plans to ask her parents for an iPod Touch for her birthday so she can use the application that will help her eat safely at other restaurants.

International Travel

Jeremy was diagnosed with celiac disease when he was seven years old, and his mother, Marin, was diagnosed soon after. Jeremy's family loves to travel, and his mother often goes abroad for work, so they made two important decisions shortly after they started living gluten free: they would not let the GFD "rule life" and they would not let it keep them from traveling or doing any of the things they wanted to do.

On a recent trip, Marin and Jeremy dined with a Londoner with celiac disease whom they met through the Celiac Listserv (to subscribe, see page xi). After discussing where to eat and buy gluten-free food in London, they enjoyed two wonderful meals with their new friend and her husband at the couple's favorite gluten-free restaurants. A few days later, at a small hotel in Paris, mother and son refused the rolls and croissants at breakfast to the shock of the waiter, who could not imagine anyone saying "pas du pain." In her limited French, Marin explained about their intolerance to "ble" (wheat) and showed him a menu card in French so the waiter would understand the situation. The next morning, the hotel chef was delighted to heat up the gluten-free baguettes the family brought to breakfast and was careful not to contaminate the baguettes during the heating. But on the return flight from Paris, when meals were served, Marin and Jeremy were given one gluten-free meal and one vegetarian meal. When they asked the flight attendant for the second gluten-free meal they had preordered, they were told, "This is what they gave us; you will have to eat the vegetarian meal." They politely declined the vegetarian meal, explaining that it is not gluten free.

While in Beijing for a scientific meeting, Marin traveled with a small group to other parts of China. The trip organizers were informed about Marin's need for gluten-free food and told Marin that they discussed the food requirements with the hotel where the group was attending a VIP luncheon with the mayor of a small town. Marin noted that some of the food served to her was different from the other diners and felt reassured that her meal was prepared to be gluten free. But, when she took a bite of the chicken dish, she became worried and asked the tour organizer to check again about whether it was gluten free. A waiter removed the dish, and an organizer told Marin that, "they thought that you would want to try this special dish even though it has wheat." Marin again had to emphasize to the tour organizer that eating even a little bit of wheat can make someone with celiac disease quite sick.

Jeremy and Marin know that traveling with a GFD can be fun if they plan ahead; it has even led to new friendships. But even when you plan ahead, things can go wrong. They have also found that it is far easier to travel in some countries, such as Norway, the United Kingdom, and Italy, than in others, such as China and Southern Germany. Even when the importance of a strict GFD is explained, they found that cultural practices can affect which food is served. For these reasons, Marin leans toward visiting China again only on a tour organized by professionals to be gluten free, such as Bob and Ruth's Travel Club (Table 2).

SELF-MANAGEMENT TIPS FOR TRAVELING GLUTEN FREE

1. **Do your homework.** This includes posting messages on the Celiac Listserv (see page xi) asking about places to eat and where to buy gluten-free food in the areas where you will be traveling. Look for the celiac-friendly Web sites for the different countries, and whenever possible find the location of health food stores. Consider that in some countries, such as in the United Kingdom, gluten-free food is sold in pharmacies.

2. **Always travel with food.** Take sufficient food to get you through the flights even when you have ordered gluten-free airline meals. This is essential because you want to feel good when you get to your destination. Airline gluten-free breakfasts can sometimes be quite minimal, such as a couple of rice cakes and some fruit. Observe what other passengers are being served and ask whether there is extra yogurt or cheese available.

3. **Confirm your gluten-free meal at every step.** Order it well ahead of your flight, confirm that it is listed when you check in, and ask the flight attendant to check to be sure they have your meal as soon as you are seated on the plane.

4. **Select hotels carefully.** When you have a choice of hotels, remember that those with full buffet breakfasts are particularly convenient because there are

usually many gluten-free foods, including yogurt, eggs, some cheeses, some meats, fruit, and nuts. Note that chefs may add wheat flour to liquid eggs that are standing on a buffet line ready to become your made-to-order omelet. If you bring your own cereal, milk is generally available.

5. **When you get to your destination, visit the grocery and health food stores for gluten-free food and snacks**. This is an exciting opportunity to try new and unusual gluten-free products. In Scandinavian countries and Europe, look for gluten-free crackers and other flatbreads and breads, gluten-free muesli cereal, and even gluten-free beers. Try Norwegian fish cakes or Swiss rostii, which is traditionally prepared with potatoes.

6. **Carry gluten-free restaurant cards in the languages of the countries that you will be visiting.** These cards make traveling much easier (Table 2), especially if you bring multiple copies to use in case you leave them behind. Learn the local language words for wheat, rye, malt, barley, and brewer's yeast.

7. **Eat early if possible and avoid "tourist" restaurants.** If you avoid crowds, you will have a better chance to talk to the chef and waiters about the food. Even if the waiter tells you they can accommodate a gluten-free meal, it is probably a good idea to ask about a specific dish or two because you get detailed feedback about the ingredients and a feel for the depth of their knowledge about the GFD. When menus and/or plastic food models are posted outside, you can decide if the restaurant has the type of food you want and identify potential gluten-free selections. Have a "default" healthy gluten-free meal in mind, such as grilled salmon, a baked potato, and a large salad with oil and vinegar dressing on the side.

8. **Be pleasant and appreciative but emphatic about your dietary requirement.** Be sure to thank the flight attendant for checking on your meal and the waiter for checking with the chef about dinner ingredients. They are helping you, and it is important to show your appreciation. At the same time, convey to them the importance of your dietary need and that you're not eating gluten free by choice but because it is essential to your health.

9. **Never hesitate to question the food or send it back.** It's valid for you to have questions about what you have been served or to ask the waiter or the chef to check that it is the right meal and that it is gluten free. If it is not correct, send it back. Be firm but insistent. Do not accept salads with evidence of croutons removed or meals where a gluten-containing item has been included. When ordering, ask what is served with the dish even if it is described on the menu. Note that foods like fried potatoes can be contaminated with wheat, so you don't want them on your plate.

10. **When you get home, share your experiences and tips.** Post a note to the Celiac Listserv informing others about the foods and restaurants that worked well for you. Having up-to-date information is one of the keys to safe and fun travel.

References

1. Cureton P. Gluten-free dining out: is it safe? *Pract Gastroenterol* 2006;XXX(11):61–67.
2. Allergy-Free Passport, Gluten-Free Passport: *Understanding Gluten and Allergen-Free Experiences Worldwide: Global Perspectives of Consumers, Hospitality & Food Service (executive summary)*. 2010. http://www.glutenfreepassport.com/pdf/ExecutiveSummary.pdf. Accessed 12/7/2009.
3. Lee A, et al. Quality of life of individuals with coeliac disease in the United States. *J Hum Nutr Diet*. In press.
4. Rashid M, et al. Celiac disease: evaluation of the diagnosis and dietary compliance in Canadian children. *Pediatrics* 2005;116:754–59.
5. Marcin G. Can gluten-free heat up your business? *The National Culinary Review* 2009; August:22–25.

Pam Cureton, RD, LDN, is a dietitian who specializes in celiac disease at the University of Maryland School of Medicine, Baltimore, in the Division of Pediatric Gastroenterology and Nutrition and the Center for Celiac Research. Her work includes clinical management of patients with celiac disease; educational programs for the celiac community, physician, dietitians, and other health care providers; and research. **Mary C. McKenna, PhD, LDN, CNS,** is an Associate Professor in the Department of Pediatrics, University of Maryland School of Medicine, Baltimore. Her primary research focus is on normal and altered brain development and neuroprotection. She and her son have both been on the gluten-free diet since 1993.

CHAPTER 27

Infant Feeding and Celiac Disease

Katrina Nordyke, BSN, RN, MPH, and Anneli Ivarsson, MD

S ara, a mother-to-be, is wondering if she should breastfeed her second child, due soon. "I've been hearing a lot about celiac disease. What is the best way to feed my baby?" Sara's older child, who was breastfed for three months, was recently diagnosed with celiac disease, and Sara wants to know if there is something she could have done to prevent it.

How we feed our infants is influenced by the current recommendations of major health organizations, cultural practices, and available resources. If you are a parent with celiac disease, or if you have a child with celiac disease, like Sara, you may be wondering whether certain infant feeding practices are connected to the development of celiac disease.

Infant Feeding Recommendations

Infant feeding recommendations and practices vary around the globe. The current recommendation of the World Health Organization (WHO) stresses the importance of breastfeeding and caregiver access to appropriate information regarding infant feeding, as well as access to skilled support during this time,[1] as breastfeeding can be a challenge for some mothers and families.

- The WHO recommends that, "As a global public health recommendation, infants should be exclusively breastfed for the first six months of life to achieve optimal growth, development and health. Thereafter . . . infants should receive nutritionally adequate and safe complementary foods while breastfeeding continues for up to two years of age or beyond."[1]
- The American Pediatric Association also recommends exclusively breastfeeding for six months and gradual introduction of foods at around that age, with continued breastfeeding for at least the first year of life.[2]
- The European society that deals with pediatric nutrition (ESPGHAN) also recommends exclusively breastfeeding for around six months and encourages continuing to breastfeed while introducing additional foods.[3]

However, only the latter recommendation addresses the possible role that infant feeding may play in the development of celiac disease. ESPGHAN suggests beginning with gluten when the infant is between four and six months old and if possible while the infant is still breastfeeding.[3]

Lessons from an Epidemic of Celiac Disease

Until the 1990s, we believed that celiac disease was unavoidable if a person had inherited the genetic risk from a parent. Then, between about 1984 and 1996, Sweden experienced an epidemic of celiac disease in children younger than two years of age. Diagnosis of celiac disease surged to levels higher than found in any other country and then sharply declined back to the previous level.[4] Clearly, genetics isn't the only thing that determines the development of celiac disease; environment and lifestyle are important factors, too.

Because the Swedish epidemic struck the youngest, many suspected that two recent nationwide changes in infant feeding practices were to blame. The first was that the national recommendation on when to introduce gluten to infants changed, from beginning at four months of age to beginning at six months of age. Note that it is during this time interval that breastfeeding often ends. The second change was that the amount of wheat in commercially prepared infant foods increased, resulting in higher gluten consumption by infants.[4]

In examining the data from the epidemic, we found that the proportion of infants introduced abruptly to large amounts of gluten while not being breastfed increased along with the diagnosis of celiac disease.[4] The risk of developing celiac disease was lower when gluten-containing foods were introduced gradually into the diet while the infant was still being breastfed, with even more protection given by prolonged breastfeeding.[4,5] Other studies have confirmed this finding.[6]

Therefore, it's important to breastfeed while introducing gluten to an infant's diet.[4,5] It's not clear exactly how breastfeeding offers this protection. It may be related to the differences in the intestinal bacteria between breastfed and formula-fed infants.[7] We need more research to understand whether breastfeeding and the way gluten is introduced actually reduces the risk for celiac disease or just modifies the symptoms, causing the disease to become apparent later in life.[7,8] An ongoing study of families with celiac disease is examining whether gradual introduction of gluten into an infant's diet, within the four- to six-month age interval, while breastfeeding protects against developing celiac disease.[8]

There may also be a critical age interval in which tolerance to gluten has a greater chance of developing. Findings suggest that the age interval of from four to six months of age may be the optimal time to begin introducing gluten into the infant's diet.[9] Also, introducing gluten-containing foods in small or medium amounts, rather than in large amounts, reduces the risk for celiac disease.[4,5] Another study is exploring whether delaying gluten introduction to up to one year of age protects against developing celiac disease.[10]

Other environmental factors have been shown to be associated with the development of celiac disease, such as seasonality in births, infections early in life, socioeconomic conditions, and gender.[7] It remains to be determined how these factors, along with other issues related to infant feeding practices, contribute to celiac disease risk. It is likely that an individual's genetic makeup interacts with environmental and lifestyle exposures to shape the immunological response to gluten. Once identified, celiac disease prevention could be possible, at least in some individuals.

What Sara Decided

Sara decided that she would introduce gluten-containing cereals to her newborn in small amounts, per her pediatrician's recommendation, starting when her baby was about four months old. She said she planned to continue to breastfeed while introducing even more foods. Because Sara's older child developed celiac disease, she will also have her new baby tested at the appropriate age (see Chapter 11 on testing strategies for children at high risk for developing celiac disease).

SELF-MANAGEMENT TIPS

☐ Genetics, environment, and lifestyle all play a role in the development of celiac disease.

☐ Breastfeeding is recommended for all newborns as a way to optimize their health, development, and psychosocial outcomes. Breastfeeding is likely to be even more important if celiac disease is in the family.

☐ The risk for celiac disease is likely to be reduced when gluten is introduced gradually and in small amounts into the infant's diet while still being breastfed.

☐ Findings suggest that the time to do this is beginning when the infant is between four and six months old.

Resources for Healthy Infant Feeding

- http:www.nal.usda.gov/fnic/pubs/bibs/gen/infnut./pdf
- http://fnic.nal.usda.gov/nal_display/index.php?info_center=4&taxlevel=2&tax_subject=358&level3_id=0&level4_id=0&level5_id=0&topicid=1612&&placement_default=0
- http://www.nal.usda.gov/wicworks/Topics/Infant_Feeding_Guide.html

References

1. WHO, UNICEF. *Global Strategy for Infant and Young Child Feeding.* Geneva: World Health Organization, 2003.
2. American Academy of Pediatrics policy statement. Breastfeeding and the use of Human Milk. *Pediatrics* 2005;115:496–506.

3. ESPGHAN (*European Society for Pediatric Gastroenterology, Hepatology, and Nutrition*) Committee on Nutrition. Complementary feeding: A commentary by the ESPGHAN Committee on Nutrition. *J Pediatr Gastroenterol Nutr* 2008;46:99–110.

4. Ivarsson A, Persson LÅ, Nyström L, et al. Epidemic of coeliac disease in Swedish children. *Acta Paediatr* 2000;89:165–71.

5. Ivarsson A, Hernell O, Stenlund H, et al. Breast-feeding protects against celiac disease. *Am J Clin Nutr* 2002;75:914–21.

6. Akobeng AK, Ramanan AV, Buchan I, et al. Effects of breast feeding on risk of coeliac disease: a systematic review and meta-analysis of observational studies. *Arch Dis Child* 2006;91:39–43.

7. Ivarsson A, Myléus A, Wall S. Towards preventing celiac disease: an epidemiological approach. *In* Fasano A, Troncone R, Branski D, Eds. *Frontiers in Celiac Disease. Pediatr Adolesc Med* Basel: Karger 2008, p. 198–209.

8. Troncone R, Ivarsson A, Szajewska H, et al. Future research on coeliac disease: a position report from the European multistakeholder platform on coeliac disease (CDEUSSA). *Aliment Pharmacol Ther* 2008;27:1030–43.

9. Norris JM, Barriga K, Hoffenberg EJ, et al. Risk of celiac disease autoimmunity and timing of gluten introduction in the diet of infants at increased risk of disease. *JAMA* 2005;293:2343–51.

10. Fasano A. Surprises from celiac disease. *Sci Am* 2009;301(Aug):54–61.

Katrina Nordyke, BSN, RN, MPH, is a doctoral candidate in the Department of Public Health and Clinical Medicine, Epidemiology and Global Health, Umeå University, Umeå, Sweden, and a nursing instructor in the Department of Nursing, College of Menominee Nation, Keshena, Wisconsin. **Anneli Ivarsson, MD,** is a pediatrician in the Department of Public Health and Clinical Medicine, Epidemiology and Global Health, Umeå University, Umeå, Sweden.

CHAPTER 28

Nutrition and Adjustment Issues for Children with Celiac Disease

Mary K. Sharrett, MS, RD, LD, CNSD

Emily was diagnosed with celiac disease at 16 months old after several months of poor growth, vomiting, diarrhea, and formula/milk changes. At the gastroenterologist's office, Emily's mom and dad were very relieved to find out finally what was causing Emily so much trouble. Emily and her parents met with the dietitian, who taught them about the gluten-free diet (GFD). Two weeks after starting the GFD, Emily was feeling better. She was no longer vomiting or having diarrhea, much to her parents' relief. At age 2, Emily was doing very well, and both her weight and height had returned to the 50th percentile, which is where she was at 6 months of age.

Shortly after Emily turned 2, her mother started working full time and began looking for a preschool. None of the schools she considered were able to accommodate Emily's GFD, however, so Mom found a private babysitter.

Emily's parents encouraged their relatives, especially Emily's two cousins, to get screened for celiac disease. Because Emily's cousins had no gastrointestinal symptoms, their parents decided not to test them. One year later, Emily's 10-year-old cousin Nate broke two bones while playing, and it was discovered that his bone density was below normal. Nate was screened for celiac disease and had a positive tissue transglutaminase (tTG) antibody level and a small intestinal biopsy consistent with celiac disease.

Emily and her cousin illustrate how different the presenting symptoms of celiac disease can be at different ages.[1-3] Emily had the classic symptoms of celiac disease, and it took a few months for her to get diagnosed. Nate had none of the typical symptoms but suffered the consequences of not absorbing calcium and vitamin D because of the damage to his small intestine.

The Parents' Role

Having a child diagnosed with celiac disease presents parents with many challenges. The first step is usually to learn about how to use the GFD to keep your child safe. The next step is to educate all of the other people who take care of your child, from babysitters to schools to coaches to relatives, about your child's requirements. Parents can expect to spend a lot of time and energy helping relatives and even health professionals learn about celiac disease and the GFD.

Emily's and Nate's parents faced many challenges with the school systems. Emily's parents could not find a preschool that was willing to work with them to keep Emily safe. The babysitter they found was familiar with celiac disease because one of her granddaughters had it. The babysitter had attended sessions on the GFD with her granddaughter's parents and had already made a gluten-free section in her kitchen for her granddaughter's frequent visits. She even made her own gluten-free version of Play-Doh from rice flour.

Nate's parents met with the school nurse, the principal, the food service director, and the school dietitian and informed them all about celiac disease (Table 1). They reviewed the school menu and decided that Nate would bring his lunch to school and they would buy a few safe items like milk and fruit cups to add to his lunch. His parents provided the school

TABLE 1. What Your Child's School Needs to Know about Celiac Disease

- The GFD eliminates wheat, rye, and barley and anything derived from these grains.
- Some foods are easily contaminated with gluten, such as oats, so they need to come from a reliable source that guarantees they are gluten free.
- Contamination can occur during food preparation. Therefore, food needs to be prepared and eaten in a gluten-free area. Tiny amounts of bread and flour can contain enough gluten to be harmful. Countertops and cafeteria tables need to be cleaned before food preparation and before eating.
- When food is prepared in the cafeteria, all utensils and equipment need to be cleaned first. Preparing the gluten-free food before gluten-containing foods will help prevent cross-contamination through the equipment.
- There are many commercially available gluten-free foods. However, all labels need to be checked. The safety of some products will vary from manufacturer to manufacturer.
- When food is prepared at home, there is potential for cross-contamination. Therefore, food from classmates' homes should not be offered to the gluten-free child unless approved by the parent.
- Ingestion of gluten may not result in an immediate reaction. However, it is important to inform the school what symptoms your child may have and allow the child to go to the restroom if necessary or to see the school nurse.
- Craft projects using products made with wheat flour, such as Play-Doh or papier maché, can be an issue for some kids because it ends up in their mouths.
- If the classroom teacher frequently provides treats for the students, it may be helpful to provide a list of safe treats or a supply of safe treats.
- Encourage the teacher or room volunteers to contact the parent in advance when special occasions are planned so that an appropriate gluten-free substitute can be provided.
- Incorporating celiac disease or the GFD into lesson plans can help the gluten-free student and the rest of the students understand why the diet is necessary.

TABLE 2. Nate's Gluten-Free Treat Choices

Microwave popcorn	Snickers bars
Envirokidz Crispy Rice Bars	Lifesavers
Small packages of gluten-free pretzels	M & Ms
Individual servings of peanut butter	Skittles

with *The Gluten-Free Diet Guide for Families* (available at www.celiachealth.org). They also gave Nate's teacher an airtight tin box with a stash of gluten-free treats so that Nate had something to eat that he liked when his classmates brought in treats that he couldn't share (Table 2).

When Nate was 12 years old, he switched schools, and his new school already had several students with celiac disease. They encouraged Nate's family to get a letter from his gastroenterologist that detailed exactly what a GFD is and how his education might be affected if he did not follow the diet. The new school worked with the family to develop a 504 plan, which specified the accommodations that the school agreed to make to ensure that Nate stayed gluten free. The school dietitian had developed a gluten-free menu and a training program for the foodservice staff to prevent cross-contamination, so Nate was able to buy a gluten-free school lunch. Details on 504 plans and sample doctor's letters are provided by the American Celiac Disease Alliance at www.americanceliac.org.

Helping Your Child Stay Gluten Free

Emily suffered from diarrhea and vomiting if she accidently ingested something with gluten in it. In grade school, she became very good at reading labels and refused to eat foods when she did not know the ingredients or the details of how the food was prepared.

Nate had no gastrointestinal symptoms when he ate gluten. He admitted to "cheating" on several occasions, especially when his friends offered him certain foods and treats. Unfortunately, Nate suffered from a third bone fracture. At that time, his level of tTG antibody was positive and his bone density was still not normal.

Several studies have shown that adolescents who develop gastrointestinal symptoms when they ingest gluten are more likely to stay gluten free than those who can cheat without getting sick.[4-7] Kids and teens are usually more focused on the present and have a harder time thinking about long-term consequences. Remember, even adults who understand what long-term damage they can do (but don't see) cheat!

Compliance varies across the world, but it's vital for you to understand that children with celiac disease who eat completely gluten free have an improved quality of life and fewer disease-related complications.[4-7] Keep this in mind when you are explaining the reasons for major changes in your child's life and your family's lifestyle.

Making Nutrition a Priority

There is no research looking at the nutritional quality of a child's GFD. However, studies have evaluated the GFDs of adults and found that their diets are frequently low in calcium, iron, B vitamins, and fiber.[8,9] Therefore, it's vital to have your child's diet reviewed by a dietitian and consider whether he or she would benefit by taking an age-appropriate gluten-free multivitamin and mineral supplement.

After eight months on the GFD, Emily had problems with constipation. A review of her typical eating plan revealed that, although she was eating gluten free, the cereals and bread products she was consuming were made from starches with little fiber in them. Emily's dietitian encouraged her parents to try products that were made with nutrient-dense and high-fiber gluten-free grains, such as amaranth, quinoa, buckwheat, flax, and millet (see Chapter 13 on gluten-free grains).

Nate's problem with bone density is very common in children with celiac disease, and osteopenia (bone loss) is often discovered at diagnosis. A strict GFD may restore bone mass back to normal.[10–13] Nate required some additional counseling and follow-up visits to convince him to maintain his GFD to help him reach optimal bone health. He was also not getting enough milk in his diet and agreed to increase his milk intake to improve his calcium and vitamin D intake. After one year of eating gluten-free and increased calcium, Nate's bone density was back to normal.

SELF-MANAGEMENT TIPS

☐ Teach your child about the GFD. Together, develop a list of gluten-free foods to guide his or her food choices at home, while eating at school or in restaurants, and from vending machines and grocery stores.

☐ Talk about situations in advance, such as adults insisting that your child eat a gluten-containing food, so your child has choices and knows what to do.

☐ Take your child to education sessions with a dietitian. The dietitian will review your child's eating plan and make suggestions as needed for improving the nutritional value or for treating problems, such as low levels of fiber or vitamin D. This will reinforce the information you are teaching and provide your child with skills, such as reading food labels, that are empowering.

☐ Your child will benefit from meeting other children who are living with celiac disease. You may be able to find local support specifically for children and their families. In support groups, you are likely to hear about new food products and places to eat that are gluten free. More information about support groups is at www.celiac.com. A list of resources is in Table 3.

☐ Be prepared to educate your child's teachers, school administrators, and other staff about celiac disease and your child's requirements. Investigate writing a 504 plan to help ensure your child's treatment at school.

TABLE 3. Resources for Families

Resources for Parents and Educators

Incredible Edible Gluten-Free Food For Kids by Sheri L Sanderson, www.woodbinehouse.com

Kids with Celiac Disease, A Family Guide To Raising Happy, Healthy, Gluten-Free Children by Danna Korn, www.woodbinehouse.com

Wheat-Free Gluten-Free Cookbook for Kids & Busy Adults by Connie Sarros, www.gfbooks. homestead.com

Growing Up Celiac by Canadian Celiac Association, www.celiac.ca

Celiac Family Health Education (DVD) by Boston Children's Hospital, www.childrenshospital.org/celiac

Gluten-Free Friends: An Activity Book For Kids by Nancy Patin-Falini, www.savorypalate.com

R.O.C.K.: Raising our Celiac Kids: www.celiackids.com

Kids Health: http://kidshealth.org/kid/nutrition/diets/celiac.html

Understanding your Student & Students with Celiac Disease by The Gluten Intolerance Group, www.gluten.net

Cel-Kids Network, Celiac Sprue Association/United States of America: www.csaceliacs.org

Kids Korner, Celiac Disease Foundation: www.celiac.org

American Celiac Disease Alliance, advocacy and school resources: www.americanceliac.org

Children's Digestive Health and Nutrition Foundation: www.celiachealth.org

Kids Corner, Celiac Disease Center at Columbia University: www.celiacdiseasecenter.columbia.edu

Books for Pre-School to School-Age Children

Eating Gluten-Free with Emily by Bonnie J. Kruszka, illustrated by Richard S. Cihlar, www.woodbinehouse.com

How I Eat Without Wheat by Karen Fine, illustrated by Russ Novak, www.authorhouse.com

No More Cupcakes and Tummy Aches by Jax Peters Lowell, illustrated by Jane Kirkwood, www.barnesandnoble.com

Bagels, Buddy and Me by Melanie Krumrey, illustrated by author, www.Baglesbuddyandme.com

The Trouble That Jack Had by Jane Pintavalle and Diane Pintavalle, http://www.chw.org/display/displayFile.asp?docid=33040&filename=/Groups/CHW/Celiac_book.pdf

Lunch With Quinn: The Story of One Child's Diagnosis and Management of Celiac Disease by Angela Porter, www.authorhouse.com

Resources for Preadolescents through College Age

The Gluten Free Kid: A Celiac Disease Survival Guide by Melissa London, www.woodbinehouse.com

Beyond Rice Cakes: A Young Person's Guide to Cooking, Eating & Living Gluten-Free by Vanessa Martin, www.celiaccentral.org

TAGS-Gluten-free Teen Support Groups: www.site.tagsatgig.com

The Gluten-Free College Blog: Gfguideny.com

Gluten Free College Student Cookbook: 201 GF/CF Recipes for Campus Cooking by Joanna Bradley, www.amazon.com

Gluten-Free–Friendly Places for Families

Contact the parks prior to your visit for the most up to date information.

Disney Parks: http://disneyworld.disney.go.com/guest-services/special-dietary-requests/; http://disneyland.disney.go.com/disneyland/en_US/help/detail?name=DiningFAQPage

Hershey Park: www.hersheypark.com/food_and_shops/ingredients/index.php

Six Flags

Sea World

Busch Gardens

Summer Camp

The Celiac Disease Foundation keeps an updated list of Summer camps: www.celiac.org

References

1. Fasano A. Clinical presentation of celiac disease in the pediatric population. *Gastroenterology* 2005;128:S68–S73.
2. Telega G, Bennet TR, Werlin S. Emerging new clinical patterns in the presentation of celiac disease. *Arch Pediatr Adoles Med* 2008;162:164–68.
3. Hill ID, Dirks MH, Liptak GS, et al. Guideline for the diagnosis and treatment of celiac disease in children: recommendations of the North American Society for Pediatric Gastroenterology, Hepatology and Nutrition. *J Pediatr Gastroenterol Nutr* 2005;40:1–19.
4. Fabiani E, Catassi C, Villari A, Gismondi P, Peirdomenico R, Ratsch IM, Coppa GV, Giorgi PL. Dietary compliance in screening-detected coeliac disease adolescents. *Acta Paediatr Suppl* 1996; 412:65–67.
5. Wagner, G, Berger G, Sinnereich, U Grylli V, Schober E, Huber WD, Karwautz. Quality of life in adolescents with treated coeliac disease: influence of compliance and age at diagnosis. *J Pediatr Gastroenterol Nutr* 2008;47:555–61.
6. Jaderesin O, Misak Z, Kolacek S, Sonicki Z, Zizic V. Compliance with gluten-free diet in children with coeliac disease. *J Pediatr Gastroenterol Nutr* 2008;47:344–48.
7. Rashid M, Cranney A, Zarkadas M, Graham ID, Switzer C, Case S, Molloy M, Warren RE, Burrows V, Butzner JD. Celiac disease: evaluation of the diagnosis and dietary compliance in Canadian children. *Pediatrics* 2005;116:754–59.
8. Thompson T. Thiamin, riboflavin, and niacin contents of the gluten-free diet: is there cause for concern? *J Am Diet Assoc* 1999;99:858–62.
9. Thompson T, Dennis M, Higgins L, Lee A, Sharrett M. Gluten-free diet survey: are Americans with coeliac disease consuming recommended amounts of fibre, iron, calcium, and grain foods? *J Hum Nutr Diet* 2005;18(3)163–69.
10. Mora S. Celiac disease in children: impact on bone health. *Rec Endocr Metab Disord* 2008; 9:123–30.
11. Tau C, Mautalen C, De Rosa S, Roca A, Valenxuela X. Bone mineral density in children with celiac disease, effect of a gluten-free diet. *Eur J Clin Nutr* 2006;60:358–63.
12. Barera G, Mora S, Brambilla P, Ricotti A, L, Beccio S, Bianchi C. Body composition in children with celiac disease and the effects of a gluten-free diet: a prospective case-control study. *Am J Clin Nutr* 200;72:71–75.
13. Jatla M, Zemel BS, Bierly P, Verma R. Bone mineral content deficts of the spine and whole body in children at time of diagnosis with celiac disease. *J Pediatr Gastroenterol Nutr* 2009; 48:175–80.

Mary K. Sharrett, MS, RD, LD, CNSD, is a clinical dietitian at Nationwide Children's Hospital in Columbus, Ohio, and the dietitian advisor to the Gluten-Free Gang.

CHAPTER 29

Teens with Celiac Disease and Gluten-Free Eating

Cecilia Olsson, RD, and Agneta Hörnell, RD

Diane, a 16-year-old, was diagnosed with celiac disease two years ago. At the time, she had iron deficiency anemia and mild symptoms of loose stool and abdominal discomfort. Since diagnosis, Diane reported that her symptoms had improved; however, her tissue transglutaminase (tTG) antibodies were still elevated, and she remained iron deficient. She was seen in clinic to evaluate her ongoing gluten exposure.

During the visit, it became clear that Diane had a very good understanding of what the gluten-free diet (GFD) required. However, she noted that she had recently changed schools and found it difficult and embarrassing to keep a strict GFD outside the home.

Being a Teen with Celiac Disease

The daily lives of people with celiac disease are more problematic than previously recognized.[1-3] Adolescence, even in the absence of a medical disorder, is a challenging period in life characterized by physical, psychological, and social development issues. Being a teen is even more demanding when you have celiac disease and have to face lifelong dietary restrictions and the everyday decision of whether or not to comply with the GFD.

It's common to choose not to adhere to the GFD, especially among teens. Factors influencing adherence are not fully understood, but they are most likely multiple and overlapping, as with other chronic diseases. Teens with celiac disease generally take one of three approaches to eating gluten free (Table 1). Their decisions are related to whether they have symptoms related to gluten ingestion; how confident they feel in their knowledge about eating gluten free; how available gluten-free food choices are; whether they like the taste of the available gluten-free foods; and when, where, and with whom they are eating.[2]

Being Different Because of Different Food

When our personal attributes, such as having a chronic disease, have the potential to influence social approval negatively, it can create a *stigma*. A stigma influences how we are viewed by others and how we view ourselves. Stigma experiences can range from actual

TABLE 1. Teens' Reasons for Adhering or Not Adhering to the GFD

Category	Gluten-Free Teen	Partially Gluten-Free Teen	Teen Not Gluten Free
Symptoms after gluten ingestion	Presence of symptoms can be a motivator for adherence	Absence of symptoms can be a reason for nonadherence	Absence or disregard of symptoms can be a reason for nonadherence
Knowledge affecting confidence in the treatment	Consideration of long-term complications promotes adherence whether symptoms are present or not	Incorrect beliefs sometimes explain nonadherence	Limited knowledge or disregard of the importance of treatment sometimes explains nonadherence
Availability of gluten-free alternatives	A matter of rationality, flexibility, and planning	Poor availability becomes an excuse for occasional nonadherence	Poor availability becomes an excuse for nonadherence
Sensory characteristics of gluten-free food	Normal food tastes better but still sticks with the GFD	Normal food tastes better so sometimes it is hard to abstain from gluten-containing foods	Normal food tastes better so I will not abstain
Social discomfort	Yes, but access to good enough motivators and social support ensures adherence	Yes, and under certain circumstances, results in nonadherence	Yes, and is often frustrating enough to result in nonadherence

discrimination to fear of social dislike. We all want to appear "normal," and if we think we have a stigma, we might use various strategies to conceal any readily apparent differences.

Keeping to the GFD can have consequences if doing so offends the social rules surrounding food and meals. For example, you might be thought impolite if you refuse the food that is offered or available. Eating the same food as everyone else can help you avoid the social consequences of not following expectations, but it has serious health consequences for you if it involves eating gluten-containing foods.

Feeling different or experiencing stigma can be a reality of everyday life for adolescents with celiac disease.[3] Having to search for and select gluten-free foods makes them visible in public. Gluten-free foods often look different and generally are not readily available, so the likelihood of appearing different is greater. The experience of stigma is more likely to happen outside the home, where teens are often challenged to improvise in various situations. Circumstances at home are more predictable, although there may still be practical, social, and personal dilemmas among family members.

Needing to find gluten-free food, or being served gluten-free foods, can place teens in the center of attention in a way that is unwelcome because it highlights their differences from others.[3] Lack of knowledge, misconceptions, and carelessness on the part of others can either diminish or amplify the importance of this treatment for celiac disease. It can be embarrassing and demanding to be thought as "special," "a victim," or "a bother" in the eyes of others.

Friends and family may have limited understanding about the potential health consequences of deviating from the GFD and challenge or neglect your need for gluten-free alternatives.[3] You may have to bring your own food to school events, celebrations, and parties to make sure that you will have something safe to eat. In school, kitchen staff may not remember the student who has celiac disease or confuse you with other students or other special diets. The requested gluten-free dish can, therefore, be incomplete, improperly prepared, or not available.

How a teen manages this stigma can vary and is to a high degree dependent on the perceived risk of stigma in a given situation.[3] Not following the GFD outside of home might be a solution if it results in a much more comfortable encounter with peers. Try to view a teen's decision to comply or not with the GFD in terms of his or her need to cope with concealing and disclosing special dietary needs.

How to Support a Teen

Adolescents with celiac disease want to pass for "normal."[2,3] This is much easier when there is social support and easy availability of tasty and normal appearing gluten-free foods outside the home. For this to happen, there must be knowledge about celiac disease and treatment with the GFD among friends and family and within society at large. We don't know if boys and girls differ in their ability to adapt to life with celiac disease and a GFD. They may use different strategies and need somewhat different types of support to make it easier to comply with the GFD.

Find ways to increase other people's awareness of and familiarity with your teen's dietary needs. This makes it easier for him or her to gain access to gluten-free alternatives with a minimum of comments or questions. In the school setting, this can often be achieved if one person among the kitchen staff is specially trained and responsible for special diets. You may need to do the training about the GFD. Restaurants could achieve this via skilled chefs with knowledge of gluten-free cooking and clear statements on menus that a meal is gluten-free or could be easily adjusted on request. Consider whether you have a family favorite restaurant where you could approach the chef about this issue.

It's comforting for teens to meet other teens who also have celiac disease.[3] This provides opportunities to share common experiences and discuss how to manage the stigma. In addition, friends with celiac disease make everyday life easier because gluten-free food is always available in their homes. And just talking things over among themselves about their condition is often empowering because it can strengthen their capacity to deal with social dilemmas. Feeling empowered is a vital trait that is especially important as a teen makes the transition to adulthood. This will ensure that your teen continues to seek out and ask for regular, appropriate medical and dietary follow-up care.

What Diane Did

It was apparent that Diane understood the GFD well and was aware of the consequences of continued gluten exposure. For this reason, the visit focused on strategies to reduce the stigma and her burden of staying gluten free outside the home. Through the local celiac disease advocacy group, Diane was able to meet a number of teens her age in her area. Her parents contacted the school cafeteria, and after some education, cafeteria staff agreed to provide gluten-free options every day for Diane.

At her follow-up visit three months later, Diane noted that, although it was sometimes still stressful, it had become gradually easier for her to keep the GFD around her peers. Diane's blood tests revealed her efforts: She now had a normal iron level and a lower tTG, which provided positive reinforcement for her efforts.

SELF-MANAGEMENT TIPS

☐ Make sure your teen is well educated about celiac disease and the importance of staying gluten free, even if he or she does not experience immediate symptoms from gluten exposure.

☐ Reducing the stigma of following a GFD is vital for helping adolescents follow it successfully.

☐ Strategies for reducing stigma focus on lessening the burden of staying gluten free, such as being supportive and making sure your teen can safely and conveniently obtain enough gluten-free foods.

☐ Meeting peers with celiac disease or related disorders, such as food allergies, can be empowering. Sharing common experiences and ideas on how to better deal with social dilemmas better prepares teens for new situations and safe ways to improvise.

References

1. Hall NJ, Rubin G, Charnock A. Systematic review: adherence to a gluten-free diet in adult patients with coeliac disease. *Aliment Pharmacol Ther* 2009; 30:315–30.
2. Olsson C, Hörnell A, Ivarsson A, Sydner YM. The everyday life of adolescent coeliacs: issues of importance for compliance with the gluten-free diet. *J Hum Nutr Diet* 2008;21:359–67.
3. Olsson C, Lyon P, Hörnell A, Ivarsson A, Sydner YM. Food that makes you different: the stigma experienced by adolescents with celiac disease. *Qual Health Res* 2009;19:976–84.

Cecilia Olsson, RD, is a Senior Lecturer, and **Agneta Hörnell, RD,** is an Associate Professor in the Department of Food and Nutrition, Umeå University, Umeå, Sweden.

CHAPTER 30

Eating Disturbances in Celiac Disease

Jessica B. Edwards George, PhD, NCSP

Emily, a 26-year-old woman diagnosed with celiac disease two years ago, was also recently diagnosed with an eating disorder. Before being diagnosed with celiac disease, Emily suffered from the "classic" gastrointestinal symptoms and was severely malnourished. At that time, Emily could eat large amounts of food without consequential weight gain, likely because of the frequent diarrhea and undetected malabsorption she was experiencing. Family and friends always remarked about Emily's "bottomless appetite" yet very slender figure.

At age 24, Emily's symptoms finally led to her celiac disease diagnosis, and she began the gluten-free diet (GFD). Within months, Emily saw a significant reduction in her gastrointestinal symptoms and began to gain weight. Family and friends starting remarking to Emily about how healthy she now looked, but Emily resented these comments and felt "fat" now that she was carrying 120 pounds on her 5-foot 4-inch frame. Emily wished she could be 95 pounds again.

Emily tried eating less and exercising more to lose weight but did not get the results she wanted. She was extremely hungry and felt deprived by not being able to eat gluten-containing treats. She got into the habit of gorging on gluten-free foods and would eat an entire box of chocolate-glazed gluten-free donuts in one sitting. Emily would tell herself that she deserved the treats because she had to stay on an "awful cardboard diet."

In time, she became aware that her eating was out of control and that she was gaining more and more weight. So Emily began to vomit the gluten-free foods that she had overindulged in to avoid weight gain. Her bingeing and purging went on for some months, and although Emily did not gain any more weight, she also did not lose any weight and always felt bloated and puffy from the overeating and vomiting cycle. Emily was very dissatisfied with her "chubby" body and began eating gluten, believing that enduring her past gastrointestinal symptoms was "worth it to be thin again."

What Is an Eating Disorder?

Eating disorders include anorexia nervosa, bulimia nervosa, and eating disorder not otherwise specified (Table 1). Mental health and medical professionals classify eating disorders into specific diagnoses using the *Diagnostic and Statistical Manual of Mental Disorders-IV-Text Revision (DSM-IV-TR)* from the American Psychological Association.

Anorexia nervosa is characterized by a patient's refusal to maintain a normal weight (15% below that expected for an individual's height and weight), misperception of size, and absence of menstrual periods in a woman of reproductive age. Two subtypes are recognized, one characterized by binge eating or purging by means of self-induced vomiting or the use of laxatives or diuretics, and the other characterized by food restriction. Bulimia nervosa is defined by episodes of binge eating, in which there is a lack of control over consumption of large amounts of food at one time, followed by vomiting or laxative use. What both eating disorders share is that the person's self-worth is greatly influenced by how he or she perceives his or her own weight and shape.

Individuals with disordered eating behaviors that resemble anorexia or bulimia but whose eating behaviors do not meet the diagnostic criteria for either disorder may be diagnosed with eating disorder not otherwise specified. This includes binge eating disorder, in which individuals binge eat but do not regularly use inappropriate weight control behaviors, such as fasting or purging, to maintain or lose weight. Binge eating may involve the rapid consumption of food with a loss of sense of control, uncomfortable fullness after eating, and eating large amounts of food when not hungry. Individuals often feel ashamed or embarrassed after bingeing and binge eating disorder is often associated with obesity. Other examples of eating disorder not otherwise specified include those who meet the criteria for anorexia but continue to menstruate or those who purge but do not binge eat.

What Causes Eating Disorders?

Disordered eating behaviors often lead to eating disorders. Disordered eating covers a variety of behavioral problems related to eating, including extreme dieting, binge eating, vomiting or laxative use, diet pill use, fasting, and excessive exercise. Each of these behaviors has been linked to the development of eating disorders.

Body dissatisfaction, the difference between body perception and body preference, seems to be one of the drivers behind disordered eating behaviors. When there is a significant difference between how you perceive your body's shape and size and your preferred body shape and size, the result is dissatisfaction with your body. The larger the difference between one's body perception and body preference, the greater the body dissatisfaction and the greater the likelihood that that individual will develop disordered eating.

Eating disorders occur in as many as 5% of adolescents and adults. They are associated with significant health and psychosocial problems and represent sometimes life-threatening forms of psychological illness, and thus are very concerning. Anorexia nervosa has the highest mortality rate, between 6% and 20%, of any psychiatric illness because of high rates of suicide and increased medical consequences. On the other hand, disordered eating behaviors are rather common.

TABLE 1. Clinical Eating Disorders

Anorexia nervosa: restricting type	■ Refusal to maintain healthy body weight and is ≤85% of normal weight; or failure to make expected weight gain during period of growth, leading to body weight less than 85% of that expected ■ Irrational fear of gaining weight or becoming fat, even though underweight ■ Absence of menstruation in girls and women of reproductive age ■ Disturbance in the way one's body weight or shape is experienced, undue influence of body weight or shape on self-evaluation, or denial of the seriousness of current low body weight
Anorexia nervosa: binge eating/purging type	All criteria for the restricting type and either of the following: ■ Binge eating—eating an amount of food that is definitely larger than most people would eat during a similar period of time and under similar circumstances—or ■ Purging (vomiting, laxative or diuretic abuse) or other compensation (fasting, overexercise) to avoid weight gain
Bulimia nervosa: purging type	■ Binge eating—eating an amount of food that is definitely larger than most people would eat during a similar period of time and under similar circumstances ■ A sense of lack of control over eating during the episode, such as feeling as if one can't stop eating or control what or how much one is eating ■ Purging (vomiting, laxative or diuretic abuse) to prevent weight gain ■ May fast or excessively exercise in addition to purging behaviors ■ Self-evaluation is unduly influenced by body shape and weight ■ Weight typically normal or high
Bulimia nervosa: nonpurging type	■ All criteria above except do not purge, but follow binges with self-starvation or compulsive exercise
Eating disorder not otherwise specified	Examples: ■ For females, all of the criteria for anorexia are met except that the patient has regular menses. ■ All of the criteria for anorexia are met except that, despite significant weight loss, current weight remains in the normal range. ■ All of the criteria for bulimia are met except that the binge eating and inappropriate compensatory mechanisms are not frequent enough or persistent enough to warrant bulimia diagnosis. ■ Normal body weight and regular use of inappropriate compensatory behavior after eating small amounts of food, such as self-induced vomiting after consuming two cookies ■ Repeatedly chewing and spitting out, but not swallowing, large amounts of food ■ Binge eating disorder: recurrent episodes of binge eating in the absence of the compensatory behaviors characteristic of bulimia

Celiac Disease and Risk for Disordered Eating

It makes sense that, because the treatment for celiac disease is dietary, there would be a risk for those with it to develop an eating disorder. Here's why.

- To be successful with the GFD, those with celiac disease must maintain a high and persistent preoccupation with and hyperawareness of food. This preoccupation may develop into a dangerous obsession that results in problems in eating behaviors.
- The GFD is a restrictive diet that must be followed for life. This chronic restriction is a challenge. When food is restricted, it's human nature to want it more. For example, children on restrictive diets may sneak food. Being restricted to a GFD may make it more likely that someone will binge on forbidden foods or on high-calorie, high-fat gluten-free treats.
- For someone used to eating foods made with wheat, gluten-free foods are often not as palatable as gluten-containing foods. They are also more expensive and not available in many restaurants and grocery stores. These factors can lead to pressure, either internal or from peers and others, to eat typical gluten-containing foods.
- Some individuals with celiac disease are underweight at diagnosis as a result of malabsorption and malnutrition. Treatment with the GFD successfully reverses this in many, so people who are in the habit of eating large amounts of food without negative consequences to their weight and shape usually need to relearn portion size and control once their intestinal villi have healed. Sometimes, this weight gain causes them to be overweight or obese (see Chapter 17 on weight gain). Weight gain may signal successful treatment of celiac disease but can also trigger disordered eating behavior. This is similar to the normal weight gain that occurs in adolescence, which often leads teens to problematic eating behaviors, such as strict dieting and fasting, and other compensatory behaviors, such as self-induced vomiting.
- Case reports demonstrate that those with celiac disease sometimes choose to ingest gluten to cause diarrhea and vomiting, specifically to avoid gaining weight.

Celiac disease and eating disorders have been linked in a number of studies and case reports. Case reports have highlighted the complex ways in which celiac disease and eating disorders interact, suggesting that patients with celiac disease and their health care providers should be vigilant in watching out for these conditions.[1] One study found higher rates of eating disorders and disordered eating behaviors in adolescents with celiac disease, especially higher rates of bulimia, compared with prevalence estimates for eating disorders in the general population of adolescents in the United States and Europe.[2] In the study, 29% had disordered eating behaviors and 14% had a current eating disorder (all individuals with an eating disorder were female). Also, celiac blood tests showed that those with an eating disorder were twice as likely to struggle with following the GFD as those without an eating disorder.

What Happened to Emily

Emily's nutritionist uncovered her disordered eating behaviors during frequent meetings with Emily to counsel her about the GFD. She referred Emily to a psychologist and a psychiatrist for further evaluation of her symptoms. Initially, Emily refused these referrals, but in time she began to feel as though her life was spinning out of control and decided to accept help.

First, Emily began working with the psychologist, with whom she developed a trusting therapeutic relationship and rapport. This allowed Emily to start to use cognitive behavioral strategies to help her modify how she was thinking and her internal self-talk. In therapy, she learned to recognize her anxiety and depression and gain some control over problematic behavior patterns caused by these symptoms. Then, Emily agreed to take antidepressant medications prescribed by a psychiatrist to treat her underlying anxiety and depression, psychiatric disorders that commonly occur with eating disorders. Emily's nutritionist was pivotal in identifying her difficulties and getting Emily into psychiatric treatment, and she continued to see her for nutritional counseling. Over time, Emily developed healthy eating habits. Although Emily continues to struggle in her relationship with food, she is managing her psychiatric symptoms and no longer eats gluten to maintain her weight.

SELF-MANAGEMENT TIPS

☐ As the celiac disease diagnosis rate continues to rise, more people are at risk for disordered eating behaviors that can lead to eating disorders. Individuals with celiac disease and their health professionals need to be aware of this association to catch problems early.

☐ Don't suffer in silence if you are having problems controlling your eating behavior. Being on the GFD can be tough. Talk with your primary care physician, gastroenterologist, or nutritionist about your concerns. They will be able to assist you in identifying a mental health professional who can further evaluate your symptoms and provide you with appropriate help.

☐ If you are a parent, recognize that balancing the support you give your child in maintaining a GFD while avoiding putting food at the forefront of your child's life can be difficult. If you notice disordered eating behaviors in your child with celiac disease, early detection, proper evaluation, and ongoing management can play a significant role in recovery and in preventing an eating disorder from progressing to a more severe or long-lasting state. Talking with your child's health care providers about your concerns is a good first step. It will help if you are nonjudgmental and patient and listen to your child, showing that you care and are trying to understand.

□ Seek help from associations that provide education, resources, and support to those with eating disorders. For example, the National Eating Disorders Association (www.nationaleatingdisorders.org) has a variety of digital toolkits for help with a variety of eating issues and for parents who are concerned about their children. In addition, local celiac support groups may also have seminars on living with the GFD and eating concerns.

References

1. Leffler DA, Dennis M, Edwards George JB, Kelly CP. The interaction between eating disorders and celiac disease: an exploration of 10 cases. *Eur J Gastroenterol Hepatol* 2007;19:251–55.
2. Karwautz A, Wagner G, Berger G, Sinnreich U, Grylli V, Huber WD. Eating pathology in adolescents with celiac disease. *Psychosomatics* 2008;49:399–406.

Jessica B. Edwards George, PhD, NCSP, is a staff psychologist at Rhode Island Hospital/Hasbro Children's Hospital, Providence, Rhode Island. She is also Adjunct Assistant Professor of Pediatrics and Psychiatry at the University of Massachusetts Medical School, Worcester, Massachusetts. Dr. Edwards George's scholarly interests are the psychological and behavioral factors of gluten-free diet adherence in individuals with celiac disease.

CHAPTER 31

Coping with and Adapting to Celiac Disease

Claes Hallert, MD, PhD, Susanne Roos, RN, MSc, and Lisa Jacobsson, RN, MSc

Mrs. Miller, a nurse who is 55 years old, was diagnosed with celiac disease six months ago after having iron deficiency anemia that responded poorly to oral iron supplementation. Although treatment with parenteral (intravenous) iron brought her blood count to normal within a few weeks, a malabsorption disorder was suspected. Celiac disease blood tests were positive, and her small intestine biopsy revealed flat mucosa typical of celiac disease. At diagnosis, Mrs. Miller displayed bitterness toward the clinician, stating "So now are you telling me I can no longer be with my friends or go anywhere and have to eat the same thing every day!"

Since starting a gluten-free diet (GFD), her blood counts and mild gastro-intestinal symptoms, which she had previously attributed to irritable bowel syndrome, had improved. However, during an exam six months later, she complained of growing tiredness and a sense of poor health despite having carefully kept to the diet. Follow-up blood testing confirmed that she was on a GFD.

As we talked, it became apparent that Mrs. Miller was having difficulties adapting to life with celiac disease. She reported that her new diet had forced her to "give up" many of her favorite activities, including eating out, traveling, and cooking. She is uncomfortable about drawing attention to herself at restaurants and has chosen not to tell her best friends, so she makes excuses not to go out with them. She also feels that it has strained her home life, because she is spending much more money on food that "nobody else wants to eat." She says that her spouse "doesn't take celiac disease seriously and thinks I'm crazy or, at the very least, that I'm taking this 'allergy thing' to an extreme. He doesn't clean up crumbs, come to my appointments, or read anything about it." Toward the end of the office visit, Mrs. Miller began to cry. "This has been so hard for me," she said.

Adapting to Life with Celiac Disease

Being diagnosed with celiac disease can come as a relief to many people, especially those who have been experiencing significant symptoms. Regardless, adapting to life with celiac disease is challenging. A serious diagnosis such as this brings on a number of emotional states for many people, including denial, anger, bargaining, depression, and finally acceptance.

Even once you've accepted, or even embraced, the diagnosis of celiac disease, hurdles remain. Emotions, relationships, and the management of daily life are considered three of the main areas in which adults living with celiac disease face dilemmas.[1, 2]

- Emotional dilemmas include feelings of isolation and being deprived, worry about being a bother, and fear of contamination.
- Relationship dilemmas include unwanted attention, feelings of neglect, avoiding disclosure of celiac disease, and risk taking with potential gluten sources.
- Management dilemmas revolve around the added work and diligence needed to follow a GFD, both in choosing and preparing foods.

Both women and men report facing these dilemmas, however, data suggest that women with celiac disease feel a greater burden of illness and report lower quality of life than do men.[3,4] Two reasons for this may be that women tend to take on greater responsibilities in managing family life and relationships and that women tend to focus on and internalize their illnesses more than men.

Although no two individuals experience celiac disease in the same way, it is important and validating to realize that almost everyone experiences some of these problems. It's perhaps even more important to know that, even though following a strict GFD may always require extra effort. Over time, many of the emotional and relationship dilemmas can be overcome. With time and the support of family, friends, and health care providers, you might find that many of your negative feelings lessen and are even replaced by positive feelings of being in control of your health and belonging to a new social network. To this end, involvement in a celiac disease support group can be incredibly helpful in making this transition. However, if you have an unusual degree of difficulty adapting to celiac disease, getting counseling from a social worker or psychologist with experience in this area can be helpful.

Nutritional Health and Ability to Cope with Celiac Disease

Complicating matters further is the coexistence of anxiety and/or depression in many people with celiac disease (see Chapter 32 on depression and anxiety). It is notable that nutritional and metabolic abnormalities related to celiac disease may directly impair your ability to overcome the challenges of celiac disease. We generally believe that depression results, at least in part, from diminished synthesis of certain compounds in the brain. For instance, the production of serotonin is critically dependent on dietary factors such as having sufficient amounts of B vitamins.

This is especially important in celiac disease because studies have shown that the GFD may be low in B vitamins and dietary fiber as well as high in fats. The positive news is that one study showed that patients on a strict GFD who took a daily B complex supplement normalized their B vitamin levels and reported significant improvement in how they viewed their health and well-being as well as less depression and anxiety[5] (see Chapter 14 on supplements).

Multidisciplinary Teams for Celiac Disease Follow-Up

Most people diagnosed with celiac disease are followed by gastroenterologists or dietitians or both. Unfortunately, we've found that many patients with celiac disease have limited confidence in information from these sources and are dissatisfied with their doctor-patient communication, which can contribute to a decreased sense of well-being.

Consider that you would be best served by a multidisciplinary care team, similar to those that exist for helping people cope with other chronic diseases like diabetes or congestive heart failure. These teams are generally led and coordinated by nurses or dietitians, but may also include social workers and physicians. These teams focus on educating patients about their disease and supporting positive self-care habits. You might find a team by working with the local celiac support group, or if one is not available, you can contact local clinicians to identify which ones treat a group of celiac patients. Regional medical centers will often provide space for support group meetings as well. Education is particularly important; the better you understand celiac disease, the more you will feel in control of your health and the less burdened you will feel by the diagnosis. The flip side is that people who feel unusually burdened by celiac disease have an increased risk for developing social phobia or depression.[6]

What Mrs. Miller Decided

We tested Mrs. Miller's nutritional status and discovered that she had abnormally low folic acid levels. She agreed to take a daily B complex vitamin, consisting of vitamin B_6, vitamin B_{12}, and folic acid for six months. Additionally, because her celiac blood tests were normal and her gastrointestinal symptoms had improved, we encouraged her to start including gluten-free oats in her diet, a food she greatly missed. We also had a frank discussion with her about the issues she was having with adapting to life with celiac disease. After our visit, she decided to join her local celiac support group and made arrangements to see a social worker.

At her next visit six months later, Mrs. Miller reported having made a variety of new friends through the celiac support group. She also was surprised to find that sharing her experiences and strategies with people even more recently diagnosed than herself made her feel great. Her husband had gone with her to some counseling sessions with the social worker, which made her feel much more supported at home. Although she still had trouble finding things to eat at some restaurants, she was eating out more and generally "beginning to enjoy life again."

SELF-MANAGEMENT TIPS

☐ Decide to take control of your celiac disease. Celiac disease can seem over-whelming at first, but with time you can adjust to this change in life as you would any other.

☐ Everyone makes mistakes. There is no way to avoid all gluten all the time. Do your best, and try not to dwell on accidental exposure.

☐ Remember that you are not alone. Celiac disease is one of the most common autoimmune and gastrointestinal disorders. Join a celiac advocacy group or reach out to others to teach and to learn about celiac disease, which can empower you and fulfil your life.

☐ Don't hide the diagnosis or your feelings from friends and family. You will likely be surprised at how much support you will get when people know what you are going through. The more you share, the more others will share with you.

☐ Eating is a key social activity. Find ways to eat out so you won't hesitate to travel or eat out (see Chapter 26 on eating out).

References

1. Sverker A, Hensing G, Hallert C. 'Controlled by food'-lived experiences of coeliac disease. *J Hum Nutr Diet* 2005;18:171–80.
2. Sverker A, Ostlund G, Hallert C, Hensing G. 'I lose all these hours . . .'—exploring gender and consequences of dilemmas experienced in everyday life with coeliac disease. *Scand J Caring Sci* 2009;23:342–52.
3. Hallert C, Granno C, Grant C, Hulten S, Midhagen G, Strom M, Svensson H, Valdimarsson T, Wickstrom T. Quality of life of adult coeliac patients treated for 10 years. *Scand J Gastroenterol* 1998;33:933–38.
4. Hallert C, Granno C, Hulten S, Midhagen G, Strom M, Svensson H, Valdimarsson T. Living with coeliac disease: controlled study of the burden of illness. *Scand J Gastroenterol* 2002;37:39–42.
5. Hallert C, Svensson M, Tholstrup J, Hultberg B. Clinical trial: B vitamins improve health in patients with coeliac disease living on a gluten-free diet. *Aliment Pharmacol Ther* 2009; 29:811–16.
6. Roos S, Karner A, Hallert C. Gastrointestinal symptoms and well-being of adults living on a gluten-free diet: a case for nursing in celiac disease. *Gastroenterol Nurs* 2009;32:196–201.

Claes Hallert, MD, PhD, is a gastroenterologist and Professor at the Norrkoping Hospital, Norrkoping, Sweden. **Susanne Roos, RN, MSc,** and **Lisa Jacobsson, RN, MSc,** are Lecturers at Linkoping University at Campus Norrkoping, Sweden

CHAPTER 32

Depression and Anxiety in Celiac Disease

Carolina Ciacci, MD

The first time I saw Anne, a 34-year-old career woman, was about three years ago. At the time, she had been suffering from fatigue and weight loss for about eight months. She felt anxious for her health and was not sleeping well, for which her doctor had prescribed a sleep aid. However, in follow-up testing, Anne was found to have anemia and low plasma cholesterol, both suggestive of malabsorption, and her immunoglobulin A tissue transglutaminase (IgA-tTG) was 80 units (less than 7 units is normal in that lab). Upper endoscopy with biopsy confirmed that she had celiac disease.

Anne started a gluten-free diet (GFD), and after 10 months, her blood tests had returned to normal, including her IgA-tTG. However, she still reported fatigue and difficulty concentrating, both of which were affecting her ability to work. Although the sleep aid she was taking helps her fall asleep, she often wakes early. She also told me that she is beginning to refuse work that requires her to travel or eat outside her home because she is afraid to worsen her health with involuntary gluten intake. Anne's responses to questions in a structured interview suggested that she is suffering from depression and that she rates her quality of life as poor. However, Anne says that she had both depression and anxiety before her diagnosis of celiac disease.

What's the Connection between Mood and Celiac Disease?

It's still common for people to live years with unrecognized celiac disease, so that at the time of diagnosis, many have had quite a long period of poor general health. This can lead to a number of mood conditions and disorders. Studies and reports describe psychiatric disorders that are part of the clinical presentation of celiac disease. Untreated celiac disease has been associated with anxiety, social phobia, fatigue, unsatisfactory sex life, and depression.[1] Of these, depression at diagnosis is very common.

Symptoms and signs suggesting depression are:

- feelings of helplessness and hopelessness
- loss of interest in daily activities, including sex
- appetite or weight changes (loss or gain)
- sleep changes, such as insomnia, early wake ups, or oversleeping
- abnormally slow or jittery movements
- loss of energy
- self-loathing or feelings of worthlessness
- concentration problems

The reasons why people with untreated celiac disease have mood alterations are unclear, but the disease itself could be the cause because of malabsorption and/or damage to the intestine. When the intestine is damaged, this causes increased permeability (sometimes referred to as a *leaky gut*), which might permit certain substances that affect brain function to get into the bloodstream from the gut. For example, the amino acid tryptophan may reduce the amount of serotonin, or other neurotransmitters, that are available for brain function. People who are depressed often have lower than normal levels of serotonin. Lack of minerals and vitamins, which can be caused by either malabsorption or a nutritionally unbalanced diet, or a combination of the two, may also impair neurological functions. Also, malabsorption can cause feelings of fatigue and of being ill, which can range from severe depression to just feeling "blah," without providing any distinct clues about what is causing it.

What Do We Know about Mood and Celiac Disease?

A diagnosis of celiac disease brings with it two immediate consequences: First, you must deal with having a chronic illness. Second, you are faced with the requirement of a GFD for life. These are major life events that most people will react to emotionally.

It's common to feel anxious because of the diagnosis and as you learn how to eat gluten free. In this regard, anxiety could be considered to be a normal reaction to the stress brought on by these changes. The feeling of anxiety will typically lessen over time as you heal and as the symptoms you've had to deal with resolve. This is not the case for depression, however, which seems to persist and may be considered a feature of celiac disease.[2] Depression was investigated in a large, population-based Swedish study of about 13,000 people with celiac disease who were compared with 66,000 individuals without the disease matched for sex and age. The study showed that those diagnosed with celiac disease in childhood had an increased risk for subsequent depression, but the reasons behind this are unclear.[3]

The perception of fatigue reported by people with celiac disease is related to depression, suggesting at least in part a psychological origin of fatigue. Depression and feelings of poor quality of life after diagnosis and after learning about the diet treatment have also been related to persisting vitamin deficiency. It has been suggested that there exists a "celiac profile" composed of two principal characteristics: *reactiveness,* the tendency to respond to events with an angry or exaggerated sense of frustration, and *pessimism,* a cluster of symptoms that all share the feeling of powerlessness.[2] Moreover, people with celiac disease often claim the desire to fit in with their social and peer group rather than stand out as needing special treatment. However, it is worth noting that all chronic illnesses influence the psychological status of the affected person, even if the disease has no symptoms or is under control, so it is expected that people will have difficulty in adapting to the chronic nature of celiac disease.

Depression also appears to be one of the main reasons why people with chronic medical diseases (not only celiac disease) often fail to follow the treatment. A recent U.S. study found that four factors, the ability to plan and organize, the presence of depression and anxiety, the presence of other food intolerances, and the presence of gluten-related symptoms, effectively predicted how well most study participants would follow a GFD.[4]

In general, people on a GFD claim that their quality of life shortly after diagnosis of celiac disease is poor[5,6] and relate their feelings to the social restrictions imposed by the GFD. The fact is that the dietary restriction is sometimes hard to accept by adults, in particular if they have a busy working and social life. However, the depressive symptoms reported in adults on a GFD are independent of how long they have been on the diet and how well they follow it.[2]

Several studies, however, have found that there is no difference in psychological behavior between individuals with and without celiac disease. Despite this, some studies have suggested that individuals with celiac disease report lower general well-being than individuals without celiac disease. This appears to be true for women more than men. The reasons for this gender difference may lie in the fact that the GFD, without question, interferes with social life. Women, more often than men, plan for and provide the food for their families and for themselves. For this reason, they may be more conscious of restrictions in shopping for food, in cooking, and in feeding their children.

So, it is conceivable that depression in celiac disease is initially a consequence of both the disease symptoms and malabsorption-malnutrition but is then sustained by the reduction in the quality of life because of the burden of living with a chronic illness. This seemed to be the case for Anne.

Treating Mood Disorders in Celiac Disease

Few studies have looked at the effectiveness of psychotherapy for mood disorders in celiac patients. One study demonstrated that patients with celiac disease and personality and/or psychiatric disorders who received psychological support at the beginning of treatment with the GFD had lower levels of depression and a better ability to keep a GFD.[6] Recently, a study showed that those with celiac disease who took vitamin B supplements had better overall health and significant improvement in feelings of well-being, with reduced anxiety and depression.[8]

It helps to have a holistic understanding of all the factors that contribute to your quality of life to see which issues you face and how to improve your well-being. This may require asking for professional help. It's easier if you have a health care provider who recognizes and knows when to evaluate patients for mood disorders and, if needed, can offer appropriate advice. As celiac disease awareness increases, more health care professionals will connect the symptoms of celiac disease, including depression at diagnosis.

What Anne Decided

I recommended to Anne that she begin both psychological and nutritional counseling. A psychologist or social worker could work with her one-on-one to develop ways to adjust to her celiac lifestyle and to handle social situations where food is involved and accept and explore new foods. A dietitian would help her learn how to replace gluten-containing foods with easy and nutritionally balanced alternatives as well as ways to eat safely outside her home.

Anne decided to begin working with both a counselor and a dietitian. At the same time, she began a trial of an antidepressant medication prescribed by her primary care physician. I saw her again eight months later. She was sleeping better and reported a couple of two-day trips away from home. During the trips, she decided to carry with her some gluten-free bread and crackers, so she wouldn't be without, and managed to have dinner in a restaurant that was identified on a celiac disease Web site as being aware of celiac disease and a provider of safe gluten-free food. Despite this progress, she was still reporting difficulty in planning her work schedule and had passed up a promotion that would have required a great deal of business travel.

SELF-MANAGEMENT TIPS

☐ Be aware that depression and anxiety are common in celiac disease and may be considered part of the symptoms. Depression is often present at diagnosis.

☐ It's normal to feel anxious about the diagnosis and that the changes to your eating habits will be a burden that negatively affects your quality of life. These feelings often recede once you learn how to control your intake of gluten and become physically healthier.

☐ Reasons for depression may include damage to the intestine that results in changes in absorption that interfere with normal brain function. Improved nutrition, including getting enough B vitamins, can lessen depression.

☐ Consider asking your doctor to screen you for mood disorders. Once a mood disorder has been identified, treatments, including psychotherapy, counseling, and/or medications, may benefit you and improve your quality of life in addition to the GFD.

References

1. Addolorato G, Leggio L, D'Angelo C, et al. Affective and psychiatric disorders in celiac disease. *Dig Dis* 2008;26(2):140–48.
2. Ciacci C, Iavarone A, Mazzacca G, De Rosa A. Depressive symptoms in adult coeliac disease. *Scand J Gastroenterol* 1998;33:247–50.
3. Ludvigsson JF, Reutfors J, Osby U, Ekbom A, Montgomery SM. Coeliac disease and risk of mood disorders: a general population-based cohort study. *J Affect Disord* 2007;99(1–3):117–26.

4. Edwards George JB, Leffler DA, Dennis MD, Franko DL, Blom-Hoffman J, Kelly CP. Psychological correlates of gluten-free diet adherence in adults with celiac disease. *J Clin Gastroenterol* 2009;43(4):301–306.

5. Hallert C, Granno C, Grant C, Hulten S, Midhagen G, Strom M, Svensson H, Valdimarsson T, Wickstrom T. Quality of life of adult coeliac patients treated for 10 years. *Scand J Gastroenterol* 1998;33(9):933–38.

6. Ciacci C, D'Agate C, De Rosa A, Franzese C, Errichiello S, Gasperi V, Pardi A, Quagliata D, Visentini S, Greco L. Self-rated quality of life in celiac disease. *Dig Dis Sci* 2003;48:2216–20.

7. Addolorato G, De Lorenzi G, Abenavoli L, Leggio L, Capristo E, Gasbarrini G. Psychological support counselling improves gluten-free diet compliance in celiac patients with affective disorders. *Aliment Pharmacol Ther* 2004;20(7):777–82.

8. Hallert C, Svensson M, Tholstrup J, Hultberg B. B vitamins improve health in patients with coeliac disease living on a gluten-free diet. *Aliment Pharmacol Ther* 2009;29(8):811–16.

Carolina Ciacci, MD, is Professor of Gastroenterology and Director of the Celiac Center at University Ferderico II, Naples, Italy. She coordinates the Campania Network for Celiac Disease, an organization that cares for more than 10,000 people with celiac disease in southern Italy.

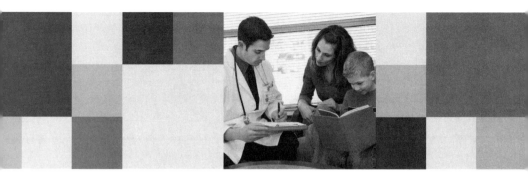

THE OBSTACLES: CONCERNS AND COMPLICATIONS

We firmly believe that celiac disease is one of the "best" diagnoses you can have. Individuals often feel much better after diagnosis and treatment than they have for years and go on to lead healthy lives. Yet, life can present obstacles. This section addresses some of the most common issues that people with celiac disease face and, wherever possible, suggests how to overcome them.

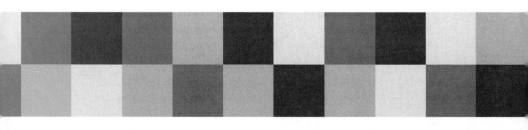

CHAPTER 33

Monitoring Celiac Disease

Daniel A. Leffler, MD, MS

S eth was diagnosed with celiac disease at age 52, when he happened to tell his gastro-enterologist about his chronic loose stools and stomach discomfort in preparation for his first screening colonoscopy. Because of these symptoms, the gastroenterologist also performed an upper endoscopy and took biopsies of the small intestine. Both the intestinal biopsies and follow-up blood tests were consistent with celiac disease. Seth received a letter in the mail saying that he had celiac disease and to go on a gluten-free diet (GFD).

Three years later, Seth visited our clinic to see whether he needed any follow-up testing. He was frustrated that his physician hadn't provided further guidance about how to live gluten free and whether his celiac disease was under control. He noted that he still had occasional episodes of loose stools. Since his diagnosis, Seth has not had any specific care for his celiac disease.

Caring for Your Celiac Disease

There are many diseases for which the recommended follow-up care is well defined by evidence and guidelines. Unfortunately, celiac disease is not one of them. Although diagnostic criteria are established, there is little agreement about which kind of specific monitoring people with celiac disease should have. For this reason, there is a great deal of variation in current practice. However, there are specific "minimum standards" that are applicable for most people. These standards were presented at an National Institutes of Health consensus conference on celiac disease[1] with a very clever mnemonic:

Consultation with a skilled dietitian
Education about celiac disease
Lifelong adherence to a GFD
Identification and treatment of nutrition deficiencies
Access to an advocacy group
Continuous long-term follow-up by a multidisciplinary team

- **Consultation with a skilled dietitian.** Immediately after diagnosis, everyone diagnosed with celiac disease needs to meet for counseling with a dietitian who has specific training in celiac disease. Although there is a concerted effort by the American Dietetic Association to increase all dietitians' ability to teach the GFD, many dietitians still lack the experience to work effectively with those with celiac disease, so *skilled* is the important word to remember. Ask your physician for a referral or seek out a celiac-skilled dietitian in your area yourself. There is a list of celiac dietitians at http://glutenfreedietitian.com/newsletter/?page_id=14 (see also Resources). You need to meet again with your dietitian after six months on the GFD and then yearly to keep your skills sharp and stay on top of new foods and other dietary advances.
- **Education about celiac disease.** Celiac disease is a lifelong disorder with many effects on your health and social life. You will be your healthiest if you learn as much as you can about the disorder and put it into action. The other key is to find health care providers with whom you can become full partners in working to keep you healthy. They will supply critical support. Reading this book is one excellent way to become informed, but there are also education classes at celiac centers or available through celiac advocacy groups and reputable Internet resources (see Resources).
- **Lifelong adherence to a GFD.** The need for strict adherence to eating 100% gluten free has been emphasized throughout this book. Simply put, it's a commitment to your health that only you can guarantee.
- **Identification and treatment of nutrition deficiencies.** One of the most controversial issues is which blood tests to use to monitor for nutrient deficiencies and when to use them. There is a great deal of variation in how this is done from one clinic to another. However, on the initial visit to consider whether someone has celiac disease, I look for celiac markers (usually immunoglobulin A tissue transglutaminase [IgA-tTG] and a total IgA level) and do a complete blood count, liver tests, and iron studies and assess levels of vitamin B_{12} and vitamin D. Depending on a patient's symptoms and severity of diarrhea, I may also test for levels of zinc, folate, calcium, vitamin B_6, selenium, carnitine, vitamin A, and parathyroid hormone. I also check thyroid function, depending on the type and severity of symptoms the individual is experiencing. Because there is a small increased risk of infectious complications in untreated or newly diagnosed celiac disease, I always consider whether the influenza and pneumonia vaccinations would be beneficial.

    After the initial visit and blood work, I ask patients to return between three and six months later. At that time, I recheck celiac blood markers and any test that was abnormal on the first visit to make sure that the adjustments made to diet and any other treatments that were needed are working. Subsequent visits are planned based on how you are doing, but at the minimum, I want to see you yearly for a "well celiac check up." At that time, I usually check celiac blood markers and get a complete blood count as well as check any abnormalities suggested by your symptoms. Additionally, an initial bone mineral density study is recommended for most adults after one year on a GFD (see Chapter 47). Follow-up endoscopies are not routinely necessary but would be needed if you are having persistent symptoms or blood test abnormalities or if your celiac blood tests were negative at diagnosis.

- **Access to an advocacy group.** Adjustment to life with celiac disease can be difficult. Many individuals with celiac disease and their family members find that participating in a celiac advocacy group, at least in the beginning, is extremely helpful. There are also data that suggest that belonging to an advocacy group improves a patient's ability to keep a strict GFD. Celiac advocacy groups are scattered across the country and are fantastic sources of information and support and increasingly are helping to raise awareness of celiac disease among physicians and government organizations.

- **Continuous long-term follow-up by a multidisciplinary team.** Celiac disease is for life and can affect nearly any part of the body. While, in general, gastroenterologists are expected to coordinate care related to celiac disease, it is often important to enlist the assistance of other health care practitioners aside from dietitians. Other physicians who may be important in your care include endocrinologists for bone and thyroid disease, dermatologists for skin disorders, allergists for concerns relating to food or environmental allergies, and gynecologists for fertility issues.

What Seth Needed

Seth had not had any blood tests since diagnosis and had taught himself the GFD. Although he said he was "mostly" gluten free, it was apparent from our discussion of his eating habits that he was having some issues with gluten contamination. He was also eating the same foods over and over because it seemed the easiest way to stay gluten free. However, this limited his nutrition intake.

So it was no surprise when his IgA-tTG came back mildly elevated and his vitamin D level tested low. I recommended that Seth begin a gluten-free multivitamin and mineral supplement without iron (supplemental iron is not generally recommended for men and postmenopausal women because of risk of iron overload, which can lead to significant health problems; see also Chapter 14 on supplements) and an extra calcium/vitamin D supplement. I referred him to a skilled dietitian and also recommended that he contact the local celiac advocacy group.

Seth returned six months later to follow up. He noted that he had learned a great deal more about living with celiac disease in the interim and had tried some new foods that had become instant favorites. Seth told me that both his energy level and bowel habits had improved. His IgA-tTG tested at a normal level at this time, and his bone mineral density was in the low-to-normal range. I am happy to report that Seth has continued to follow up with me and his dietitian once a year.

SELF-MANAGEMENT TIPS

- ☐ You need health care professionals, including a physician and a dietitian, who are knowledgeable about celiac disease on your team.
- ☐ Have your celiac markers and other blood tests, individualized to your health needs, checked after the diagnosis and monitored until they have normalized.
- ☐ If you are an adult, have your bone mineral density measured after one year on a GFD (see Chapter 47 on bone disease). Children and adolescents who are diagnosed and treated appropriately so that normal bone mineral density may be attained do not routinely need to have their bone mineral density measured.
- ☐ You generally won't need a routine follow-up endoscopy if your celiac disease was diagnosed with both blood tests and biopsy unless problems arise.
- ☐ Educating yourself about celiac disease and participating in a celiac advocacy group are important steps in adjusting to your life with celiac disease.

Reference

1. James SP. This month at the NIH: final statement of NIH Consensus Conference on celiac disease. *Gastroenterology* 2005;128(1):6.

CHAPTER 34

Nonresponsive Celiac Disease

Shailaja Jamma, MD, and Daniel A. Leffler, MD, MS

R uth, now 50, was diagnosed with celiac disease eight years ago. Her primary symptoms were abdominal pain, diarrhea, and anemia. Although during the first few years, she "cheated" when she wanted a bagel or a "real" piece of toast, for the last 5 years, she has been vigilant about eating gluten free. For the most part, her symptoms have resolved, but she tells us she has mild episodes of loose stools and abdominal discomfort on about a monthly basis. Ruth thought that she could trace some of these episodes back to gluten exposure, but many came "out of nowhere." She also noted having some issues with constipation that were longstanding.

Recently, however, her symptoms have become worse, with loose stools almost on a daily basis. Her weight has been stable, and she's been able to carry out her daily activities as usual and without any serious incidents. Ruth is understandably concerned about why her symptoms have recently returned and would like to be sure nothing "serious" is going on.

What Is Nonresponsive Celiac Disease?

Nonresponsive celiac disease (NRCD) is a general term clinicians use to describe people with celiac disease for whom the gluten-free diet (GFD) does not appear to resolve all the symptoms or problems that were initially attributed to the celiac disease. It is important to recognize that NRCD is not a diagnosis itself; it is just a description that is used until we can find the root of the problem and make a firm diagnosis. You would need to be on a GFD for at least 6 months without significant improvement before we would decide that you were not responding and look for other reasons. There is a great deal of variability in how long it takes people to feel fully better on a GFD, so as long as there is some continual improvement, even if it seems very slow, a full evaluation for NRCD is usually unnecessary.

As we discuss below, there are many reasons for NRCD. The first step is often to get confirmation that you do indeed have celiac disease. Many people are aware that celiac disease can be mistaken for other disorders such as irritable bowel syndrome. But you may be surprised to know that the reverse often occurs as well, that is, celiac disease can be mistakenly diagnosed when the true problem is something else. If you are having continued symptoms on a GFD and either blood tests or intestinal biopsy were normal before going on GFD, you should talk to your doctor about the possibility that you do not actually have celiac disease.

Finding the Cause of NRCD

The evaluation for NRCD is individualized, based mostly on your symptoms and medical history. As with most medical problems, unintentional weight loss is generally felt to be the most concerning symptom; it generally prompts us to look for refractory celiac disease with endoscopic evaluation. Typically, however, your physician will begin with blood tests and a thorough history and exam.[1]

In addition, many people are asked to visit a dietitian skilled in celiac disease to help assess accidental gluten exposure. For some, this seems unnecessary or even irritating; after all, you may have many years of experience keeping a strict GFD. But gluten exposure is the most common cause of NRCD. Gluten can slip in where you least expect it, such as with a change in formulation of a medication or trusted food. By taking a fresh look at potential gluten sources with a trained dietitian, we can often root out gluten, avoiding more burdensome and often invasive testing. Finally, we have no test to discriminate between the most common kind of refractory celiac disease (type 1; see Chapter 43) and gluten exposure. For this reason, evaluation by a dietitian is also included when looking for refractory celiac disease.

When it seems unlikely that you are exposing yourself to gluten, your physician will work to determine the best next step in evaluation based on the most likely cause (Table 1). Most often, more than one test is necessary, and possible causes must be ruled out before a definitive diagnosis is made.

Treating NRCD

Because there are so many causes of NRCD, treatment must be based on the final diagnosis. However, if symptoms are very severe, your doctor may try some nonspecific treatment while the evaluation is ongoing.

What Ruth Decided

We explained to Ruth that it is very common for people with celiac disease to have persistent or recurrent symptoms and/or blood test abnormalities despite continuing to maintain a GFD. We informed her that it is usually possible to find a specific reason for symptoms, but that it may take several tests before we can arrive at a confident answer. Ruth felt reassured that, because she wasn't losing weight, a diagnosis like refractory celiac disease or cancer was very unlikely.

TABLE 1. Causes of Nonresponsive Celiac Disease

Cause	Typical Features/Tests	How Common
Gluten exposure (see Chapter 20)	Evaluation by dietitian skilled in celiac disease	Very common
Irritable bowel syndrome (see Chapter 38)	None	Very common
Lactose intolerance or fructose malabsorption (see Chapter 37)	Trial of lactose or fructose restriction; lactose or fructose breath testing	Somewhat common
Microscopic colitis (see Chapter 39)	Biopsy of colon	Somewhat common
Small intestinal bacterial overgrowth (see Chapter 40)	Breath testing and or a response to antibiotic therapy	Somewhat common
Refractory celiac disease (see Chapter 43)	Biopsy of small intestine	Rare
Eating disorder (see Chapter 30)	None	Rare
Inflammatory bowel disease	Biopsy of small or large intestine, imaging studies of intestine	Rare
Pancreatic exocrine insufficiency	Stool levels of chymotrypsin or elastase	Rare
Motility disturbances (too slow or too fast movement of food through the intestine)	Gastric emptying study, intestinal transit testing	Rare
Food allergy (see Chapter 35)	Allergy testing (skin or blood)	Very rare
Cancer	Endoscopy, imaging studies of intestine	Very rare

From references 2 and 3.

Ruth's initial blood tests were normal, except for a mildly elevated immunoglobulin A tissue transglutaminase (IgA-tTG) of 26 units (normal is less than 20 units). Ruth met with a dietitian, and together they identified a few possible sources of gluten, including a medication that had recently been changed from a known gluten-free brand to a generic preparation. After beginning a gluten-free version of the medication, her symptoms improved and her IgA-tTG decreased to 14 units.

However, Ruth continued to experience constipation with occasional episodes of abdominal discomfort and diarrhea, especially around periods of stress. We discussed performing an endoscopy and biopsy with Ruth, but she decided to wait to do this, because her symptoms were mild and there was no evidence of blood test abnormalities. However, the connection between stress and symptoms led us to discuss the possibility that Ruth had mild irritable bowel syndrome, coexisting with her celiac disease. She responded well to adding more gluten-free fiber sources to her diet and taking fiber supplements in addition to learning some stress management techniques, including deep, relaxing breathing.

References

1. Krauss N, Schuppan D. Monitoring nonresponsive patients who have celiac disease. *Gastrointest Endosc Clin N Am* 2006;16:317–27.
2. Leffler DA, Dennis M, Hyett B, Kelly E, Schuppan D, Kelly CP. Etiologies and predictors of diagnosis in nonresponsive celiac disease. *Clin Gastroenterol Hepatol* 2007;5:445–50.
3. Abdulkarim AS, Burgart LJ, See J, Murray JA. Etiology of nonresponsive celiac disease: results of a systematic approach. *Am J Gastroenterol* 2002;97:2016–21.

Shailaja Jamma, MD, is a Research Fellow at Beth Israel Deaconess Medical Center. She is part of the Celiac Center team and works in a variety of clinical and research areas related to celiac disease.

CHAPTER 35

Food Allergies and Intolerances

Sheila E. Crowe, MD, AGAF, FRCPC, FACP, FACG

Rebecca, a 38-year-old mother, came to me soon after her daughter was diagnosed with celiac disease at age 10. Rebecca's symptoms included frequent bowel movements, abdominal bloating, cramping, and hives after eating certain foods. She reported some wheezing after eating but had no history of weight loss, anemia, or miscarriages. She was following a lactose-free diet but was uncertain that it was helping. Given her daughter's diagnosis, Rebecca was tested for celiac disease. Her celiac antibodies were not elevated, and genetic testing showed she was not susceptible to celiac disease. As it turned out, her husband's brother was recently diagnosed with celiac disease, indicating that her husband was the likely genetic link to their daughter's celiac disease.

A review of Rebecca's gastrointestinal symptoms suggested a possible food allergy because not all meals resulted in symptoms and her complaints included wheezing, some itching around her mouth, and hives, consistent with an allergic tendency. Recently, she had noticed that latex rubber gloves caused itching and a rash. Rebecca also had family members with allergic disorders, including eczema, asthma, and allergic rhinitis. Rebecca began to keep a food diary so we could identify any specific associations.

When Rebecca returned several weeks later, she had experienced two mild episodes of hives, both of which occurred soon after eating bananas. She also reported wheezing and diarrhea after eating kiwi fruit. Because I suspected a latex-food allergy syndrome, I referred Rebecca to an allergist to be tested for this. Her skin test panel to common food allergens resulted in positive reactions to bananas, kiwi, and avocado along with the histamine test control (histamine control is done to make sure that an individual produces the expected welt-like reaction). Based on these evaluations and her clinical picture, the allergist and I concluded that she had a latex-food allergy. The allergist recommended that she carry epinephrine to inject if her symptoms ever progressed beyond wheezing and wear a bracelet that identifies her as latex allergic. Rebecca met with a knowledgeable dietitian and also found helpful information at the Food Allergy and Anaphylaxis Network (www.foodallergy.org).

What Are Food Allergy and Food Sensitivity?

Adverse reactions to food (ARF) are common around the world, with 25% or more of various populations reporting food-induced symptoms. Most ARF are classified as food sensitivity or food intolerance. The rest are because of an abnormal response to a food protein that prompts an immune-mediated response—in other words, a food allergy. Food allergies and other immune-mediated ARF are rarer than the nonimmune reactions; they affect 6–8% of children younger than age 10 and 3–4% of adults.[1] It's important to consider both food allergies and food intolerances when evaluating patients complaining of diet-induced gastrointestinal symptoms, including those with celiac disease (Table 1).

Immune-Mediated Reactions

An immune-mediated reaction that involves immunoglobulin E (IgE) and causes the release of inflammatory chemicals from (degranulates) mast cells and basophils is a type I food hypersensitivity or food allergy. IgE-mediated reactions cause classic food allergy symptoms, affecting the skin and the respiratory tract. When allergic reactions affect the digestive tract, nausea, vomiting, diarrhea, cramping, and abdominal pain may result. Gastrointestinal symptoms are reported in 30–70% of people experiencing food allergy.[1] The foods primarily responsible for this type of food allergy include cow's milk, eggs, nuts, seafood, and fish. However, with the globalization of eating habits, new allergens are emerging and food allergy and allergic reactions are increasing worldwide, particularly in urban populations.[2]

Oral allergy syndrome or pollen-food allergy syndrome occurs when ingested plant proteins cross-react with specific inhaled antigens, particularly from birch, ragweed, and mugwort.[3]

TABLE 1. Types of Adverse Reactions to Food or Food Additives

Immune-mediated reactions
- IgE-mediated food allergy
  - Gastrointestinal food allergy
  - Oral allergy syndrome
  - Latex-food allergy syndrome
  - Anaphylaxis
- Eosinophilic gastrointestinal disorders
- Food protein–induced enterocolitis syndromes
- Celiac disease

Food intolerance (nonimmune-mediated reactions)
- Food toxicity or poisoning
- Pseudoallergic reactions
- Pharmacological reactions
- Carbohydrate intolerances
- Physiological reactions
- Psychological reactions

Foods that cross-react with birch pollen include raw potatoes, carrots, celery, apples, pears, hazelnuts, and kiwi. Individuals who are allergic to ragweed pollen may react to fresh melons and bananas. Grass pollen allergies can be associated with tomato allergy. The cross-reaction may lead to itching; tingling and/or swelling of the tongue, lips, mouth, or throat; and occasionally trouble breathing or a whole-body (systemic) reaction, a life-threatening condition called anaphylaxis.

In the latex-food allergy syndrome or latex-fruit syndrome, food antigens cross-react with various latex antigens. Natural rubber latex contains more than 200 proteins, some of which bind IgE and cross-react with a variety of food antigens including kiwi, potato, tomato, avocado, chestnut, and banana. When exposed to any of these foods, latex-sensitive individuals can develop itching, eczema, oral-facial swelling, asthma, gastrointestinal complaints, and anaphylaxis. Worldwide, banana, avocado, chestnut, and kiwi are the most common causes of food-induced symptoms associated with latex allergy.[4]

Other immune-mediated food reactions involve T-cells as in celiac disease, the generation of immune complexes, and/or the activation of white blood cells called *eosinophils*. Eosinophilic gastroenteritis is a rare condition in which about half with the disease also have evidence of food allergies. Food protein–induced enterocolitis syndromes, including food protein enteropathy, are food reactions that occur almost exclusively in very young children. Symptoms include bloody or nonbloody diarrhea, vomiting, and failure to thrive. The most common causative foods are milk and soy. These are not IgE-mediated like true food allergies and typically resolve by the age of three.

Nonimmune-Mediated Reactions

Food toxicity or food poisoning is generally the result of eating food contaminated by toxins, such as staphylococcal enterotoxin, or pathogens, such as *Campylobacter, Salmonella, Shigella,* or *E. coli.* These reactions can be distinguished from other ARF because they usually do not recur and have fairly characteristic symptoms. Occasionally, an infection, even though cured, may result in irritable bowel syndrome (IBS).

Anaphylactoid or pseudoallergic reactions to food result from foods that mimic the effects of mast cell degranulation (inflammatory chemical release) but do not involve antibodies. Strawberries and shellfish may cause this type of ARF. Certain food additives, such as salicylates, benzoates, and tartrazine, can induce pseudoallergic reactions.

Pharmacological or drug reactions to naturally occurring elements in food or food additives, such as caffeine, may produce symptoms of tremors and are a relatively common type of ARF. Most of these reactions cause symptoms outside of the gastrointestinal tract that include headaches, rashes, and respiratory complaints.

Globally, the most common adverse physiological reaction to a specific food is lactose intolerance. Most cases result from declining levels of intestinal lactase, the enzyme that breaks down lactose (the natural sugar in milk), late in childhood or in early adult life. Most of the world is lactose intolerant because of this genetically controlled decline in lactase, and even in populations of northern European origin, where milk drinking is common, the frequency of lactose intolerance in adults is around 30%. Symptoms of lactase deficiency are usually related to the amount ingested and include bloating, flatulence, and diarrhea. Another cause of lactase deficiency is loss of the lactase-expressing cells of the small intestinal villi because of viral gastroenteritis, radiation enteritis, Crohn's disease, or untreated celiac disease.

Individuals with lactose intolerance do not suffer severe or life-threatening complications from ingesting lactose, and most are able to consume naturally lactose-free dairy products, including hard cheese and yogurt, without problems. This is different from cow's milk allergy, in which individuals may suffer anaphylactic or asthmatic reactions to dairy products and must avoid all foods containing the culprit cow's milk protein allergen, usually casein or β-lactoglobulin. Many well-meaning physicians place patients with lactose intolerance on a dairy-free diet instead of a lactose-free diet. This unnecessarily restricts their diets and reduces calcium intake, which increases the risk for bone disease.

Individuals who suffer gastrointestinal symptoms after eating most types of dairy products, including those with very little lactose, but do not have symptoms that suggest allergy, such as swelling of the mouth, rash, or wheezing, may have an underlying form of a functional gastrointestinal disorder such as IBS, functional dyspepsia, or functional bloating (the term *functional* is used when symptoms occur in the absence of any objectively observable reaction or inflammation). The long-chain fat content of whole milk and cream and foods made from them, including butter, ice cream, cheese, and yogurt, may be a factor in perceived dairy intolerance in patients with functional gastrointestinal disorders and other conditions, including some patients with celiac disease.[5]

Lactose is not the only sugar that can cause gastrointestinal complaints. Fructose and related products (fructans) as well as sorbitol can cause diarrhea and bloating in some individuals. There is growing recognition that a large group of dietary carbohydrates referred to as FODMAPs (fermentable oligosaccharides, disaccharides, monosaccharides, and polyols) can cause gastrointestinal symptoms in certain populations (see Chapter 37 on fructose intolerance). FODMAPs have been studied primarily in those with IBS but could play a role in celiac disease, particularly in those with an IBS component to their illness.

One of the most common forms of ARF results from physiological reactions to food components or additives. Starches such as raffinose, found in legumes, promote the production of gas by colonic flora as do many other foods associated with gas, including onions, cabbage, and bran fiber. Certain foods and food additives affect the lower esophageal sphincter, and foods high in fat delay gastric emptying, both of which result in symptoms of heartburn and stomachache. Usually, the best advice for patients who suffer from these ailments after eating is to limit the volume of food and beverage they consume at one time, especially for their evening meal, and reduce high-fat foods, which can make symptoms of functional gastrointestinal syndromes worse.

Finally, in certain individuals, reactions to food may be psychological. Symptoms such as nausea, abdominal pain, and diarrhea can occur because a particular food is associated with a traumatic experience.

Rebecca's Outcome

After learning about latex rubber protein and its cross-reactivity with a number of foods, Rebecca eliminated the culprit foods from her diet and replaced all items in her home containing latex. At follow-up a few months later, she was happy to report that her complaints had resolved.

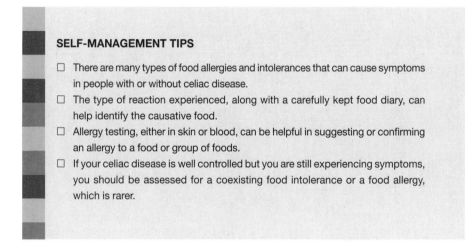

SELF-MANAGEMENT TIPS

☐ There are many types of food allergies and intolerances that can cause symptoms in people with or without celiac disease.

☐ The type of reaction experienced, along with a carefully kept food diary, can help identify the causative food.

☐ Allergy testing, either in skin or blood, can be helpful in suggesting or confirming an allergy to a food or group of foods.

☐ If your celiac disease is well controlled but you are still experiencing symptoms, you should be assessed for a coexisting food intolerance or a food allergy, which is rarer.

References

1. Bischoff S, Crowe SE. Gastrointestinal food allergy: new insights into pathophysiology and clinical perspectives. *Gastroenterology* 2005;128(4):1089–113.
2. Sicherer SH, Leung DY. Advances in allergic skin disease, anaphylaxis, and hypersensitivity reactions to foods, drugs, and insects in 2008. *J Allergy Clin Immunol* 2009;123:319–27.
3. Hofmann A, Burks AW. Pollen food syndrome: update on the allergens. *Curr Allergy Asthma Rep* 2008;8:413–17.
4. Blanco C. Latex-fruit syndrome. *Curr Allergy Asthma Rep* 2003;3:47–53.
5. Mishkin S. Dairy sensitivity, lactose malabsorption, and elimination diets in inflammatory bowel disease. *Am J Clin Nutr* 1997;65:564–67.

Sheila E. Crowe, MD, AGAF, FRCPC, FACP, FACG, is a gastroenterologist specializing in immune-mediated disorders including celiac disease, food allergies, and inflammatory bowel disease at the Digestive Health Center of Excellence, Division of Gastroenterology and Hepatology, Department of Medicine, University of Virginia, Charlottesville, Virginia. She is Director of the University of Virginia Celiac Disease Center.

CHAPTER 36

Elimination Diets and Rechallenge Trials

Melinda Dennis, MS, RD, LDN

"I'm already avoiding gluten. If it's not gluten, what could be bothering me?" asked Jessie, a 44-year-old patient. A few months after her diagnosis, Jessie was worried about the return of the gas and bloating after meals, along with general indigestion. A year earlier, she had been diagnosed with celiac disease by bloodwork and biopsy. Jessie had quickly adjusted to her new gluten-free diet, and her initial complaints of diarrhea, gas, and bloating resolved. Within months, her immunoglobulin A tissue transglutaminase antibodies had fallen into the normal range

In addition to the gastrointestinal problems, Jessie also got frequent headaches and felt more fatigued than she thought she should for her age. She told me that she had been feeling this way "for as long as I can remember." She started a food record to see if something she was eating was the problem, but she never seemed to be able to track down the trigger. One day it seemed to be one food, the next day another; sometimes she was just fine eating a particular food, and then another time, she would get a stomachache and gas the day after eating the same food. Jessie was frustrated, and food had lost a lot of its charm. She wondered, "What else could be causing my symptoms? Could it be food allergies or food intolerances?"

Food Allergy vs. Food Intolerance

A food allergy provokes a classic immune response in the body, stimulating a cascade of activity that ends with an allergic reaction in the person eating the food. Food allergy reactions generally occur within a few minutes after eating the offending food; can include any number of reactions in the ears, nose, eyes, throat, and skin; and can sometimes be fatal. Foods are usually identified through a combination of clinical history, including diet records; physical exam; allergy skin prick tests or RAST blood tests; and an elimination diet with oral challenges done under medical guidance.[1] Once identified, the individual then strictly avoids specific trigger foods. If pursued under physician supervision, follow-up testing can confirm whether the person is still allergic to the particular food. The eight most common allergenic foods are egg, cow's milk, fish, shellfish, tree nuts, peanuts, soy, and wheat (see Chapter 35 on food allergies).

Food intolerances or sensitivities are much more common in the American population than food allergies. They occur when a trigger food or food additive produces symptoms that develop without involving an immune reaction.[2] Food intolerances may cause a *wide* variety of symptoms that sometimes occur days after the exposure, which makes it more difficult to track. Symptoms such as headache, migraine, coughing, sore throat, hoarseness, frequent throat clearing, runny or stuffy nose, postnasal drip, ear infections, sneezing attacks, hay fever, excessive mucus formation, dark circles under eyes, difficulty sleeping, insomnia, irregular heartbeat, asthma, bronchitis, constipation, diarrhea, indigestion, bloating, stomach pain, cramping, heartburn, mood swings, muscle/joint aches, arthritis, psoriasis, eczema, food cravings, fatigue, and poor concentration can occur.[3] Because many health conditions can also cause these symptoms, it takes professional evaluation to sort through the symptoms that may link them to specific foods.

Detecting Food Intolerance

Standard food allergy testing will not detect food intolerance. However, blood tests for some types of food intolerance exist outside of traditional medical practice. In conjunction with guided dietary modifications, these may be helpful in outlining which foods you are unable to tolerate. A few of the companies that offer this kind of testing include Metametrix (www.metametrix.com), Genova Diagnostics (www.genovadiagnostics.com), Signet Diagnostic (www.nowleap.com), and ALCAT Labs (www.alcat.com). Speak to your health care provider for more details. If avoided for a period of time, typically 3–4 months, some foods that were previously poorly tolerated can be reintroduced into the diet. A suspected environmental sensitivity, such as a reaction to trees, pollen, animals, or chemicals, would be investigated separately.

One of the reliable methods to determine the presence of a food intolerance, or even a previously undetected food allergy, is the elimination diet and rechallenge trial (also called *reintroduction or provocation test*). This is a sometimes lengthy and challenging undertaking that, nonetheless, can target foods poorly tolerated by an individual. There are several types of elimination diets: directed ones that target one or more foods, extreme ones eliminating most allergenic foods, and even stricter ones using amino acid–based formulas alone or along with a few proven safe foods thus eliminating virtually any potential allergen.[1] The choice of which one to use is based on clinical judgment of the individual situation.

A standard elimination diet process takes place in three stages. First, you stop eating every food suspected of causing a problem, which allows your symptoms to calm down. Usually, the foods that end up being the most provocative are the foods that we eat the most on a consistent basis. Which foods to eliminate are often the most common trigger foods (the common food allergens) and/or the foods that are suspicious to that particular person. These trials are very individualized. After a 7- to 28-day elimination (this time frame varies among practitioners), the second step is to reintroduce each food one by one a few days apart (this also varies by practitioner) and note any reactions. In the last stage, the poorly tolerated foods are identified and taken out of the diet for about 4–6 months, giving the body more time to heal. Then the foods are reintroduced—unless they caused a dangerous or immune-mediated food allergy reaction—one by one, noting the return of symptoms. If they are tolerated, they remain in the diet.

Not everyone has a smooth road from there. Certain people who are highly sensitive to foods based on food intolerance (not allergy) find that eating one food or another consistently bothers them. These people can benefit from a rotation diet, in which they eat their newly tolerated foods only at regularly spaced intervals of between 4 and 7 days (exact intervals are not critical).[4] Although this method is restrictive and a bit complicated to arrange, it often allows you to continue eating certain foods occasionally. As an added bonus, because different food "families" offer different carbohydrates, proteins, fats, vitamins, and minerals, it is beneficial to rotate foods in a structured fashion as part of a well-balanced diet.

What Jessie Decided

It's important to eliminate food allergies as the cause of symptoms before undertaking food intolerance testing. Jessie visited the allergist and was tested for *food allergies*. As she suspected, the results for all foods tested by skin prick were negative. Jessie's next visit was to the dietitian to find out if she could target one or more *food intolerances* that were causing distress.

The dietitian took a detailed history, which included the type and quantity of food and beverages, food preparation, possibility of cross-contamination with gluten or other allergens to which Jessie might be sensitive, type and consistency of symptoms, and the timing between food or beverage ingestion and the appearance of symptoms.[2]

Jessie's Food Record for a Typical Day

BREAKFAST: 1 cup of cold gluten-free (GF) rice cereal with extra sugar, milk, banana, and coffee with cream and sugar; gassy 20 minutes later

SNACK: GF pretzels; fuzzy headed, slight headache 30 minutes later

LUNCH: sandwich on GF bread with turkey, lettuce, tomato, and mayonnaise; orange slices, water, small GF candy bar; fatigue, gas, bloating 30 minutes later

SNACK: soy yogurt; gassy 20 minutes later

DINNER: miso soup, grilled salmon, mixed stir-fry vegetables, GF dinner roll, milk; gassy, bloated all evening after dinner, slight headache continued

The dietitian noted that Jessie's diet was largely composed of soy and dairy, with significant amounts of yeast and sugar. Soy is in soy yogurt, miso soup contains tofu (made from soy) and miso (soy) paste, and stir fry is often made with soy sauce. She uses milk in her cereal, as her beverage of choice, and in her coffee; milk is often an ingredient in bread and rolls with significant amounts of yeast, such as sandwich bread, pretzels, dinner rolls. Jessie also uses extra sugar in her cereal and coffee and gets more in her yogurt and candy bar. Soy is commonly a poorly digested protein-carbohydrate food that can cause gas and bloating. Milk can cause gas and bloating in someone lacking sufficient enzymes to digest the milk sugar (lactose) (see Chapter 37 on fructose, lactose, and related carbohydrates). Yeast, a common ingredient in baked products, can cause headaches and fatigue if someone is sensitive to it. Sugar, in moderate to large quantities, can cause shifts in blood glucose levels that can lead to fatigue.

The dietitian suggested that Jessie eliminate soy, dairy, yeast, and sugar and provided lists of foods to choose and foods to avoid. They discussed how to find these particular foods and ingredients on food labels, what questions to ask when dining out, and the best ways to prevent accidental exposure.[1] As you might imagine, Jessie was already well-versed on how to avoid gluten. Fortunately, the food labeling laws have made identification of major allergens much simpler and for that, we are fortunate, because the key is to follow the elimination diet fully. There is no such thing as a day off or a meal off, because that would greatly skew the results.

Although soy, milk, yeast, and sugar are common sources of food intolerance, individuals may react to many different foods. A few of them are listed in Table 1.

Practically any food or ingredient can be the source of food intolerance. Although some people are sensitive to a great number of foods, most of us are only sensitive to between two and five foods.[3]

Common Concerns about Food Elimination Diets

Most people feel better each day that they are on an elimination diet as their body slowly rids itself of the foods that are causing undesirable symptoms. But it is also common to feel increased fatigue, headaches, food cravings, or muscle aches as the body slowly withdraws from the foods it normally consumes. People avoiding yeast, sugar, or caffeine may experience fatigue or irritability. Although this is unpleasant, it is expected and will pass. It helps to eat meals spaced throughout the day so that your blood glucose level remains fairly stable. Don't overeat, yet don't use this trial as a time to focus on losing weight.

You will reach the point at which you feel well and are satisfied with your digestion, usually between one and four weeks (this varies among individuals). That's when you and your health care provider can agree on how you will reintroduce the foods (usually one at a time) and note any symptoms.

What Jessie Found

Jessie carefully avoided soy, dairy, yeast, and sugar for a full month. In place of soy and dairy, she drank gluten-free rice, almond, hazelnut, or hemp milk. Avoiding yeast and sugar meant avoiding bread and processed foods and sweets, so she relied on gluten-free cooked whole grains and simply prepared meals. She made sure to eat plenty of fresh, dark green, leafy vegetables and fruit of different colors (particularly dark ones, such as berries) for extra vitamins, minerals, and antioxidants. Because she was already preparing most foods from scratch, Jessie was able to easily control the ingredients. She found that she preferred using olive oil, lemon, balsamic vinegar, garlic, salt, freshly ground pepper, and fresh herbs for her dressings and her marinades rather than store-bought alternatives, which included ingredients she did not recognize.

TABLE 1. Foods/Ingredients Often Eliminated during Elimination Diets

Grains/starches/grasses: corn, oats, millet, buckwheat, amaranth, rice, quinoa, and gluten-containing grains (wheat, rye, barley)
Alcohol
Caffeine: coffee and tea
Carbonation
Chocolate and cocoa
Vinegar
Sulfites/sulfates
Preservatives (BHA, BHT)
Coloring/flavoring
Eggs
Shellfish and fish
Milk
Soy
Tree nuts
Peanuts
Legumes (lentils, soybeans)
Citrus (orange, grapefruit)
Artificial sweeteners
Sugar-free sweeteners and foods
Histamines: in strawberry, tomato, spinach, salami, very ripe cheese
Tyramines: in aged, fermented and/or spoiled meats and cheeses; sauerkraut; fermented soybean products; beer/ale
Colorings, flavorings, preservatives, flavor enhancers, stabilizers and other additives

One Day of Jessie's Elimination Diet

BREAKFAST: hot buckwheat cereal with gluten-free almond milk and berries, hot tea

LUNCH: Cooked quinoa* with black beans and vegetables roasted in olive oil, garlic, pepper, and salt; water; sliced mangoes or kiwi fruit

SNACK: banana with cashew or almond butter

DINNER: grilled salmon, sweet potato, broccoli or other dark, leafy green vegetable, fresh mixed berries for dessert

*Eating vitamin-rich vegetables, such as broccoli, tomatoes, and bell peppers, with quinoa and beans increases absorption of the iron from the quinoa and beans (nonheme sources of iron; see Chapter 49 on anemia).

Not only did Jessie's gas, bloating, and indigestion resolve, but she reported feeling much more energy in the morning and throughout the day. On her food and symptom log, she described having a clearer head and did not "droop" in midafternoon.

Like Jessie, many of my patients, especially the ones who follow an elimination diet that removes processed foods, sugar-free foods, soda, sugar, alcohol, caffeine, and their individual trigger foods, find that they feel *much* better in general. They report better energy, healthier looking skin, more stable moods, and fewer cravings, to name a few benefits. Although weight loss is not an intended outcome, numerous patients tell me that they were able to either lose weight in a healthy way or maintain their weight much more easily when they followed a diet that was "closer to the earth," with whole, unprocessed foods.

You do not need a reason to eliminate processed food from your diet. When a food is processed, it loses nutrients, protective antioxidants, and polyphenols, which are, ironically, the exact nutrients that your body needs to fully digest and use processed foods. Eating whole, unprocessed foods provides your body with the nutrients it needs to maximize cellular function. Your body will thank you for this healthy and wise decision.

Table 2 (slightly condensed for the purposes of this chapter) provides a list of the foods that would be allowed on a comprehensive elimination diet—one in which all processed foods and the major allergens are removed, including gluten. If you decide at some point to undergo an elimination diet, you will want to collaborate with a dietitian who will help

TABLE 2. Foods to Eat on a Comprehensive Elimination Diet

Fresh fruits: whole, unsweetened, frozen or water-packed canned fruits (no oranges or orange juice)	Dairy substitutes: gluten-free rice, hemp, nut (almond, hazelnut), and coconut milks (high in saturated fat; use sparingly); oat milk (only if guaranteed to be gluten free)
Vegetables: raw, steamed, sautéed, juiced, or roasted (no corn)	Nuts/seeds: sesame, pumpkin, and flax seeds; hazelnuts, almonds, walnuts, pecans, cashews, nut butters (no peanuts or peanut butter)
Grains and starch: brown rice, gluten-free oats, millet, quinoa, amaranth, teff, buckwheat, sorghum (no gluten-containing grains)	Oils: cold-pressed or virgin olive oil and flax seed, safflower, sesame, almond, sunflower, walnut, canola, pumpkin, grapeseed oils
Animal protein: fresh or water-packed fish, wild game, lamb, duck, organic chicken and turkey (no eggs)	Drinks: filtered or distilled water, decaffeinated herbal teas, seltzer or mineral water (no caffeine or sodas)
Vegetable protein: split peas, lentils, (black beans, kidney beans, and other cooked dried beans) (no soy or peanuts in any form)	Condiments/sweeteners: vinegar (except malt vinegar), all spices and herbs, brown rice syrup (unless it contains barley), agave nectar, Stevia, fruit sweetener, black strap molasses (no refined sugar, honey, maple syrup, corn syrup, or high-fructose corn syrup)

Adapted from Lipski E. Comprehensive Elimination Diet. Applying Functional Medicine in Clinical Practice Tool Kit. The Institute for Functional Medicine, 2004.

you decide exactly how expansive or restrictive your individual diet will be. This chart can be modified in many different ways depending on your needs.

Jessie gave some serious thought to maintaining her new healthy, balanced diet, but ultimately, she was curious to know which foods were giving her trouble. She began the rechallenge phase.

Rechallenge Trial

One at a time, Jessie added each of the four foods back into her diet using the purest form of the food possible. If you use the plainest, purest form of the food and you develop a symptom, you will know that it is from the food itself, not another ingredient. She made certain to have at least two normal-sized portions of the trial food per day (at breakfast and lunch) for 2–3 days (serving sizes and number of days varies among practitioners). Jessie waited at least two days in between each trial—called the *washout period*—to be certain that she did not have any residual symptoms from the last food tried. Washout periods vary between 2 and 7 days.

Jessie's Food Trial Results

> Soy (unsweetened, gluten-free soy milk, plain tofu); gassy, bloated (but less than before)
>
> Milk (cow's milk); no symptoms
>
> Yeast (gluten-free bread containing yeast); headache, bloated
>
> Sugar (white table sugar); no symptoms

Jessie decided to introduce milk back into her diet, but not every day. She reintroduced cow's milk but also continued drinking gluten-free rice, hazelnut, almond, and hemp milk on occasion. Because soy continued to give her symptoms, Jessie eliminated it from her diet for 4–6 months to give her body time to heal. She focused on other ways of getting protein: lean turkey, chicken, and fish; dried beans and hummus; amaranth and quinoa (both very high in protein); and nuts and seeds. She also avoided yeast and, by doing so, she automatically reduced her sugar intake because she was eating fewer baked goods.

Six months later, Jessie reported that she has successfully reintroduced soy into her diet but does not eat it as much as before the trial. She is eating minimal yeast because, to her delight, she is enjoying the unintentional weight loss that came with eating less bread and fewer baked goods and processed foods.

A formal food elimination diet and rechallenge trial should be done under the supervision of a trained health care professional. Although protocols vary somewhat, it is important to be guided through the process to ensure a balanced diet of key nutrients, both during the trial and after completion. You will need advice about what to do if you react to foods during your trial, when and how to introduce well-tolerated foods, how to rotate foods (if necessary), how to find healthy substitutions, and whether you need to permanently or temporarily avoid certain foods. If you suspect that certain foods may be bothering you, start a food and symptom log so that at your first appointment with your provider you can provide helpful detailed information to guide the elimination diet. For more information on additional supportive nutrients, such as aloe (historically used as a soothing agent for the gut), glutamine (an amino acid that is the preferred source of food for the cells lining the intestine), and probiotics (beneficial bacteria) that may be used to help heal the intestine, consult with your dietitian.

Acknowledgement

Elizabeth Lipski, PhD, CCN, Director of Doctoral Studies at Hawthorn University, on faculty at the Institute for Functional Medicine, and author of *Digestive Wellness* and *Digestive Wellness for Children,* assisted in the preparation of this chapter.

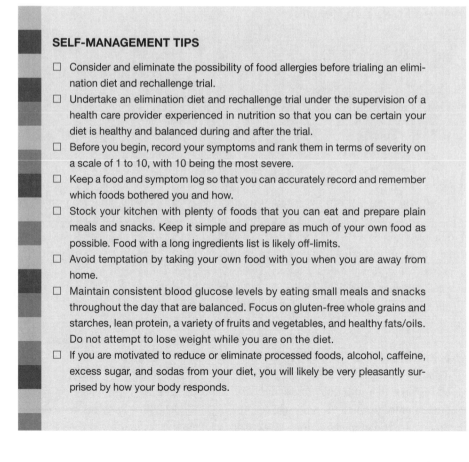

SELF-MANAGEMENT TIPS

☐ Consider and eliminate the possibility of food allergies before trialing an elimination diet and rechallenge trial.

☐ Undertake an elimination diet and rechallenge trial under the supervision of a health care provider experienced in nutrition so that you can be certain your diet is healthy and balanced during and after the trial.

☐ Before you begin, record your symptoms and rank them in terms of severity on a scale of 1 to 10, with 10 being the most severe.

☐ Keep a food and symptom log so that you can accurately record and remember which foods bothered you and how.

☐ Stock your kitchen with plenty of foods that you can eat and prepare plain meals and snacks. Keep it simple and prepare as much of your own food as possible. Food with a long ingredients list is likely off-limits.

☐ Avoid temptation by taking your own food with you when you are away from home.

☐ Maintain consistent blood glucose levels by eating small meals and snacks throughout the day that are balanced. Focus on gluten-free whole grains and starches, lean protein, a variety of fruits and vegetables, and healthy fats/oils. Do not attempt to lose weight while you are on the diet.

☐ If you are motivated to reduce or eliminate processed foods, alcohol, caffeine, excess sugar, and sodas from your diet, you will likely be very pleasantly surprised by how your body responds.

References

1. American College of Allergy, Asthma & Immunology. Food allergy: a practice parameter. *Ann Allergy Asthma Immunol* 2006;96(3 Suppl. 2):S1–68.
2. Lied GA. Gastrointestinal food hypersensitivity: symptoms, diagnosis and provocation test. *Turk J Gastroenterol* 2007;18(1):5–13.
3. Lipski E. *Digestive Wellness,* 3rd Edition. New York: McGraw-Hill, 2004, p. 91.
4. Brostoff J, Gamlin L. *Food Allergies and Food Intolerances: The Complete Guide to Their Identification and Treatment.* Rochester, VT: Healing Arts Press, 2000.

Further Reading

- Melina V, Stepaniak J, Aronson D. *Food Allergy Survival Guide.* Summertown, TN: Healthy Living Publications, 2004.
- Fenster C. *Cooking Free: 220 Flavorful Recipes for People with Food Allergies and Multiple Food Sensitivities.* New York: Avery/Penguin Group, 2007.

CHAPTER 37

Malabsorption of Fructose, Lactose, and Related Carbohydrates

Melinda Dennis, MS, RD, LDN, and
Jacqueline Barrett, PhD, BSc(Biomed)(Hons), MND, APD, RNutr

Jill, a 22-year old college student, came to the nutrition clinic seven months after being diagnosed with celiac disease. Despite following a gluten-free diet (GFD), she was bothered by nearly continuous burping, along with painful gas and bloating, followed by cramping and loose stools. Jill told us that this happened after eating. Also, she said she was eating less food than usual before feeling very full.

Our first step was to perform a celiac blood test for immunoglobulin A tissue trans-glutaminase (IgA-tTG), which was slightly elevated at 23 units (less than 20 units is normal) but down from 74 units at diagnosis. The large drop in tTG suggested that she was doing a good job on the GFD and that her celiac disease was becoming less active.

We then talked about the types of foods she had been eating by going over her food diary. She did not seem to be inadvertently ingesting gluten. A closer look at her food records showed that the timing of her symptoms appeared to be associated with meals or snacks that included orange juice, apples, soft drinks, onions, candies, and sugar-free gum. All of these items contain high levels of fructose and other poorly absorbed sugars, known as *FODMAPs*.

What Are FODMAPs?

The human intestine's ability to absorb fructose and several other short-chain carbohydrates is relatively limited. These carbohydrates include fermentable oligosaccharides, disaccharides, monosaccharides, and polyols (FODMAPs). The FODMAPs are fructose (found in apples, pears, honey), fructans (wheat, rye, garlic, onions), galactans (cabbage, legumes), lactose (milk, milk products), and polyol sweeteners that include sorbitol (peaches, plums, apricots, nectarines, cherries), xylitol, mannitol (cauliflower, mushrooms), and isomalt, which are also found in many sugar-free products.

It is normal to not absorb FODMAPs well. However, when you have a gastrointestinal disorder such as celiac disease or irritable bowel syndrome, this incomplete absorption can cause gastrointestinal symptoms. Undigested FODMAPs pass through the digestive tract and reach the colon. There they are rapidly fermented by bacteria, producing gas and short-chain fatty acids, which typically cause bloating, gas, cramping, and diarrhea.

We see many patients with celiac disease who appear to be following a strict GFD but have persistent symptoms that are related to ingesting FODMAPs. Fortunately, these symptoms can often be relieved by making specific dietary changes.

We reviewed Jill's food diary to identify any dietary factors that might be related to her symptoms. First, we ruled out inadvertent or unintentional gluten exposure, which is the most common cause of the persistent symptoms that she was experiencing. She also said she had no problems when eating lactose or foods with soy, but she had a significant intake of high-fructose, fructan, and polyol foods.

Finding FODMAP Culprits

To determine whether FODMAPs are involved in causing symptoms, you need to avoid eating all types of FODMAPs for 6–8 weeks. Then, add each individual FODMAP (fructose, lactose, fructans, galactans, and polyols) back into your diet one at a time to see if your symptoms return. For most people, sticking to a FODMAP-free diet is not necessary, which is helpful because FODMAPs are found in the majority of our food supply. Limiting, rather than completely avoiding, FODMAP foods should reduce your FODMAP intake sufficiently so that your symptoms improve.

We can use breath tests to investigate whether two of the FODMAPs, fructose and lactose, might be triggering your gastrointestinal symptoms. Breath testing involves drinking the test sugar (either fructose or lactose) and breathing into a bag every 15–30 minutes for 2–3 hours. If you do not absorb the sugar, we will detect a rise in breath hydrogen and/or methane that results from the fermentation of the sugar by intestinal bacteria. This is a useful test if you are experiencing symptoms and want to know if you will benefit from excluding fructose or lactose from your diet.

The remaining FODMAPs—fructans, galactans, and polyols—cannot be formally investigated. This is because they are always poorly absorbed in the human small intestine. If you are suffering from the effects of excessive fermentation, with symptoms of bloating, abdominal pain, gas, and altered bowel habits, you will need to omit these from your diet, then reintroduce them slowly to find your tolerance level. Most people manage to eat small amounts of these problem foods, and this usually does not require strict adherence, unlike the GFD.

Problem Foods in Fructose Malabsorption

If you are suffering from problems related to fructose malabsorption, you don't need to follow a fructose-free diet and eliminate all sources of fructose. There are other ways to deal with it. For instance, eating fructose at the same time as another natural sugar, glucose, improves fructose absorption. You will probably be able to tolerate foods that contain equal amounts of fructose and glucose, such as oranges and bananas. Only foods that contain more fructose than glucose trigger symptoms, such as honey, apples, and pears. Table 1 shows how much of these sugars are in a typical serving of these foods; the higher the excess fructose, the harder the food is to digest. Remember that fructose and high-fructose corn syrup are often used as sweeteners in the commercial food industry, so check food labels for these sugars.

TABLE 1. Foods with High Fructose Content

Food	Average Serving	Glucose (g)	Fructose (g)	Excess Fructose (g)
Apple	1 whole, 6 oz.	2.46	2.69	0.23
Asparagus	4 spears, 2.5 oz.	1.76	2.02	0.26
Watermelon	1 large slice, 4 oz.	2.00	2.70	0.73
Mango	1 whole, 7 oz.	2.85	3.82	0.97
Honey	1 tablespoon	6.80	8.20	1.40
Sugar snap peas	½ cup, 2 oz.	0.35	2.00	1.64
Asian pear	1 whole, 4 oz.	2.92	4.92	2.00
Peach, clingstone	1 whole, 5 oz.	1.89	7.22	5.32
Pear	1 whole, 6 oz.	5.35	11.46	6.11

Another thing to be aware of is the concentration of fructose in a food (its fructose load), regardless of glucose content. Even fruits that are well tolerated, such as oranges and bananas, can provoke symptoms if you eat them in large quantities or as concentrated forms such as fruit juice and dried fruit. Consider the portion size of one orange compared with how much "orange" you get in orange juice. People with fructose malabsorption can usually tolerate eating an orange but might notice gas, cramping, and loose stool after drinking orange juice. That's because a typical cup of orange juice contains the fructose of 4–5 squeezed oranges.

High-fructose corn syrup (HFCS) is an inexpensive sweetener widely used in food manufacturing to improve sweetness, texture, and shelf life. Because it's found in a variety of foods, this could be the source of your gastrointestinal symptoms. HFCS contains both fructose and glucose but the ratio varies (from 40:60 to 80:20) depending on the product. It's too confusing to determine the ratio and thereby predict whether you would tolerate it; it's better for people aiming for a low-fructose diet to avoid HFCS altogether.

Sucrose, also known as table sugar, contains fructose and glucose in a 50:50 concentration. You will likely be able to tolerate it in small amounts, but ingesting it in concentrated fruit sources, such as orange juice, can cause symptoms. If you are following a low-fructose diet, minimize your intake of high-sucrose foods such as sweetened drinks, sweets, and candies.

Don't confuse fructose malabsorption with hereditary fructose intolerance. This is a disorder that presents in infancy usually at about the age that infants move from drinking only breast milk to eating food. Fructose intolerance occurs when the specific enzyme responsible for digesting fructose is lacking or completely absent. Symptoms of hereditary fructose intolerance are recurring low blood glucose levels (hypoglycemia) and vomiting.

Managing Lactose Malabsorption

In patients with newly diagnosed celiac disease, lactose malabsorption, or intolerance, is very common because of loss of lactase, the enzyme that digests milk sugar, along the lining of the small intestine. Lactose is the sugar present in cow's milk products. If you aren't absorbing lactose, it might be because your lactase levels are too low. If you are having symptoms of gas, bloating, and diarrhea or loose stool, it might be useful to have a lactose breath test (described above) or trial a low-lactose diet. Because most people produce at least a small amount of lactase, managing lactose intolerance does not usually require complete avoidance of lactose.

Studies have shown that limiting ingestion to 4–7 grams of lactose per day can help you avoid symptoms (Table 2). This is the amount found in ⅓ cup of cow's milk and 3–4 oz. of yogurt. You can probably tolerate regular milk in small amounts when added to food, such as a cup of tea, scrambled eggs, or mashed potatoes. Soft cheeses such as ricotta and cottage cheese have greater amounts of lactose and are best consumed in small amounts.

TABLE 2. Lactose Content of Common Foods and Beverages

Food or Beverage	Serving Size	Lactose (g)
Acidophilus milk	1 cup	11
Buttermilk	1 cup	10
Chocolate milk	1 cup	11
Evaporated milk	1 cup	24
Low-fat milk	1 cup	11
Nonfat dry milk powder, unreconstituted	1 cup	62
Nonfat milk	1 cup	11
Sweetened condensed milk, undiluted	1 cup	40
Whole milk	1 cup	11
Light cream	½ cup	4
Half-and-half	½ cup	5
Sour cream	½ cup	4
Whipping cream	½ cup	3
Butter	1 tsp.	Trace
Oleomargarine	1 tsp.	Trace
American cheese	1 oz.	2
Blue cheese	1 oz.	1
Cheddar cheese, sharp	1 oz.	0–1
Cottage cheese, creamed	½ cup	3
Cottage cheese, uncreamed	½ cup	2
Cream cheese	1 oz.	1
Parmesan cheese, grated	1 oz.	1
Swiss cheese	1 oz.	1
Ice cream	½ cup	6
Ice milk	½ cup	9
Sherbet, orange	½ cup	2
Yogurt, low fat	1 cup	5

Used with permission from the University of Virginia Digestive Health Center of Excellence.

Hard cheeses, such as cheddar and parmesan, as well as butter and margarine, are so low in lactose they are considered almost lactose free. Goat and sheep milks also contain lactose but tend to be better tolerated by some people with lactose intolerance. So, don't focus on having a dairy-free diet but instead work toward a low-lactose diet. This involves replacing large amounts of milk and yogurt with lactose-free alternatives and continuing to eat cheeses and spreads. The assessment of Jill's diet showed that she consumes only small amounts of milk and has cheese daily, so she is not ingesting lactose at levels likely to cause symptoms.

What about Other FODMAPs?

If you have fructose and/or lactose malabsorption, it is not always the complete answer to what is causing your symptoms. Because they are so poorly absorbed, fructans, galactans, and polyols are always likely culprits if you are suffering from gastrointestinal symptoms. Restricting these FODMAPs might also be necessary.

Table 3 outlines the foods high in fructans, galactans, and polyols that you can totally avoid and then slowly add to your diet, noting changes in your symptoms. You can do this in addition to a fructose- and/or lactose-restricted diet or as a separate dietary strategy if fructose and lactose malabsorption have been excluded as causes of your problems.

What Jill Decided

Because Jill's symptoms were typical for fructose malabsorption and her food diary showed that symptoms occurred after fructose intake, we suggested she start a trial period on a low-FODMAP diet, without restricting her lactose intake. Already avid about following her GFD, Jill didn't want to restrict her diet further. She needed some convincing that we were on the right track for helping her get rid of her symptoms. So she elected to undergo a formal breath test for fructose. Her results are shown in Table 4 and indicate malabsorption of fructose. People who absorb fructose completely should not have a rise in hydrogen or methane more than 10–20 parts per million above the baseline reading.

With these results in mind, Jill proceeded with fructose restriction and also limited her intake of the other FODMAPs, fructans, galactans, and polyols. She received instruction on what to look for on food labels. Jill was also asked to check her medications and supplements for fructose, sorbitol, and other polyol-containing ingredients.

Following the low-FODMAP diet without replacing those fruits and vegetables can result in very low fiber intake. Jill learned to include "intestinal friendly" fruits and vegetables (Table 5), aiming for 2–5 servings of each type of food per day. She also experimented with more of the gluten-free whole grains, which are also rich in fiber (see Chapter 13 on grains).

Outcome

In addition to her GFD, Jill has been avoiding orange juice, honey, candies, onions, garlic, and high-fructose corn syrup. She has been much less troubled with burping and gas, and her diarrhea is gone. At the end of eight weeks, she will introduce small amounts of FODMAPs into her diet and note how well she tolerates each one.

TABLE 3. Foods with Fructans, Galactans, and Polyols

Food	Average Serving	Fructans/Galactans (g)	Polyols (g)	Total (g)
Pear	1 whole, 6 oz.	0	7.4	7.4
Artichoke, Jerusalem	½ cup, 2 oz.	7.3	0	7.3
Blackberry	⅓ cup, 2.5 oz.	0	3.4	3.4
Asian pear	1 whole, 4 oz.	0	2.8	2.8
Cauliflower	½ cup, 2 oz.	0	1.8	1.8
Peaches	1 whole, 5 oz.	0.2	1.3	1.5
Artichoke, globe	1 medium, 4 oz.	1.4	0	1.4
Onion, shallot	1 Tbsp., ½ oz.	1.4	0	1.4
Nectarine	1 whole, 5 oz.	0	1.3	1.3
Apple	1 whole, 6 oz.	0	1.2	1.2
Legumes	½ cup, 3 oz.	1.1	0	1.1
Mushrooms	½ cup, 1.5 oz.	0	1.0	1.0
Watermelon	1 large slice, 4 oz.	0.4	0.3	0.7
Snow peas	½ cup, 1 oz.	0.2	0.4	0.6
Peas	½ cup, 2.5 oz.	0.5	0	0.5
Garlic	1 clove, 3 g	0.5	0	0.5
Avocado	½ medium, 3 oz.	0	0.5	0.5
Beetroot	1 whole, 4 oz.	0.5	0	0.5
Cabbage	1 cup, 4 oz.	0.4	0	0.4
Broccoli	4 flowerettes, 1.5 oz.	0.4	0	0.4
Asparagus	4 spears, 2.5 oz.	0.3	0	0.3
Onion, white/brown	1 Tbsp., ½ oz.	0.3	0	0.3
Onion, Spanish	1 Tbsp., ½ oz.	0.3	0	0.3
Fennel	½ cup, 2 oz.	0.2	0	0.2
Leek	1 Tbsp., ½ oz.	0.2	0	0.2
Brussels sprouts	1 sprout, 2 oz.	0.2	0	0.2

TABLE 4. Jill's Fructose Breath Test Results

Time	Hydrogen (parts per million)	Methane (parts per million)
Baseline	1	1
30 minutes	3	1
60 minutes	20	1
90 minutes	38	1
120 minutes	40	1
150 minutes	102	1
180 minutes	65	1

TABLE 5. Guidelines for Fruits and Vegetables

Intestinal-Friendly Fruit	Eat Cautiously
Pineapple, strawberry, raspberry, blueberry, lemon, lime, orange, mandarin, banana, rhubarb, honeydew melon, rockmelon, kiwifruit, passionfruit	Large servings of intestinal-friendly fruits or concentrated sources such as jam/jelly, dried fruit, fruit juice
Intestinal-Friendly Vegetables	Eat Cautiously
Green peppers,* leafy greens, celery, potatoes, spinach, green beans, cucumber,* pumpkin, carrot, alfalfa sprouts, tomatoes, chives, sweet corn, sweet potato	Large servings of tomatoes, i.e., tomato soup, tomato juice

*Potentially gas producing.

SELF-MANAGEMENT TIPS

☐ The most common symptoms of fructose or FODMAP malabsorption—gas, bloating, and loose stool/diarrhea—mimic those of gluten exposure.

☐ If you are experiencing these symptoms, especially after eating, and gluten exposure is ruled out, consider fructose or lactose malabsorption and an overall intolerance to FODMAPs.

☐ Two options for diagnosis include fructose and/or lactose breath tests or a dietary trial involving avoidance of most sources of FODMAPs (honey, apples, pears, peaches, fruit juice, dried fruit, soft drinks, sugar-free foods containing polyols, onions, garlic, and the ingredients fructose, corn syrup and high fructose corn syrup) for at least 6–8 weeks and note any change in your symptoms.

☐ If the diagnosis is made through breath testing, consider restricting fructose and/or lactose and limiting your intake of the remaining FODMAPs for approximately 6–8 weeks.

☐ You need the guidance of a registered dietitian when starting a low-FODMAP diet. Your dietitian can ensure you maintain a balanced and healthy diet and may be able to provide more insight if you do not have complete relief of your symptoms.

☐ If your symptoms improve, after 6–8 weeks you can begin slowly to add back small amounts of FODMAPs to test your own tolerance level.

☐ If your symptoms do not improve, it is unlikely that you will gain much by continuing restriction of FODMAPs. You might find, however, that although you feel your symptoms did not resolve on the diet, you notice that reintroducing fructose and other FODMAPs makes your existing symptoms worse. If so, the diet may still be helpful for you.

Further Reading

- Barrett JS, Gibson PR. Clinical ramifications of malabsorption of fructose and other short-chain carbohydrates. *Pract Gastroenterol* 2007;XXXI(8):51–65.
- Gibson PR, Newnham E, Barrett JS, Shepherd, Muir JG. Fructose malabsorption and the bigger picture (review). *Aliment Pharmacol Ther* 2007;25:349–63.
- Choi Y, Johlin F, Summers R, Jackson M, Rao S. Fructose intolerance: an under-recognized problem. *Am J Gastroenterol* 2003;98(6):1348–53.
- Shepherd S, Gibson P. Fructose malabsorption and symptoms of irritable bowel syndrome: guidelines for effective dietary management. *J Am Diet Assoc* 2006;106:1631–39.
- Ali M, Rellos P, Cox TM. Hereditary fructose intolerance. *J Med Genet* 1998;35(5):353–65.
- Rao S, Attaluri A, Anderson L, Stumbo P. The ability of the normal human small intestine to absorb fructose: evaluation by breath testing. *Clin Gastroenterol Hepatol* 2007;5(8):959–63.

Jacqueline Barrett, PhD, BSc(Biomed)(Hons), MND, APD, RNutr, is an Australian dietitian in private practice who specializes in gastrointestinal disorders (www.dietsolutions.net.au) and Lecturer at Monash University, Eastern Health Clinical School, Victoria, Australia. Her research in dietary management of gastrointestinal conditions focuses on FODMAPs, intestinal microbiota, irritable bowel syndrome, and related gastrointestinal conditions.

CHAPTER 38

Irritable Bowel Syndrome and Celiac Disease

Filippo Cremonini, MD, MSc, PhD, and Anthony Lembo, MD

Rita is a 38-year-old accountant who has been struggling with frequent gassy cramps in her lower abdomen and loose stools since her teenage years. She reports that her symptoms are worse when she gets stressed at work, during which time she can have up to 10 small, loose bowel movements a day, with an urgent need to get to a toilet. Her cramps get better right after she passes stools. Occasionally, she also gets constipated, and this may make her gassy pain worse. She has never noticed blood in her stools, although she is worried because her father died of colon cancer at age 68. She is on no medication, although she uses loperamide (Imodium) when her bowel movements are so frequent that she cannot work, with some improvement.

Four years ago she was diagnosed with celiac disease because of iron deficiency anemia that was not responding to standard supplementation. She has been on the gluten-free diet (GFD) since then, and her anemia has resolved and her immunoglobulin A tissue transglutaminase (IgA-tTG) has normalized. However, she has not seen any change in her symptoms. Because of this, Rita's gastroenterologist evaluated her for nonresponsive celiac disease (see Chapter 34 on nonresponsive and Chapter 43 on refractory celiac disease). Her complete blood count, thyroid function tests, and electrolyte, glucose, and IgA-tTG levels are all normal. Her C-reactive protein (a marker of inflammation) is also within normal limits. Rita had a colonoscopy with random biopsies of her colon to rule out microscopic colitis (see Chapter 39) and an upper endoscopy with duodenal biopsies, both of which revealed no abnormalities. A small bowel follow-through X-ray showed a normal contour of her entire small bowel.

Her gastroenterologist explained to Rita that her celiac disease is well controlled and her symptoms are probably because of irritable bowel syndrome (IBS). After a review of these tests, Rita's primary care physician also tells her that she has IBS. She wonders what caused this problem.

What Is Irritable Bowel Syndrome?

IBS is the most common diagnosis in the gastroenterologist's office. It is defined as abdominal discomfort or pain that is relieved with bowel movements, with this discomfort accompanied by change in the frequency or in the form of stools (Table 1). For IBS,

TABLE 1. Rome III Criteria for Diagnosis of Irritable Bowel Syndrome

Abdominal pain or discomfort, which began at least 6 months prior to the visit, is recurrent and is present at least 3 days per month in the last 3 months and is associated with 2 or more of the following:

    Improvement with defecation
    Onset associated with a change in frequency of stool
    Onset associated with a change in form (appearance) of stool

Adapted from Reference 3.

we first consider stool consistency (whether the patient has predominantly looser or harder stools), then frequency, considering diarrhea to be more than three stools per day and constipation to be fewer than three stools per week. Some people with IBS have predominantly diarrhea, others have predominantly constipation, and still others alternate between the two. Symptoms can change over time, so that those who initially complained of diarrhea might become constipated and vice versa.[1,2]

For a diagnosis of IBS, these disturbances must be ongoing and have been present at least three days a month in the last three months. There can be no visible abnormalities that explain such symptoms on endoscopy, imaging, or laboratory tests. In the case of celiac disease, symptoms must persist despite apparent healing of the intestine to be attributed to IBS.

IBS is common, and we believe that 5–20% of the general U.S. population suffers from the symptoms of IBS. A lot of conditions have symptoms in common with IBS and may mimic it (Table 2), including celiac disease, so it is important to have a careful, thorough diagnosis. Only recently has testing for celiac disease become a standard recommendation when evaluating patients with suspected IBS.

How Are IBS and Celiac Disease Related?

A small but significant number of people initially thought to be suffering from IBS eventually receive a diagnosis of celiac disease. The prevalence of celiac disease in individuals who also have IBS has been estimated to be approximately 4-fold higher than in the general population or about 4%. Reaching the diagnosis of celiac disease is important because avoiding gluten often leads to resolution of symptoms and may prevent future complications (see Chapter 45 on complications). It is important to note that IBS can coexist with any other gastrointestinal disorder, including celiac disease and inflammatory bowel disease. It can often be quite difficult to sort out which symptoms are because of which disease, and there may actually be interaction where inflammation in the intestine can cause or worsen IBS.

What Causes IBS?

IBS is the result of a complex interaction between the brain and gut via the brain-gut axis and thus involves both physiological and psychological factors. The two physiological factors that are affected are the sensory function and the motor function. The sensory function

TABLE 2. Differential Diagnoses of IBS by Predominant Bowel Habit

Diarrhea-Predominant IBS	Constipation-Predominant IBS
Celiac disease (and tropical sprue in selected populations)	Slow transit
Inflammatory bowel disease (ulcerative colitis, Crohn's disease)	Pelvic floor dysfunction (paradoxical contraction of pelvic muscles during defecation making stool passage more difficult)
Neoplasms	Obstruction and pseudo-obstruction of the gastrointestinal tract (non-cancer)
Microscopic (lymphocytic or collagenous) colitis	Neoplasms, colorectal cancer
Lactose intolerance	Endocrine disorders: diabetes, hypothyroid, hypokalemia, hypercalcemia
Sugar malabsorption and excessive ingestion of nonabsorbable sugars (e.g., sorbitol)	Central and peripheral neurogenic disorders such as Parkinson's disease or peripheral or diabetic neuropathy
Small intestinal bacterial overgrowth	Small and large intestine smooth muscle disorders
Whipple's disease	Hirschprung's disease
Parasitic infection	Pregnancy
Medications	Anorexia nervosa
	Medications

is the way the bowel perceives pain, gas, and other sensations. Problems with this can lead to hypersensitivity, where sensations that people without IBS feel are normal are perceived as painful by those with IBS. The motor function is the way the bowel propels contents through it. Problems with this can lead to faster movement of gut contents, with diarrhea and explosive bowel movements, or to slower contractions, leading to constipation. Sensation and motor function are finely regulated by a complex system of neurons that constitute the so-called enteric nervous system. The enteric nervous system resides in the layers of gut, yet contains more nerve cells than the entire brain! The enteric nervous system works closely with the brain for the transmission of sensation to the brain and the reception of signals from it.

The autonomic nervous system is also involved in regulation of digestion and sensation of the gut. It controls the way the pancreas secretes digestive hormones and how information is processed by the gut sensory nerves. Other major regulators are the immune system and hormones, some of which are produced right in the gut and change the motility and sensation of the stomach and small and large intestine. Certain bacteria in the gut can elicit immune responses that can affect sensory and motor function and also produce excess gas, which is linked to IBS. This complicated, multipronged interaction between the brain and gut is the reason why physical or mental stress, trauma, and acute and chronic illnesses can cause bowel symptoms. We are still debating whether problems in sensory and motor functions are brought on by environmental or dietary causes, inheritable causes, or acute/chronic infections.

How Is IBS Treated?

Although there is no one-size-fits-all treatment plan, we usually try to improve the predominant bowel problem—either diarrhea or constipation—with antidiarrheals such as loperamide or laxatives such as polyethylene glycol or a combination for those with alternating symptoms. Fiber-containing laxatives such as psyllium and methylcellulose can make constipation and bloating worse and so are typically avoided.[4]

If these simple, first-line measures fail, we can target the motor function for those with constipation-predominant IBS with prokinetics that accelerate gut transit, antispasmodics that can reduce the abdominal cramping associated with bowel spasm, and drugs that increase secretion in the gut lumen that loosens and speeds up stool. In those with diarrhea-predominant IBS, we can use anticholinergic drugs such as dicyclomine or non-narcotic opioid medications, such as diphenoxylate or loperamide that slow overall and colonic transit.

There are also medications that target pain, such as nonnarcotic pain medications and low-dose antidepressants. For instance, amitriptyline can be used at doses that improve pain and discomfort from IBS without changing mood. Narcotic analgesics should not be used to treat IBS because they interfere with gastrointestinal motility and there is a high potential for users to develop tolerance and addiction.

Probiotics—live bacteria, such as *Lactobacilli* and *Bifidobacteria*, that rebalance gut flora when it is unbalanced—are effective in IBS (see Chapter 41 on probiotics). Oral antibiotics that are not absorbed but remain primarily in the gut lumen are also sometimes effective, as they may correct bacterial flora imbalances.

Is There a Diet for IBS?

Food can make IBS symptoms worse. However, despite the overwhelming amount and variety of dietary advice about the best IBS diets, there are no high-quality data on dietary treatments in IBS.

Some have advocated a diet limited in poorly absorbed carbohydrates, such as lactose and/or fructose (see Chapter 37). Generally, high-fiber diets are thought to treat constipation, but the benefit of fiber may be minimal, and insoluble fiber (such as broccoli, cauliflower, and other rough vegetables) may increase symptoms of bloating, distention, and pain. You may need to learn the difference between soluble and insoluble fiber and to choose foods accordingly (see Chapter 16 on constipation). Some individuals may have intolerance to specific foods, prompting testing for allergies, but continued testing to rule out false positives is not practical for most patients. It is more reasonable to try an elimination diet and gradually reintroduce suspected foods or classes of food into your meals. Some foods commonly eliminated and reintroduced are chocolate, carbonated beverages, caffeine, sugar, fatty foods, processed foods, alcohol, sugar-free foods, and high-gas-producing foods (see Chapter 36 on elimination diets).

GFDs have not been formally tested in IBS, although some evidence suggests that the IBS symptoms in those with gluten intolerance, rather than celiac disease, improve after going gluten free (see Chapter 8 on gluten intolerance).

What Rita Decided

Rita was given a "toolkit" for her IBS that consists of an antispasmodic medication to be used as needed and a schedule for escalating doses of Imodium when her diarrhea gets worse. She started using an over-the-counter probiotic that has helped with her gas (see Chapter 41 on probiotics). Although she feels in better control of her bowel movements, pain remains an occasional issue.

Rita has discussed with her gastroenterologist starting low-dose amitriptyline as the next step. She has been successful at staying on a strict GFD but wonders if she should be avoiding anything else, although she does not feel there is a particular food that makes her symptoms better or worse. Rita plans to visit a dietitian to improve her knowledge about and confidence with her diet and to ensure that her choices are nutritionally adequate.

Patients like Rita often try additional alternative or complementary approaches for treating their IBS. Practices such as cognitive behavioral therapy, hypnotherapy, and acupuncture have been shown to provide some additional symptom relief in clinical trials. Although not formally recommended by IBS treatment guidelines, these approaches are generally safe in expert hands.

SELF-MANAGEMENT TIPS

☐ IBS is a disorder of gut function that is defined by pain or discomfort in the abdomen, associated with bowel habit changes, that is relieved by bowel movements. In addition to pain, diarrhea, constipation, or both are the primary symptoms.

☐ IBS is very common in the general population and occurs in people with celiac disease.

☐ IBS symptoms can mimic celiac disease, but these two conditions can be distinguished by blood tests and endoscopy. Gastrointestinal symptoms that persist despite a strict GFD are often because of IBS, but other causes of nonresponsive celiac disease should be ruled out.

☐ In contrast to celiac disease, there is no specific diet to treat IBS. However, consider meeting with a dietitian to assess your need for an elimination-reintroduction diet to assess the roles various foods can play in your symptoms.

References

1. Mayer EA. Clinical practice: irritable bowel syndrome. *N Engl J Med* 2008;358(16):1692–99.
2. Drossman DA, Camilleri M, Mayer EA, Whitehead WE. AGA technical review on irritable bowel syndrome. *Gastroenterology* 2002;123(6):2108–31.
3. Longstreth GF, Thompson WG, Chey WD, et al. Functional bowel disorders. *Gastroenterology* 2006;130(5):1480–91.
4. Lembo AJ. A 54-year-old woman with constipation-predominant irritable bowel syndrome. *JAMA* 2006;295(8):925–33.

Filippo Cremonini, MD, MSc, PhD, is a Clinical Fellow in gastroenterology and **Anthony Lembo, MD,** is Associate Professor of Medicine at Beth Israel Deaconess Medical Center and Harvard Medical School, Boston, Massachussetts.

CHAPTER 39

Microscopic Colitis and Celiac Disease

Joseph A. Murray, MD, and Alberto Rubio-Tapia, MD

When Kelly, a 65-year-old woman, came to the Celiac Clinic, she had been through two months of persistent watery diarrhea (about 6 bowel movements per day without blood or fat) and bloating. She was diagnosed with celiac disease 10 years ago and had been without symptoms for the last 10 years by following a gluten-free diet (GFD). Kelly's past medical and family histories showed no reason for the diarrhea, and she had not recently traveled internationally. She said she had not had fever, weight loss, or abdominal pain and was still eating completely gluten free.

Kelly had normal temperature, pulse, and blood pressure. When palpated, she didn't have pain in her abdomen, and her liver and spleen felt normal. Her blood work was normal (hemoglobin 14), and the blood test for immunoglobulin A tissue transglutaminase antibodies was 2 units (normal is less than 20 units), which showed that she was eating gluten free.

Because of the recent onset of persistent diarrhea, Kelly was evaluated for other causes of nonresponsive celiac disease. An upper endoscopy showed that her small intestine was normal. Intestinal biopsy specimens were normal, and no bacteria were detected after analysis of intestinal fluid. The normal appearance of the small intestine also confirmed Kelly's gluten-free lifestyle. Kelly had a colonoscopy, during which the surface of the colon appeared normal. However, random biopsies of the large intestine showed severe inflammation highly suggestive of microscopic colitis (in this case, lymphocytic colitis subtype).

For this reason, Kelly was instructed to take an anti-inflammatory drug for the gut called budesonide.

What Is Microscopic Colitis?

Microscopic colitis is an inflammatory disorder of the large intestine that causes watery diarrhea.[1] The term *microscopic* is used because the diagnosis is confirmed by microscopic examination of a biopsy of the normal-looking large intestine. There are two types of colitis, collagenous colitis and lymphocytic colitis, although some experts believe that they are different phases of the same disease. Microscopic colitis is more common in older adults.

The cause of microscopic colitis is unknown.[2] The use of certain medications may increase the risk of microscopic colitis in some people. Therefore, it is very important to tell your doctor about all prescription and over-the-counter medications that you are taking (Table 1). In patients with drug-induced microscopic colitis, the symptoms disappear once the drug causing the problem is stopped. People with microscopic colitis often have additional immune-mediated disorders such as thyroid disorders, arthritis, diabetes, and celiac disease.

Microscopic colitis has been linked to other medications but the associations have not been proven through research.

The association between microscopic colitis and celiac disease is not new and has been extensively reported. However, the exact reasons why this condition can occur in celiac disease, or vice versa, are unknown. They may have "shared" immune and/or genetic factors. One study demonstrated a 70-fold increased risk for individuals with celiac disease to have microscopic colitis compared with the general population.[3] Most are diagnosed with celiac disease first, but some have both conditions diagnosed together or have microscopic colitis diagnosed first. Microscopic colitis is one of the reasons for persistent or recurrent diarrhea in individuals with celiac disease treated with a GFD. The presence of microscopic colitis is not only a cause of symptoms but may also make it more difficult for your body to absorb nutrients from food. Those with celiac disease and microscopic colitis may have more severe destruction of the finger-like projections lining the small intestine (called *villous atrophy*) compared to those with only celiac disease.[3]

Finding Microscopic Colitis

The most frequent symptoms of microscopic colitis are watery diarrhea, nonspecific abdominal pain, and weight loss.[1,2] The diagnosis of microscopic colitis requires a biopsy of your large intestine. During the biopsy, small samples of the tissue from your colon are removed.

TABLE 1. Drugs Commonly Associated with Microscopic Colitis

Drug	Use	Prescription Required?
Nonsteroidal anti-inflammatory drugs (such as ibuprofen or aspirin)	Pain relievers	No
Lansoprazole	Peptic ulcer disease, gastro-esophageal reflux disease	Yes
Ranitidine	Peptic ulcer disease, gastro-esophageal reflux disease	No
Acarbose	Diabetes mellitus	Yes
Sertraline	Depression	Yes
Cyclo3 fort	Venous insufficiency	Not available U.S.
Ticlopidine	Prevent blood clotting	Yes

Then the samples are evaluated using a microscope because the inflammation that results from microscopic colitis is not visible to the naked eye. This analysis can also differentiate between the two types of microscopic colitis: lymphocytic colitis is characterized by inflammation alone but collagenous colitis has inflammation plus an increase in the thickness of collagen (a normal protein of the gut) just below the colon surface.[2]

Blood and urine tests are usually normal and not helpful to diagnose microscopic colitis.[2] However, your doctor may request a blood test for celiac disease when microscopic colitis is diagnosed, especially when your symptoms don't improve with the treatment or there is evidence of fat in your stool, unexplained weight loss, or other condition that suggest you may also have undiagnosed celiac disease.

Treatment

Strict GFD is the most effective treatment for celiac disease but does not treat microscopic colitis. So, if you have both celiac disease and microscopic colitis, you will continue the GFD but require additional treatment. The first step is to discontinue any medications and foods that can cause diarrhea, such as caffeine and alcohol.[2] If you are using a drug thought to cause microscopic colitis, your doctor may eliminate or replace it, if possible. There are many drugs that might help control the symptoms of microscopic colitis, but their effectiveness varies by individual (Table 2).[1,2] The treatment for lymphocytic colitis and collagenous colitis is the same.

Your doctor may select the most appropriate treatment based on the severity of your symptoms. Microscopic colitis usually responds to treatment, and the currently available medications may control the symptoms in the majority of the patients. Microscopic colitis can be chronic although the course of the disease is highly variable—it can wax and wane.[2] In some circumstances, your doctor may recommend a prolonged treatment (called *maintenance therapy*), usually with a lower dose than that used as initial medication, to keep the disease under control.[4] Patients with microscopic colitis associated with the use of certain drugs

TABLE 2. Medications for Microscopic Colitis

Drug	Comment
Antidiarrheals (such as loperamide)	Safe, good control of mild diarrhea, well tolerated
Bismuth subsalicylate (Pepto-Bismol)	Safe, beneficial for many patients
Cholestyramine	Safe, poor tolerance
Budesonide	Expensive, effectiveness proved by clinical trials
Mesalamine/sulfasalazine	Usually safe, weak evidence of effectiveness
Prednisone	Use reserved for severe cases, potential of severe side effects
6-Mercaptopurine, azathioprine	Use reserved for severe cases, potential of severe side effects

are likely to remain well forever if they don't use that medication again. Thus, it is advisable that you remember the generic name of the medication that caused your symptoms and tell your doctors about it, to avoid accidental prescription of a similar drug. Surgery is reserved for very rare patients with severe symptoms that do not improve with any medication.

Outcome

Kelly's diarrhea disappeared after just a few days on the medication. Two months later, she was feeling good and without diarrhea using only one capsule of budesonide a day. The plan is to stop the medication in the near future.

SELF-MANAGEMENT TIPS

☐ Microscopic colitis is often associated with celiac disease and can be a cause of persistent or recurrent diarrhea after treatment with a GFD.

☐ The most frequent symptoms of microscopic colitis are watery diarrhea, non-specific abdominal pain, and weight loss.

☐ The diagnosis of microscopic colitis requires a colonoscopy or flexible sigmoidoscopy to take a biopsy of the large intestine.

☐ The GFD does not treat microscopic colitis; additional treatment is necessary.

☐ There are many medications available to control the symptoms of microscopic colitis. Your doctor may select the most appropriate treatment based on the severity of your symptoms.

References

1. Rubio-Tapia A, Martinez-Salgado J, Garcia-Leiva J, et al. Microscopic colitides: a single center experience in Mexico. *Int J Colorectal Dis* 2007;22(9):1031–36.
2. Pardi DS. Microscopic colitis: an update. *Inflamm Bowel Dis* 2004;10(6):860–70.
3. Green PH, Yang J, Gheng J, et al. An association between microscopic colitis and celiac disease. *Clin Gastroenterol Hepatol* 2009;7:1210–16.
4. Miehlke S, Madisch A, Bethke B, et al. Oral budesonide for maintenance treatment of collagenous colitis: a randomized double-blind placebo-controlled trial. *Gastroenterology* 2008;135(5):1510–16.

Joseph A. Murray, MD, is Professor of Medicine and Immunology and **Alberto Rubio-Tapia, MD,** is Assistant Professor of Medicine in the Division of Gastroenterology and Hepatology of the Department of Medicine of the Mayo Clinic College of Medicine in Rochester, Minnesota. Dr. Murray is Director of the Celiac Disease Research Program at the Mayo Clinic. Dr. Rubio-Tapia is also a member of the Celiac Disease Research Program and the Gastrointestinal Research Unit at the Mayo Clinic.

CHAPTER 40

Small Intestinal Bacterial Overgrowth

Daniel A. Leffler, MD, MS

I first saw Rose, an 82-year-old woman, two years ago. At the time, she was suffering from anemia, diarrhea, and weight loss. After her intestinal biopsies came back consistent with celiac disease, she was diagnosed and immediately began a strict gluten-free diet. At first, Rose's gastrointestinal symptoms improved, and she returned to her baseline weight. Her initial celiac blood test for immunoglobulin A tissue transglutaminase (IgA-tTG) was 112 units and over the first year of treatment decreased to 28 units, which suggested that she was doing a good job keeping to her gluten-free diet and that her celiac disease was becoming less active.

But a recent blood test at Rose's regular follow-up clinic visit showed that her tTG was slightly elevated at 25 units (less than 20 units is the normal level). Rose reported that, over the past few months, she has had more bloating and gas with occasional loose stools. She has had several visits with a dietitian skilled at treating celiac disease to discuss her diet and symptoms, and together they have not been able to identify any source of gluten exposure.

Because of her symptoms and persistently elevated tTG, Rose followed up with her gastroenterologist, who performed an EGD with duodenal biopsy. The endoscopy looked normal, but the biopsies revealed mildly increased numbers of white blood cells in the lining of the small intestine and patchy damaged villi. The combination of symptoms, blood, and biopsy results without any apparent gluten exposure suggested small intestinal bacterial overgrowth (SIBO).

What Is SIBO?

SIBO is being increasingly recognized as a complication of multiple gastrointestinal disorders, including irritable bowel syndrome, gastrointestinal surgery, and Crohn's disease as well as long-standing diabetes. If you are following a gluten-free diet but still having symptoms that mimic either gluten exposure or refractory celiac disease (see Chapter 43), it's possible that SIBO is behind it. If it goes untreated, SIBO can lead to persistent damage to villi (enteropathy) and elevated celiac blood tests.[1-3]

Most people have between 300 and 500 different bacterial species in their gastro-intestinal tracts. These are primarily in the middle and last parts of the small intestine and colon, because fewer bacteria can survive the muscular contractions and acidic environment of the stomach and first part of the small intestine of a healthy person. They perform functions that assist in keeping us healthy, including producing vitamin K and folate and converting certain foods into short-chain fatty acids that serve as fuel to the cells that line the colon.

Although the reasons that SIBO occurs in some people are unclear, for some it appears that abnormal intestinal motion and lowered immune defense allow large numbers of bacteria to grow in the upper small intestine (duodenum and/or jejunum), which normally contain very few bacteria. Bacteria and other organisms cause symptoms by digesting nutrients before your body can, which can cause vitamin deficiencies (especially vitamin B$_{12}$) and produce gas, which causes bloating and abdominal discomfort. Bacteria also may injure the intestinal lining (mucosa) leading to malabsorption, gastrointestinal symptoms, and abnormal biopsy results.[4]

Testing for SIBO

Recommendations for diagnosis and treatment of SIBO in celiac disease come from studies in other diseases. The standard test for SIBO is the lactulose or glucose breath test. In this test, the patient drinks a solution of either lactulose or glucose (both sugars), and the breath is tested to see if bacteria are digesting the sugar. Rose's lactulose breath test was positive because it showed a significant rise, more than 20 parts per million above baseline within the first 60 to 90 minutes. Although most bacteria produce hydrogen, some only produce methane, so for that reason, both gases are measured (Table 1). A high baseline level is also considered positive. Test results are often borderline or otherwise difficult to interpret, and so the decision to treat is based on type of symptoms and pattern of test results.

TABLE 1. Rose's Lactulose Breath Test Results

Time	Hydrogen (parts per million)	Methane (parts per million)
Baseline	4	1
15 minutes	8	1
30 minutes	39	1
45 minutes	48	2
60 minutes	51	2
75 minutes	41	1
90 minutes	32	1

Treating SIBO

Although SIBO breath testing is imperfect, it is safe and easy and can be very helpful in guiding therapy of what can be a chronic or recurring condition. For this reason, I generally perform breath testing to help decide on the treatment. Antibiotics are typically used for the treatment of SIBO, although the development of bacteria resistant to antibiotics is a concern. Various antibiotic regimens can be used.

Medicines that stimulate intestinal movement have also been used, although there are few data on these and they tend to have more side effects than antibiotics. Prebiotics and probiotics have also been used. These are safe but may take longer to work than antibiotics. They can be used as primary treatment in mild SIBO or with antibiotics to prevent or delay recurrence. Depending on the cause of the SIBO, people may have recurrences and need to be treated intermittently.

Given Rose's dramatic elevation in exhaled hydrogen levels along with typical symptoms, I started her on antibiotics. I generally begin treatment with a traditional antibiotic such as penicillin but will use newer antibiotics such as rifaximin and nitazoxanide when other antibiotics don't work or are causing unacceptable side effects.

Outcome

Rose got an initial 10-day course of amoxicillin–clavulanic acid (500 mg, 3 times/day), which improved her gas and bloating but resulted in a few days of antibiotic-associated diarrhea. But she got better and had three months of complete remission, after which she began to notice the return of symptoms. Repeat breath testing was again positive. She went on another 10-day course of rifaximen (400 mg, 3 times/day), and so far her symptoms have been gone for 8 months.

SELF-MANAGEMENT TIPS

☐ SIBO is a common complication of celiac disease that produces persistent symptoms of gas, bloating, and diarrhea and damages the intestinal lining.

☐ You can be evaluated for SIBO with a lactulose or glucose breath test.

☐ SIBO is a clinical diagnosis depending on symptoms, breath test results, and whether you respond to antibiotics.

☐ If you have SIBO, you will respond promptly to the appropriate antibiotics.

☐ It's very common for SIBO to recur, so you may need to treat it several times or with different methods for sustained relief.

☐ Because antibiotics can alter the natural flora of the intestine, taking probiotics once the antibiotic course ends may be beneficial.

References

1. Ghoshal UC, Ghoshal U, Misra A, Choudhuri G. Partially responsive celiac disease resulting from small intestinal bacterial overgrowth and lactose intolerance. *BMC Gastroenterol* 2004;4:10.
2. Tursi A, Brandimarte G, Giorgetti G. High prevalence of small intestinal bacterial overgrowth in celiac patients with persistence of gastrointestinal symptoms after gluten withdrawal. *Am J Gastroenterol* 2003;98:839–43.
3. Leffler DA, Dennis M, Hyett B, Kelly E, Schuppan D, Kelly CP. Etiologies and predictors of diagnosis in nonresponsive celiac disease. *Clin Gastroenterol Hepatol* 2007;5:445–50.
4. Quigley EM, Quera R. Small intestinal bacterial overgrowth: roles of antibiotics, prebiotics, and probiotics. *Gastroenterology* 2006;130:S78–90.

CHAPTER 41

Probiotics in Celiac Disease

Stefano Guandalini, MD, and Lina M. Felipez, MD

Cathy, a 19-year-old female, visited our clinic to discuss her continued symptoms of mild gas, bloating, and some alternating loose stool with constipation. She had been diagnosed more than a year earlier with celiac disease and she said that she had been carefully following a gluten-free diet since then. But she had seen no improvement in her symptoms and had even tried a lactose-free diet and limiting her fructose intake. Because of the persistence of these symptoms, we repeated the endoscopy, something we don't typically do, to confirm the diagnosis. Her recent endoscopy showed a well-healed small intestine, and all of her blood tests were normal. Cathy wanted to discuss whether probiotics might help her resolve some of these bothersome symptoms. She had heard claims that probiotics, in general, were beneficial in regaining gut health and was wondering if this was true.

What Are Probiotics?

Probiotics, also commonly referred to as "healthy bacteria" or "good bacteria," are living microbial food ingredients that, when ingested in adequate amounts, are beneficial to health. Even though the science behind them is relatively new, their use goes back to ancient times when, in many areas of the Roman Empire, people used products fermented by bacteria with the assumption they would be beneficial to health. But it was Metchnikoff[1] in the early 1900s who hypothesized that fermented products "seed" the gastrointestinal tract with healthy bacteria that fight harmful bacteria, preventing illness and especially gastrointestinal infections.

The use of "friendly bacteria," ingested most commonly in yogurts but also in other dairy products, bars, supplements, and other forms, to improve the health of the gut is being advertised by many food manufacturers. They are said to be beneficial in a myriad of ways, including making us more resistant to infections, improving our digestion, and even helping us live longer. Are these claims justified?

Scientists have long considered probiotics to be a popular remedy devoid of any real effect. But in the last 15 years, they have been the focus of ever-expanding research, both in laboratory and clinical investigations. As a result, we now have identified a number of microorganisms, especially *Lactobacilli* and *Bifidobacteria,* that possess the capacity of favorably affecting a number of functions, mostly, but not exclusively, related to intestinal health. Table 1 lists the best known agents.

It is important to realize that not all probiotics are created equal. First, not all preparations on the market contain microorganisms that have been studied, such as the ones listed in Table 1. In addition, no probiotic (even those listed in Table 1) is effective for every circumstance. For instance, *Lactobacillus rhamnosus* GG (commonly referred to as *LGG*) has been shown to be effective at reducing the duration of acute infection of the intestine[2] but has minimal use in controlling symptoms of irritable bowel syndrome. LGG and *Saccharomyces boulardii,* but not *L. acidophilus,* are effective in reducing the incidence of antibiotic-associated diarrhea.[3] Therefore, the choice of the proper probiotic should always be based on evidence of effectiveness for a specific problem, not just based on hype. For an accessible, comprehensive, and authoritative review of probiotics, visit www.usprobiotics.org/basis.asp, hosted by the nonprofit organization USprobiotics.

Probiotics are available in many forms and shapes: in foods and as dietary supplements, capsules, tablets, and powders. Some foods that contain live bacteria (and therefore are potential probiotics) are fermented milk, miso, tempeh, raw kimchi, raw sauerkraut, kefir, and some juices and soy beverages. Yogurts are, of course, one of the best known food sources of probiotics. However, note that the two strains of bacteria that all real yogurts contain (*L. bulgaricus* and

TABLE 1. Probiotics with Health Benefits

Strain	Type
Lactobacilli	*Acidophilus**
	Bulgaricus*
	Casei*
	Rhamnosus GG
	Johnsonii
	Paracasei
	Plantarum*
	Reuteri
	Salivarius
Bifidobacteria	*Animalis*
	Bifidum
	Breve*
	Infantis*
	Lactis
	Longum*
Escherichia coli	Nissel 1917
Streptococci	*Salivarius* subsp. *Thermophilus**
Enterococci	*Faecium*
Yeasts	*Saccharomyces boulardii*

*Active on its own but also present in combination preparation called *VSL#3.*

S. Thermophilus) typically do not possess all features of probiotics, as they tend to be present in low amounts. Some yogurts are supplemented with bacterial strains that can be considered adequate as probiotics. Only by carefully reading the food label to learn the strain(s) contained and their concentration can you be certain that yogurt or any other foods that claim to contain probiotics actually have them.

Usefulness of Probiotics in Celiac Disease

One of the most important functions of the intestine is to prevent ingested toxins and antigens from crossing the lining and passing into the bloodstream. This barrier function is largely the job of the tight connections between adjacent cells of the mucosal lining (called *tight junctions*). In untreated celiac disease, tight junctions are somewhat loosened, thus the intestine becomes more permeable to foreign molecules[4] (see Figure 3, page 6). Although this permeability is generally restored once a person is on a strict gluten-free diet, the intestine can remain "leaky" for quite some time after beginning the diet.[5] In addition, inadvertent exposure to gluten is likely to cause a flare-up of the inflammation with increased leakiness.[4] There is also evidence that gluten itself (via its main protein component gliadin) may directly be toxic to the lining of the intestine, causing or contributing to the increased permeability.

Here is where probiotics may be beneficial. Most probiotics, in fact, are able to affect the intestinal barrier function favorably, increasing its tightness and reducing the inflammation.[6] And there is also experimental evidence that some probiotics (especially *Bifidobacteria*) are capable of preventing the gliadin-induced toxicity to the intestinal lining.[7] In addition, research has shown that children with celiac disease differ from their healthy counterparts in the composition of the kinds and amounts of naturally occurring intestinal bacteria (microflora). They have lesser numbers of some species (again, especially *Bifidobacteria*) in their small and large intestines, and their content of bacteria is, in general, less diverse, with fewer strains present.[8] Also, research showed that bacteria in stool samples from treated or untreated patients with celiac disease can stimulate inflammation in the intestine.[9] When some *Bifidobacteria* are added to such preparations, there is much less inflammatory effect.

Can Probiotics Replace the Gluten-Free Diet?

No. Although there is evidence supporting the beneficial role of probiotics in celiac disease, there is no research showing that adding any probiotic would allow an increased tolerance to gluten. Thus, strict adherence to the diet is the only treatment for celiac disease. However, probiotics could in the future be positioned to play exciting roles in prevention and treatment of celiac disease. Note that these proposed roles for probiotics are speculative and have not yet been validated by adequate research studies.

- The composition of the intestinal microflora is largely determined during the very first few months of life and remains remarkably constant afterward. If it is true, as it would seem, that individuals with celiac disease develop a microflora composition that is different from their healthy counterparts and assuming additionally that such a difference plays a role in the onset of the disorder, it might be possible to influence the composition of the microflora of the infant at risk for celiac disease, such as babies born into a family with celiac disease, by providing them with plenty of "good bacteria."

- Adding probiotics to the diet could be beneficial for those few people who fail to show a full response to gluten-free diet. This gives the diet that extra "push" to support a more complete recovery of the intestinal inflammation. Furthermore, probiotics administered immediately after the diagnosis could possibly help speed up the recovery of the small intestine mucosa and, thus, a clinical recovery.

What Cathy Decided

We told Cathy that she was likely suffering from irritable bowel syndrome with alternating diarrhea and constipation, a condition quite common in the general population that often coexists with celiac disease (see Chapter 38). Her normal blood levels of celiac antibodies and the normal repeat endoscopy supported this conclusion. We told Cathy that IBS is a condition where probiotics could be beneficial, as there is now a growing body of reputable medical literature to show this. A recent guideline states that probiotic therapies show a trend for being efficacious in IBS and also that probiotic combinations improve symptoms in IBS patients.[10] Thus, we recommended that Cathy begin taking one of the two preparations that have been shown to be effective in this regard: either *Bifidobacterium infantis* 35624 (marketed under the name Align in the U.S.)[11] or the preparation VSL#3 that contains eight different probiotic strains.[12,13] Cathy followed our advice and at a follow-up appointment three months later reported a marked improvement in her symptoms, especially the abdominal bloating.

SELF-MANAGEMENT TIPS

☐ It is safe to enjoy your probiotic-enriched, gluten-free yogurt. For continued benefits, probiotics must be ingested on a daily basis and for a period of at least several weeks. Whether they should be taken indefinitely is not clear from available evidence, but the general consensus is that they are safe and their ongoing intake should pose no risk in those with a normally healthy immune system.

☐ On the other hand, if you experience no benefit at all after at least several weeks on a well-chosen probiotic, there is probably no reason to continue it.

☐ Should you suffer from other gastrointestinal disorders unrelated to celiac disease, note that probiotics may also be beneficial, either for short- or long-term use[14] and speak with your health care provider.

☐ Discuss your situation and specific symptoms with your doctor or dietitian and decide whether you might benefit from probiotics. Remember to always pay strict attention to the product you select: It must be gluten-free!

References

1. Metchnikoff E. *Optimistic Studies.* New York: Putman's Sons, 1908.
2. Guandalini S. Probiotics for children with diarrhea: an update. *J Clin Gastroenterol* 2008;42(Suppl 2.):S53–57.
3. Johnston BC, Supina AL, Ospina M, et al. Probiotics for the prevention of pediatric antibiotic-associated diarrhea. *Cochrane Database Syst Rev* 2007(2): CD004827.
4. Visser J, et al. Tight junctions, intestinal permeability, and autoimmunity: celiac disease and type 1 diabetes paradigms. *Ann N Y Acad Sci* 2009;1165:195–205.
5. Duerksen DR, Wilhelm-Boyles C, Parry DM. Intestinal permeability in long-term follow-up of patients with celiac disease on a gluten-free diet. *Dig Dis Sci* 2005;50(4):785–90.
6. Whelan K, Myers CE. Safety of probiotics in patients receiving nutritional support: a systematic review of case reports, randomized controlled trials, and nonrandomized trials. *Am J Clin Nutr* 2010;91(3):687–703.
7. Lindfors K, Blomqvist T, Juuti-Uusitalo K, et al. Live probiotic Bifidobacterium lactis bacteria inhibit the toxic effects induced by wheat gliadin in epithelial cell culture. *Clin Exp Immunol* 2008;152(3):552–58.
8. Collado MC, Donat E, Ribes-Koninckx C, et al. Specific duodenal and faecal bacterial groups associated with paediatric coeliac disease. *J Clin Pathol* 2009;62(3):264–69.
9. Medina M, De Palma G, Ribes-Koninckx C, et al. Bifidobacterium strains suppress in vitro the pro-inflammatory milieu triggered by the large intestinal microbiota of coeliac patients. *J Inflamm (Lond)* 2008;5:19.
10. Brandt L. et al. An evidence-based systematic review on the management of irritable bowel syndrome. *Am J Gastroenterol* 2009;104(Suppl. 1):S1–35.
11. Whorwell PJ, et al. Efficacy of an encapsulated probiotic Bifidobacterium infantis 35624 in women with irritable bowel syndrome. *Am J Gastroenterol* 2006;101(7): 1581–90.
12. Guandalini S, et al. VSL#3 improves symptoms in children with irritable bowel syndrome: a multicenter, randomized, placebo-controlled, double-blind, cross-over study. *J Pediatr Gastroenterol Nutr* In Press.
13. Kim HJ, et al. A randomized controlled trial of a probiotic combination VSL# 3 and placebo in irritable bowel syndrome with bloating. *Neurogastroenterol Motil* 2005;17(5):687–96.
14. Floch MH, et al. Recommendations for probiotic use—2008. *J Clin Gastroenterol* 2008;42(Suppl. 2): S104–108.

Stefano Guandalini, MD, is Professor of Pediatrics and Chief of the Section of Gastroenterology, Hepatology and Nutrition of the Department of Pediatrics, University of Chicago. He is also the founder and Medical Director of the University of Chicago Celiac Disease Center. His primary research and clinical focus is currently on celiac disease and on the use of probiotics in disorders of the GI tract in children. **Lina M. Felipez, MD,** is a pediatrician and a second-year Fellow in pediatric gastroenterology at The University of Chicago Comer's Children Hospital, where she does also clinical research on the IBD population with infliximab failure.

CHAPTER 42

Balancing Your Gut: Functional Medicine in Celiac Disease

Diana Noland, MPH, RD, CCN, and Guy F. Pugh, MD

Fran is a 56-year-old woman who was diagnosed with celiac disease two years ago. She went on a gluten-free diet immediately after diagnosis and, in general, her gastrointestinal symptoms improved and her blood tests normalized. However, she continues to struggle with fatigue, insomnia, and intermittent stomach discomfort she describes as bloating and "gurgling." With her celiac disease diagnosis, Fran's gastroenterologist also diagnosed her with irritable bowel syndrome. Fran was not content with the therapies suggested for her symptoms and decided to visit a functional medicine clinic to address her symptoms in a different way.

What Is Functional Medicine?

Over the past few decades, there has been increasing interest in a variety of medical approaches that lie outside of the usual experience of most doctors and hospitals. One approach to health care, called *functional medicine,* is rapidly gaining appreciation as an alternative or add-on treatment for many chronic diseases or conditions. Functional medicine is a "systems biology" approach that assesses and addresses whole systems and underlying root causes rather than focusing on a single organ. Similar disciplines are known as alternative medicine, natural or naturopathic medicine, holistic medicine, complementary medicine, complementary and alternative medicine, and integrative medicine, among others. The unique value that functional medicine brings is a disciplined architecture that organizes the patient's whole story. This provides the framework needed to identify patterns of the system dysfunction and priorities for treatment.

The functional medicine model includes a thorough physical evaluation followed by the development of a plan that supports your body's natural mechanisms to restore balance and health. This plan may include conventional medicine as well as the use of foods, supplements, and lifestyle changes; in celiac disease, the plan includes maintaining a completely gluten-free diet to support the body's tremendous potential to heal the intestine. The goal in functional medicine is to get at the "root cause" of the disturbance causing the illness, rather than simply treating the symptoms, and to call on the body's ability to self-heal.

A Functional Medicine View of the Gastrointestinal Tract

The gastrointestinal tract is the main component of the body through which nutrients enter and wastes and toxins are eliminated. Many functional medicine practitioners view the gastrointestinal tract as much more than this: it is the major interface we have with our environment. Also, the gut contains about 70% of our immune system. For our bodies to be healthy throughout life, it is critical to keep the gut healthy and functioning.

Chronic inflammation from gluten exposure and other assaults can damage the gut, and the immune system suffers, weakening the ability of the body to defend itself from infections or autoimmune diseases. Many types of assaults other than gluten may add to the damage, such as poor diet, poor sleep, medications, emotional stress, and infections. When these assaults are prolonged under gluten-sensitive conditions, there is continual risk for damage to the gut. This disrupts the connections between the gut, the immune system, and the nervous system that are critical for health. Therefore, problems in the gastrointestinal tract can be related to many problems and symptoms elsewhere in the body—from rashes and joint pains to fatigue and "mental fog."

Functional medicine provides an alternative guide to restoration of the gastrointestinal tract called the *four Rs*. They stand for:

- Remove offending pathogens and toxins, such as yeast overgrowth
- Replace or replenish digestive enzymes, nutritional whole foods, and digestive factors that may be lacking
- Reinoculate by reintroducing the desirable bacteria normally in a healthy gut
- Repair by reducing inflammation and healing gut lining

What Conditions Are Commonly Treated in Functional Medicine?

Patients who visit a functional medicine practitioner may be bewildered by a variety of new conditions that might have never been discussed or addressed by their gastroenterologist or primary care physician. Common functional medicine diagnoses of the gastrointestinal tract include:

- achlorhydria (too little stomach acid)
- digestive enzyme deficiency
- leaky gut syndrome
- bacterial dysbiosis
- yeast (*Candida*) overgrowth
- parasites
- food intolerance or sensitivity

These conditions are based on medical knowledge about how the gastrointestinal system works but are traditionally overlooked as clinically unimportant. This trend is changing, and there has been growing acceptance of their involvement in gastrointestinal dysfunction.

Many health care practitioners have found these diagnoses useful in directing therapy that yields health benefits for patients, particularly people with celiac disease.

Achlorhydria or Hypochlorhydria

Achlorhydria or hypochlorhydria describes the condition of too little stomach acid. In the normally functioning gastrointestinal tract, after a brief encounter with saliva in the mouth and esophagus, food enters the stomach, a dramatically different environment. The pH of the stomach is extraordinarily low. This strongly acidic environment is important for:

- stimulating your pancreas, stomach, and small intestine to produce the digestive enzymes and bile necessary to further break down the carbohydrates, proteins, and fats in your food
- breaking down proteins into amino acids, nutrients that your body needs to stay healthy
- preventing disease by killing pathogenic bacteria and yeast normally present in food

As we age, stomach acid generally becomes less strong—the pH rises. In addition, many medications given for gastrointestinal complaints block the production of stomach acid. The stomach of someone taking an ulcer medication such as omeprazole or ranitidine may have secretions similar in pH to water.

Functional medicine practitioners may feel that this lack of stomach acid is unnatural and should be counteracted to restore normal digestive function. Symptoms that may be attributed to low stomach acid include bloating, belching, and flatulence after meals; heartburn (can be because of either low or high stomach acid) or indigestion; diarrhea or constipation; chronic *Candida* yeast infections; undigested food in stools; vitamin deficiencies; dry skin; rectal itching; acne; multiple food allergies; and chronic fatigue.

Use of acid-blocking medication may be discouraged for certain individuals. To improve digestion, functional medicine practitioners may recommend taking acid-containing supplements (hydrochloric acid tablets) with meals to lower the pH (increase acidity in stomach). Patients should consider this recommendation in consultation with their gastroenterologist or physician. When indicated, acid-blocking medications have a long and well-established track record for effectively treating high acid-related diseases with very few significant side effects. These diseases, including ulcers, can be very serious and even life-threatening.

There is some evidence that the acid barrier of the stomach plays a role in sterilizing our food and preparing food nutrients for digestion. Long-term use of acid blockers may have subtle effects on our ability to absorb certain nutrients, especially calcium, B_{12}, and iron. Therefore, it is important that your practitioner monitor your nutrition status if you are taking acid blockers long term so any deficiencies can be treated.

Digestive Enzyme Deficiency

Digestive enzymes are made in your body and are released by the salivary glands, stomach, pancreas, and glands in the small intestine. Digestive enzymes, in addition to bile from the liver and gallbladder, are powerful secretions that help break down proteins and fats into absorbable molecules. Digestive enzymes have two primary functions. The most obvious job is the digestion of food. The other very important function is digesting and recycling old cells throughout the body. This process is called *autophagy* (self-eating). These enzymes break down excess mucus and attack the walls of old cells and pathogens, such as yeast cells, to destroy them.

Through various tests, usually stool tests, the functional medicine practitioner may diagnose digestive enzyme deficiency and recommend or prescribe specific replacement enzymes. Some people have insufficient output of digestive enzymes, for example, because of chronic pancreatic disease. This is usually detected when the stool has high quantities of fat or there are obvious signs of malnutrition of fat-related vitamins.

Adding digestive enzymes, such as papain, bromelain, or lipase, is a safe intervention that may help some patients decrease indigestion, bloating, and undigested food in stool. Table 1 provides examples of digestive enzyme formulas available in drug and health food stores.

Leaky Gut Syndrome

The intestine is lined with a thin but very effective layer of cells that form a functional lining. These cells release mucus that protects the gut and also allows transport of small molecules—amino acids, electrolytes (chemicals and minerals), water, and other nutrients—into the bloodstream to be used by the body.

When this layer of cells is disrupted or inflamed, such as in celiac disease, larger molecules that would normally be blocked can enter the bloodstream. Some of these large molecules or antigens may stimulate the immune system to generate antibodies that may contribute to an inflammatory response by the body as it protects itself from these larger molecules.

TABLE 1. Enzyme Formulas Available Over-the-Counter

Bromelain (from pineapple)
Papain (from papaya)
Bromelain and papain combination

Starch, protein, and fat digestive enzymes combination:
  Bromelain, papain (protein, anti-inflammatory)
  Amylases (starch)
  Proteases (such as chymotrypsin,* trypsin*)
  Lipases (fat)

Protease combination
  Bromelain, papain
  (vegetarian protein enzymes, anti-inflammatory)
  Proteases
  (glandular-animal protein, chymotrypsin,* trypsin*)

*Contraindicated for alpha-1-antitrypsin deficiency, a rare genetic disease.

It is normal for small numbers of these antigens to pass into the bloodstream and be handled by the immune system. However, when the gut lining is damaged and large numbers of antigens pass into the bloodstream, the immune system is activated excessively and produces symptoms all over the body. When the intestines permit excessive amounts of antigens to enter the bloodstream, it is called the *leaky gut syndrome.*

Leaky gut may be demonstrated using specialized lab tests, sometimes a series of intestinal permeability tests or similar. Because of the loss of intestinal villi, people with celiac disease are at high risk for leaky gut syndrome. This condition may be the reason why some people with celiac disease have symptoms outside the intestine, including other autoimmune conditions, neurological deficits, and allergies.

The most important treatment for leaky gut is to remove the cause of the problem. Avoiding gluten allows the intestine to repair itself and resolves the problem. Some practitioners also recommend helping to restore gut function with probiotics, enzymes, and balanced gluten-free nutrition.

A specific approach is to supplement the diet with the amino acid L-glutamine. Glutamine is a major source of energy for the cells that line the intestine, and it is appealing to imagine that "feeding the gut cells" would lead to a more rapid recovery from celiac disease or other intestinal diseases. Your individual need for glutamine can be determined by testing plasma amino acids or with a simple 1- to 2-day trial of glutamine to see if it is well tolerated. Signs of intolerance might be headache or anxiety. Also, glutamine should not be taken for anyone with an MSG allergy or sensitivity. Most people benefit from glutamine supplementation during a "healing phase." A dose of three grams daily is sometimes suggested. If glutamine is not tolerated, other agents are available to sooth the gut lining and promote healing, such as acetyl glucoseamine, zinc carnosine, quercitin (a bioflavonoid), and ginger.

Bacterial Dysbiosis

The vast majority of bacteria found in and around the human body are in the gastrointestinal tract, especially the large intestine. Although some of these bacteria are harmful pathogens that cause illness, other bacteria appear to be helpful, preventing the growth of harmful bacteria, helping detoxify waste products, and producing nutrients for the intestinal cells.

However, there exist many strains of bacteria that are harmless to most people but appear to cause problems for others. When the balance of harmful, beneficial, and other bacteria is disturbed, this is known as *bacterial dysbiosis.* Symptoms of bacterial dysbiosis can include diarrhea, constipation, bloating, and abdominal pain. Bacterial dysbiosis is the source of many people's intestinal symptoms, including irritable bowel syndrome.

Bacterial dysbiosis is usually diagnosed by sending stool samples to a lab to measure the levels of good, neutral, possibly harmful, and harmful bacteria. If there appears to be a lack of beneficial bacteria, a practitioner may recommend adding probiotics such as *Lactobacillus* (the bacteria found in most yogurt). If high levels of possible pathogens are seen, herbal remedies such as oil of oregano, garlic, or berberine might be recommended to suppress the growth of these pathogens.

The concept of bacterial dysbiosis has gained wider acceptance among conventional practitioners and gastroenterologists in recent years. Some intestinal diseases, such as Crohn's disease, which are not seen as primarily caused by infection, are sometimes treated with antibiotics to change the balance of bacteria. Probiotics are another choice that may be recommended by many practitioners of all kinds to promote overall bowel health.

For people with celiac disease, the diagnosis and treatment of bacterial dysbiosis is complicated. Although the symptoms of celiac disease and dysbiosis may be quite similar, such as indigestion, abdominal pain, and bloating, celiac is a disease of the small intestine. Dysbiosis is usually considered a problem of the lower small intestine and large intestine, where most bacteria reside. When we test stool for dysbiosis, our findings may not reflect the bacterial populations of the small intestine.

On the other hand, it appears that probiotics such as *Lactobacillus acidophilus* and *Bifidobacteria,* as well as live-culture yogurt, are safe and well-tolerated and may promote overall gut health in a way that helps people with celiac disease (see Chapter 41 on probiotics). It is essential to check that any supplements or foods are gluten free.

Yeast (Candida) Overgrowth

Fungi, including yeasts, are part of our environment and live in, around, and on all surfaces of the body. Yeast grows in warm, damp, dark places in the presence of sugars. Under certain conditions, they can become so numerous that they cause infections. Of the twenty species of *Candida* yeast that infect humans, *Candida albicans* is the most common.

Yeasts are responsible for familiar, minor infections such as toenail infections, thrush (yeast in the throat), vaginal yeast infections, and skin rashes in damp areas. Symptoms are usually itching, cracking, and bleeding of the skin and sometimes pain. When the immune system is compromised, yeast can overgrow and become a serious health problem. In some cases, with severely health-compromised patients, an overwhelming yeast infection can be fatal.

Between these extremes (minor infection and fatal illness) lies the yeast overgrowth syndrome. The idea is that in some circumstances people with normal or minimally compromised immune systems may have yeast in high numbers that then produce a variety of symptoms. Symptoms of excess yeast are intestinal gas and bloating as well as non-intestinal symptoms caused by yeast byproducts or toxins, such as headaches, mental fog, fatigue, rashes, and joint pains. The diagnosis of yeast overgrowth is sometimes made based on symptoms and examination. Some lab tests, including antibody tests for anti-*Candida* antibodies, may also be used by some practitioners to support the diagnosis. A person with celiac disease may have symptoms that overlap with those caused by yeast overgrowth.

Risk factors for the yeast overgrowth syndrome include use of antibiotics, which suppress good, protective bacteria; use of steroids, which depress the immune system; and uncontrolled diabetes or a high-sugar diet, because sugar encourages yeast growth. Women seem to have a higher risk of yeast overgrowth than men. It may make sense to consider the role of yeast if there are clear signs of yeast-related conditions such as thrush or recurrent vaginal yeast infections or if you have other risk factors for yeast growth, such as diabetes or excessive use of antibiotics.

Therapy directed at yeast overgrowth includes:

- eliminating the risk factors
- re-establishing healthy gut bacteria, including the use of probiotics like *Lactobacillus acidophilus, Bifidobacteria,* and *Saccharomyces boulardii*
- suppressing yeast growth with natural antifungal supplements and/or prescription antifungal medications

A yeast-free diet is also usually recommended. This may include eliminating foods containing yeast as well as foods thought to promote yeast growth, including sugars and simple carbohydrates (Figure 1).

For the most part, treatment of yeast overgrowth involves improving the diet and making healthy choices. However, for some patients, the dietary restrictions for a yeast-free diet may mean weight loss. For those with celiac disease, who may be at low body weight to begin with, the focus is on getting adequate calories to maintain a healthy weight. Counseling by a registered dietitian will help you understand how to optimize your nutrition.

Food Sensitivities

There is considerable confusion and miscommunication between practitioners and patients on the topics of food allergies and food sensitivities. Those with celiac disease may have been told that they are "allergic" to gluten but not to other foods. You may see a holistic practitioner, have a series of blood tests, and be told you are "allergic" to a wide array of foods.

Let's specify the terminology. A food allergy is an immunoglobulin E (IgE) antibody–mediated immune response to a specific food that is usually immediate and dramatic. A common example is allergy to peanuts or shellfish. For those with an allergy, contact with

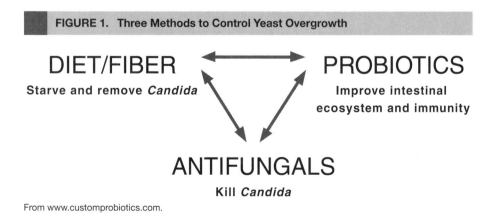

FIGURE 1. Three Methods to Control Yeast Overgrowth

DIET/FIBER
Starve and remove *Candida*

PROBIOTICS
Improve intestinal ecosystem and immunity

ANTIFUNGALS
Kill *Candida*

From www.customprobiotics.com.

even a small amount of the food produces a dramatic allergic reaction, including hives, swelling, and in severe cases, difficulty breathing or swallowing.

This is different from celiac disease, which is an autoimmune disorder characterized by a reaction to gluten. The autoimmune reaction to gluten exposure may take some time to develop. There may be few symptoms at first, but once the reaction is established, the gastrointestinal tract and immune system may take weeks or months of gluten avoidance to return to normal.

A third type of reaction to food is called *intolerance* or *sensitivity*. When exposed to an offending food, you may have a delayed reaction, perhaps hours or even days later. This reaction may be gastrointestinal, or symptoms may be seen elsewhere in the body. Common symptoms attributed to food sensitivities include fatigue, headache, rashes (including acne), and joint pains.

Immunological tests, which measure other antibodies (IgG, IgM, and IgA) to foods, are available and are used by some practitioners to diagnose food intolerances or sensitivities. When interpreting these tests, it is important to keep in mind what is being measured. If a test shows the presence of high levels of IgG antibodies to almond, for instance, this could mean that the patient

- eats a lot of almonds, causing increased exposure
- is sensitive to almonds and overreacts to small amount

To make matters more complicated, some people have high levels of all antibodies, whereas others react less overall. Furthermore, the levels of antibodies do not reliably predict the severity or type of symptoms from exposure to the food.

The most reliable way to tell if you have a negative reaction to a particular food is to eliminate it from the diet to see if the target symptom improves. However, skin or blood testing for food intolerances or sensitivities may help provide some ideas about which food(s) may be best tolerated and which ones may most likely be the source of a problem.

Because untreated celiac disease damages the intestinal lining, which may allow large molecules to get into the bloodstream and cause immune reactions (see "Leaky Gut," page 290), large numbers of antibody-positive foods can be detected with IgG-based tests. These are the best tests to reflect the result of the leaky gut allowing particles of the foods you eat to enter the blood and trigger an IgG antibody response. This is usually not an allergic reaction, rather a food sensitivity reaction. When gut health is restored, the antibody response usually subsides. Until the integrity of the gut is restored, it may be helpful to minimize or avoid foods to which you are sensitive for at least two months, or as directed by your physician or dietitian. It is important to seek the counsel of a clinician who can both help to interpret the testing for you and plan an appropriate, individualized and balanced diet (see Chapter 35 on food allergies and Chapter 36 on elimination diets).

It is particularly important not to use these antibody tests as a guide to eating if they contradict the advice of your gastroenterologist in managing your celiac disease. It is quite possible that food sensitivity testing may show little or no antibodies to wheat or other gluten-containing foods. If you have been avoiding these foods, we would expect these levels to be low. This does not mean that you are "no longer sensitive" to gluten or that you can resume eating gluten-containing foods.

What Fran Decided

Fran addressed her remaining health complaints, especially the fatigue that interfered with her quality of life, with her functional medicine practitioner. The functional assessment of Fran's condition identified three top priorities to begin treating her underlying root causes of fatigue.

- Magnesium deficiency. Magnesium is the primary cofactor for the production of the energy molecule, ATP, in all cells. It is also a "relaxing" mineral and can contribute to better sleep. Fran's treatment included 200 mg of magnesium glycinate twice a day with meals and one dose daily of a multivitamin/chelated mineral/antioxidant.
- Insomnia/poor sleep. Sleep of good quality and duration (7–8 hours per night) is one of the most anti-inflammatory factors known and improves immune and hormonal strength for all systems of the body. Sleep is one of the strongest "de-stressors" to improve health. In addition to the magnesium, Fran's treatment included 1.5 mg melatonin before bed and bedtime by 11 p.m. to ensure she received 8 hours of sleep.
- Low levels of digestive enzymes. Because of her continued complaints of intermittent stomach discomfort and bloating and "gurgling" even after probiotic therapy, Fran probably had low levels of digestive enzyme production. A stool sample tested low in pancreatic elastase, indicating poor production of pancreatic enzymes, and low in bile salts; also there was excess fat, implicating poor fat digestion. Fran's treatment included taking two capsules of digestive enzyme supplement just before meals until her next follow-up, at which time this therapy would be reevaluated.

Fran's Outcome

Within three days of taking the digestive enzymes with meals, Fran reported reduced stomach discomfort. At her two-week follow-up appointment she reported no stomach discomfort for one week, so Fran decided to continue taking the enzymes for another six months. After four weeks of working to improve her sleep, Fran reported waking refreshed with much improved energy during the day. At six weeks, she reported energy enough to begin 30 minutes of walking exercise daily.

Fran continued her plan of lifelong gluten-free diet. In addition, she committed to a one-year lactose- and casein-free diet while her gastrointestinal mucosa heals. She also took probiotics recommended by her gastroenterologist during the functional medicine treatment regimen. Fran appreciated the collaboration between her gastroenterologist and functional medicine practitioner that resulted in elimination of her stomach discomfort and her improved feeling of well-being and quality of life.

Diana Noland, MPH, RD, CCN, is a registered dietitian who operates a clinical functional nutrition practice (www.nolandnutrition.com). She is also an international speaker, educator, and author, serves on the faculty of the Institute for Functional Medicine (IFM), and is the lead author of *Functional Nutrition Therapy: Principles of Assessment,* to be published by IFM. **Guy F. Pugh, MD,** is a primary care physician and former Medical Director of the Marino Center for Integrative Health in Cambridge, Massachusetts. His practice combines conventional with evidence-based alternative therapies and uses functional medicine as a framework when conventional approaches prove inadequate. Dr. Pugh has lectured on yeast overgrowth and alternative approaches to thyroid disease and is participating in a national study of EDTA chelation therapy for heart disease.

CHAPTER 43

Refractory Celiac Disease

Christophe Cellier, MD, PhD

We first saw Madeline, a 67-year-old woman, 5 years ago. At the time, she had been suffering from diarrhea, bloating, and episodes of abdominal pain for 10 years, and she had previously been diagnosed with irritable bowel syndrome. Her initial celiac blood test for immunoglobulin A tissue transglutaminase (IgA-tTG) was 224 units (normal is less than 20 units). Her intestinal biopsies showed damage consistent with celiac disease: total villous atrophy together with an increased number of intraepithelial lymphocytes.

Madeline began a gluten-free diet (GFD), and her symptoms improved. Over the first year of treatment, her IgA-tTG level returned to normal, suggesting that she was doing a good job staying on the GFD. However, four years later, she developed progressively more severe diarrhea and anemia and lost 20 pounds in 3 months. Madeline's IgA-tTG level was always in the normal range, and she was referred to a dietitian skilled at treating celiac disease. Together, they could find no evidence of gluten in her diet or environment.

What Is Refractory Celiac Disease?

Refractory celiac disease (RCD), also called *refractory sprue*, occurs when symptoms and villous atrophy persist or come back despite a patient's scrupulousness in following a GFD. Approximately 5% of adults with celiac disease have primary RCD, in which there is no response to removing gluten from the diet, or secondary RCD, in which there is initial improvement on a GFD but it fails to continue. The symptoms that usually develop include diarrhea and weight loss and recurrence of malabsorption, abdominal pain, and anemia. Low blood protein level and ulcers in the small intestine (ulcerative jejunitis) often arise as well.[1]

RCD is classified into two types:

- type 1, in which there is normal development of intraepithelial lymphocytes (white blood cells found in the lining of the intestine that produce antibodies to attack infected and cancerous cells) that carry on their surface both CD3 and CD8 proteins

- type 2, in which there is expansion of abnormal intraepithelial lymphocytes that carry CD3 but not CD8 proteins on their surface

Another test can be performed on T-cells (another kind of white blood cell different from the intraepithelial lymphocytes) to look for abnormalities in the T-cell receptor (TCR). Normally, different T-cells have different T-cell receptors. If a large number of T-cells have the same T-cell receptor (known as *clonality*), this is abnormal and may suggest either RCD type 2 or even an early lymphoma. It is important to distinguish RCD type 1 from RCD type 2 because RCD type 1 has a good long term prognosis, whereas RCD type 2 is associated with a high risk of ulcerative jejunitis, which can progress to a severe form of cancer known as enteropathy-associated T-cell lymphoma. The risk of lymphoma in RCD type 2 is high: 30–40% after 5 years.[2]

Diagnosing Refractory Celiac Disease

If you develop new symptoms, such as weight loss, abdominal pain, or fever, or if you develop diarrhea despite following a GFD, consult your physician for an evaluation. The first step is to reassess the initial diagnosis of celiac disease, because villous atrophy is not exclusive to celiac disease. The next step is to address the likelihood that you are voluntarily or inadvertently ingesting gluten, which would appear to be the case if you have positive celiac blood tests (higher than normal IgA-tTG or -EMA levels) after a year or more of eating gluten free. Inadvertent gluten exposure is the most common cause of unresponsive celiac disease, and it's important to discover why this is happening and understand how to prevent it. You may need to consult a dietitian skilled at treating celiac disease to find the hidden gluten in your diet. If you are having trouble adjusting to the gluten-free lifestyle, connecting with a celiac support group may be helpful. However, there are several other causes of persistent symptoms in patients on a GFD (Table 1).

If the dietary causes for your symptoms can be ruled out, you and your physician should consider more serious complications of celiac disease, like intestinal lymphoma, small intestinal adenocarcinoma, or refractory sprue. It may require extensive investigations to discover the source of your new symptoms or recurring diarrhea.

In Madeline's case, the first step was a colonoscopy with multiple biopsies, which were normal, and then an endoscopy that clearly showed damage to the duodenum. The small intestine biopsies confirmed that she still had total, severe villous atrophy with increased intraepithelial lymphocytes. Her physician then ordered a computed tomography (CT) scan with enteroclysis, in which imaging is performed after a large volume of contrast material is infused into the small intestine. Madeline's small intestine appeared normal. The next investigation was videocapsule enteroscopy, for which Madeline swallowed a small "pillcam" that takes 2–3 pictures per second. This allows good visualization of the entire small intestine and is actually the most accurate tool for diagnosing complications of celiac disease or ulcerative jejunitis. This confirmed Madeline's villous atrophy and also showed that she had multiple large ulcers in the proximal part of the small intestine. These ulcers were biopsied, and lymphoma was ruled out.

TABLE 1. Causes of Unresponsive Celiac Disease

Incorrect diagnosis
Gluten ingestion (intentional or unintentional)
Microscopic colitis
Lactose intolerance
Pancreatic insufficiency
Bacterial overgrowth
Intolerance of foods other than gluten (fructose, milk, soy)
Inflammatory bowel disease
Irritable bowel syndrome
Anal incontinence
Collagenous sprue
Autoimmune enteropathy
Refractory celiac disease (type 1 or type 2, with or without clonal T cells)
Enteropathy-associated T-cell lymphoma

When investigating suspected RCD, it's vital that a pathologist extensively analyze the specimens collected during the small intestine biopsy. This should include assessing whether someone has RCD type 1 or type 2 because the two types have different developmental courses and risks. When Madeline's intraepithelial lymphocytes were studied, most of the lymphocytes expressed CD3 but not CD8, indicating that Madeline had RCD type 2.

Treating Refractory Celiac Disease

Treatment of RCD involves close medical monitoring and nutritional support with the goal of gaining weight (including intravenous nutrition if necessary) and replenishing vitamins and minerals, plus a GFD. Most people require treatment with steroids, which control symptoms by decreasing inflammation. Immunosuppressive drugs may be beneficial but should be used with caution because of the risk of lymphoma, particularly in RCD type 2. Given this high risk of lymphoma, it's vital that we find ways to assess new treatments, such as stem cell transplantation or blocking interleukin-15. This will require international cooperation given the rarity of this disease.

Madeline's Treatment

Madeline was initially treated with steroids and improved significantly. After 6 months, however, she developed small bowel obstruction, and double-balloon enteroscopy revealed multiple narrowed areas (strictures) of the jejunum requiring surgery. During surgery, it was discovered that Madeline had T-cell lymphoma. She is currently undergoing chemotherapy.

SELF-MANAGEMENT TIPS

☐ RCD is a rare complication of celiac disease, defined as persistent symptoms and villous atrophy despite a GFD.

☐ If symptoms such as diarrhea recur or if you have new symptoms such as weight loss, abdominal pain, fever, or intestinal bleeding when you are following a GFD, consult your physician.

☐ The most common cause of persisting symptoms when you are on a GFD is voluntary or inadvertent gluten exposure. Consult a dietitian skilled at treating celiac disease to review your diet and consider participation in a support group.

☐ If gluten exposure is ruled out, your physician may require a new work-up, including duodenal biopsies during upper endoscopy, to search for evidence of RCD type 1 or 2.

☐ Treatment of RCD primarily involves medical monitoring, enhancing nutrition and medications to control inflammation.

References

1. Green PH, Cellier C. Celiac disease. *N Engl J Med* 2007;335:1731–43.
2. Cellier C, Delabesse E, Helmer C, et al. Refractory sprue, coeliac disease, and enteropathy-associated T-cell lymphoma. *Lancet* 2000;356:203–208.

Christophe Cellier, MD, PhD, is Professor of Gastroenterology, University René Descartes, European Georges Hospital, Paris, France.

CHAPTER 44

Autoimmune Diseases and Celiac Disease

Daniel A. Leffler, MD, MS

John is an 18-year-old student who was recently diagnosed with celiac disease. He is otherwise healthy, but several autoimmune diseases, including type 1 diabetes, thyroid disease, and ulcerative colitis, run in his family. He knows that celiac disease is an autoimmune disease and wonders if he is at risk for developing other autoimmune disorders. If so, John wants to know if he can lower his risk and which tests he can have to look for other diseases.

What Is Autoimmune Disease?

Disorders in which the immune system mistakenly attacks healthy body tissue are autoimmune disorders or diseases. There are about 100 known autoimmune disorders targeting almost every part of the body. Note that autoimmune diseases, such as celiac disease, are different from allergic disorders. In allergic reactions, the target of the immune system is a foreign substance, such as pollen, taken into the body. When various body parts are affected by allergic reactions, they are actually innocent bystanders, and collateral damage is caused by immune reactions that are nonspecific or just too strong. In autoimmune diseases, the target of the attack is a part of your own body.

Why Autoimmune Disorders Occur

The relationship between celiac disease and other autoimmune disorders is complex and is the subject of much ongoing research and speculation. On the most basic level, there appear to be a number of genes that can predispose an individual to celiac disease and to other autoimmune disorders. The best example of this is the fact that the human leukocyte antigen genes HLA-DQ2 and HLA-DQ8, which must be present in order for celiac disease to develop (see Chapter 6 on genetic testing), are also risk factors for type 1 diabetes, adrenal insufficiency, and certain thyroid disorders. A variety of other genes that help regulate the immune system (which code for interleukins, chemokines, and cell-signaling molecules) may also provide the link between celiac disease and thyroid disease, type 1 diabetes, and rheumatoid arthritis.[1]

It appears that it was once advantageous to have certain hereditary traits that we now consider diseases. For instance, sickle cell trait protects against malaria, mild forms of cystic fibrosis make cholera infection less severe, and hemochromatosis, a disorder where the body accumulates too much iron, may either protect against anemia and/or confer resistance to infections. There is clearly no advantage to having an autoimmune disease, however, so we have to wonder why these disorders are so common. While there is no certain answer to this question, investigators have come up with some reasonable suggestions.

Although autoimmune diseases are common now, they were rare less than 100 years ago, and conversely, many infections that were once common are now rare (Figure 1). This observation suggests two possibilities, both of which may be true. The first is known as the "hygiene hypothesis."[2] Simply put, this states that the immune system was built to be very busy keeping lots of infections at bay, including parasites (such as worms or amoeba), bacteria, and viruses. In modern society, we have almost no parasites and fewer severe bacterial infections. Without enough to do, the immune system can escape normal regulation and begin to attack things randomly, which leads to allergies and autoimmune diseases.

The second theory developed as we realized that many people with autoimmune diseases share specific genes. For the vast majority of human existence, the main threat to survival has been infection. For that reason, having a relatively aggressive and nonselective immune system may have allowed some people to fight off new infections faster than others. However, the same lack of selectivity that made these genes so good at quickly reacting to new infections now increases the chance that they will react to proteins from the environment or your own body that are not a threat, which causes allergies or autoimmune disorders, respectively.

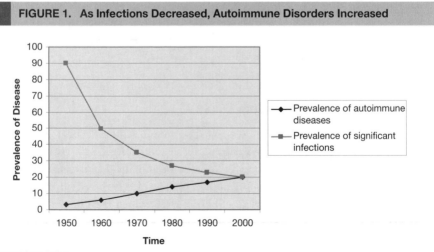

FIGURE 1. As Infections Decreased, Autoimmune Disorders Increased

Adapted from Ref. 2.

We do understand that, for whatever reason, many autoimmune disorders are associated with celiac disease and may present before, after, or at the same time as celiac disease. A list of autoimmune diseases more commonly associated with celiac disease can be found in Table 1.[3-5]

Although a number of autoimmune disorders occur more commonly in people with celiac disease, there is little reason to test for them unless you have symptoms that suggest a particular disorder. In most cases, tests for these other diseases are not very accurate so you would not start any treatment in the absence of symptoms. The two exceptions are thyroid disease and liver disease. These are common, relatively easy to test for, and may not have obvious symptoms. In general, both thyroid-stimulating hormone (TSH), and liver function tests should be checked at diagnosis of celiac disease and every few years afterward. Further testing would be done if these are abnormal. Other than this, tell your doctor about any new symptoms you have been experiencing, and decisions can be made on an individual basis regarding further testing.

The question of whether following a gluten-free diet prevents the development of future autoimmune diseases is being debated. Theoretically, either constant immune stimulation or intestinal damage (leaky gut) could predispose a person to developing autoimmune diseases. However, a number of well-conducted studies have reached opposite conclusions, some finding that the later celiac disease is diagnosed, the greater the chance of developing other autoimmune diseases, and still others finding that it made no difference. For

TABLE 1. Autoimmune Diseases Associated with Celiac Disease

Likely
- Raynaud's disease
- Vitiligo
- Microscopic colitis
- Type 1 diabetes
- Autoimmune thyroid disease
- Autoimmune liver diseases
- Inflammatory bowel disease

Possible
- Psoriasis
- Rheumatoid arthritis
- Sarcoidosis
- IgA nephropathy
- Sjogren's syndrome
- Alopecia areata (hair loss)
- Autoimmune anemia, thrombocytopenia, neutropenia
- Systemic lupus erythematosus
- Addison's disease
- Atrophic gastritis

Adapted from Refs. 2–5.

various reasons, this is actually a very difficult area to study and a conclusive answer is unlikely in the near future. The bottom line, however, is that a lifelong gluten-free diet is beneficial for those with celiac disease and it may possibly prevent development of other autoimmune diseases.

Outcome

After discussion with his physician, John did not seem to have any symptoms other than those directly related to his celiac disease. He had liver function tests and TSH level checked, and both were in the normal range. He plans on returning for a follow-up visit in one year, or sooner if new symptoms develop.

SELF-MANAGEMENT TIPS

☐ Several autoimmune diseases are more common in people with celiac disease.
☐ The gluten-free diet may decrease the risk of developing other autoimmune diseases, but this is uncertain.
☐ Liver and thyroid tests should be done routinely in patients with celiac disease.
☐ Evaluation for other autoimmune disorders is based on suggestive symptoms or laboratory results.

References

1. Hunt KA, van Heel DA. Recent advances in coeliac disease genetics. *Gut* 2009;58:473–76.
2. Bach JF. The effect of infections on susceptibility to autoimmune and allergic diseases. *N Engl J Med* 2002;347:911–20.
3. Garud S, Leffler D, Dennis M, Edwards-George J, Saryan D, Sheth S, Schuppan D, Jamma S, Kelly CP. Interaction between psychiatric and autoimmune disorders in coeliac disease patients in the Northeastern United States. *Aliment Pharmacol Ther* 2009;29:898–905.
4. Ventura A, Magazzu G, Greco L, SIGEP Study Group for Autoimmune Disorders in Celiac Disease. Duration of exposure to gluten and risk for autoimmune disorders in patients with celiac disease. *Gastroenterology* 1999;117:297–303.
5. Sategna Guidetti C, Solerio E, Scaglione N, Aimo G, Mengozzi G. Duration of gluten exposure in adult coeliac disease does not correlate with the risk for autoimmune disorders. *Gut* 2001;49: 502–505.

CHAPTER 45

Celiac Disease–Related Diseases and Complications

Jonas F. Ludvigsson, MD

Most of the severe complications discussed in this chapter are rare. It is important to realize that having an autoimmune disease increases your risk for other autoimmune diseases and certain conditions. This chapter covers type 1 diabetes, thyroid disease, osteoporosis, infection, cancer, and premature death. If you take the approach that learning about these conditions can help you get proper treatment early (if you should need it), then you are doing a lot to live well with your celiac disease.

Diabetes

David was 6 years old when his parents noted that he was very thirsty. His mother immediately suspected why. David's uncle had suffered from abnormal thirst just before being diagnosed with type 1 diabetes mellitus. David's parents alerted his pediatrician, and David's high blood glucose level confirmed that David also had developed type 1 diabetes. Unlike many people with newly diagnosed type 1 diabetes, David had not lost weight and showed no signs of fatigue or illness. His mother's early recognition of symptoms was fortunate. In many cases of newly diagnosed type 1 diabetes, severe electrolyte imbalances and even early signs of shock may occur.

In the first few days, the physician aimed to reduce David's blood glucose levels, which are brought to normal slowly to reduce the risk of brain swelling. In this period, it also becomes clear how much insulin the patient needs to keep his blood glucose near normal levels (often between 5 and 10 units of insulin). In type 1 diabetes, the pancreas stops making insulin, so replacing insulin is the only way to decrease blood glucose levels and treat the diabetes.

During his one-week stay in the hospital, David met with the diabetes team, including a diabetes nurse educator, physicians, dietitian, and a social worker. The family learned the basics of the disease and how to perform blood tests, administer insulin injections, and adjust the insulin dose based on what David ate at meals and his physical activity. These huge changes were very stressful, especially for David's mother, who had many questions. Why did David get type 1 diabetes? Would he have it for life? And how would it affect his everyday life and long-term health?

As part of the initial investigation, David was tested for thyroid disease and celiac disease. The screening for thyroid disease was negative, but both endomysial antibodies and tissue transglutaminase antibodies were detected. A subsequent small intestine biopsy showed damage to the villi, and David was diagnosed with celiac disease. David's mother was surprised and told the physician that David had never had any gastrointestinal problems. Could it really be that he had two diseases at the same time?

Like celiac disease, type 1 diabetes mellitus is an autoimmune disease.[1] In type 1 diabetes, an individual's immune system destroys the insulin-producing cells in the pancreas, which prevents the body from making insulin. This hormone is essential to the process of allowing glucose, primarily from digested food, to enter cells for use as fuel. Without insulin, blood glucose levels increase, which can upset the electrolyte and pH balances over the short term and also cause long-term complications. Type 1 diabetes occurs in approximately 1 in 400 children in the Western world, in contrast with type 2 diabetes, which occurs more often in adults and affects 20 million Americans. Type 2 diabetes in children is linked to obesity.

The most likely explanation for the association between celiac disease and type 1 diabetes is a shared genetic susceptibility. Human leukocyte antigen (HLA) is a part of a person's genetic makeup that responds to infectious attacks against the body. Certain HLAs, such as HLA-DQ2, are associated with both celiac disease and type 1 diabetes. So, a person at genetic risk of celiac disease is automatically also at increased risk of type 1 diabetes. Some people develop celiac disease first and type 1 diabetes later, and others have just the opposite experience.

Thyroid Disease

At age 16, David became tired and depressed. His mother worried that this was the result of David wandering from the gluten-free diet or not taking his insulin properly. She had read that many teenagers with celiac disease are sometimes careless with their diet, so she took David to a pediatric gastroenterologist. David said he occasionally consumed gluten and also that he had some problems with constipation. His blood test revealed an increased level of thyroid-stimulating hormone (TSH) and peroxidase autoantibodies and low thyroxine (T4) levels. David had developed chronic autoimmune thyroiditis, resulting in low thyroid function, and was prescribed levothyroxine. His health improved over the following few weeks.

The thyroid gland produces two hormones, thyroxine and triiodothyronine. These are released into the bloodstream and carried to tissues in the body where they control the speed of activity of the cells. Too little of the hormones (hypothyroidism) means that the cells work at a slower rate than normal, whereas too much of the hormones (hyperthyroidism) causes them to work faster than normal. Common symptoms of hypothyroidism are goiter, tiredness, depression, constipation, and weight gain. Symptoms of hyperthyroidism are usually goiter, tiredness, weight loss, racing heartbeat, and diarrhea.

The most common causes of both hypothyroidism and hyperthyroidism are autoimmune. Autoimmune thyroid disease is associated with other autoimmune diseases, so that if you have been diagnosed with an autoimmune disease, you are at an increased risk to develop autoimmune thyroid disease. People with celiac disease are nearly four times more likely to develop thyroid disease.

Osteoporosis

Allan, 54, is a nonsmoker and regular exerciser who does not drink alcohol. So when Allan had a hip fracture, everyone was surprised. At the emergency department, he had blood tests and underwent a bone scan (densitometry). His blood tests were normal, but his bone density was reduced. He had a T-score below −2.5, fitting the diagnosis for osteoporosis. As part of the extended investigation, Allan was screened for celiac disease. The blood tests for celiac antibodies were positive, and Allan had a small intestine biopsy that confirmed his diagnosis of celiac disease. After one year on a gluten-free diet, his bone density had increased but not normalized (never fully recovered). When his wife accompanied him to one of his regular checkups, she thanked the physician and said that Allan's spirits had also improved as a result of the gluten-free diet.

Osteoporosis is a skeletal disease that is characterized by loss of bone mineral density. As a consequence, the bone is more fragile, and fractures occur more easily. About 1–3% of individuals with osteoporosis also suffer from celiac disease (see Chapter 47 on bone disease).[2] This is consistent with a twofold increased risk of fractures in those with celiac disease. Although a gluten-free diet increases bone mineral density in people with celiac disease and osteoporosis, it may not always reduce fracture risk. In fact, research has shown that there is a twofold increased risk of hip fractures both *before* and *after* a celiac disease diagnosis and that this increase remains at least 20 years after diagnosis. Children with celiac disease also seem to be at increased risk of fractures, although serious fractures are very uncommon in children. The connection between osteoporosis and celiac disease may be because of the chronic intestinal inflammation, the malabsorption of calcium and vitamin D, and perhaps the generation of autoantibodies that target and neutralize a hormone important for bone health.[3]

Infection

Anne, 44, had severe pneumonia 10 years ago. She was diagnosed with celiac disease three years ago but never strictly followed the gluten-free diet. Now she was coughing and had a temperature. She went to her physician, who referred her to the emergency department. Her C-reactive protein was increased, suggesting inflammation somewhere in her body, and an X-ray showed pneumonia. Anne quickly became much more ill, and she was transferred to the intensive care unit where she was given intravenous antibiotics. A blood test later confirmed that she had a pneumococcal infection. People with celiac disease are at increased risk of pneumonia and severe infections (sepsis), especially because of the bacteria pnemococci, for reasons described below. Anne was lucky and recovered fully.

Studies have shown a clear relationship between celiac disease and certain types of infections. Impaired function of the spleen (called *hyposplenism*) is more common in those with celiac disease, which makes them more sensitive to encapsulated bacteria, including pneumococci.[4] In those with both celiac disease *and* type 1 diabetes, reduced ability of white blood cells to attack and digest bacteria adds to hyposplenism, increasing the risk of infectious disease even more. This is the reason that in certain countries, people with celiac disease are immunized against pneumococci (with the pneumonia vaccine or pneumovax). Another possible explanation for increased risk of infection is that the intestinal lining is damaged causing increased permeability (sometimes referred to as *leaky gut*), which might allow more intestinal bacteria to enter the body.

People with celiac disease are also at increased risk of tuberculosis. This may be because of vitamin D malabsorption. Vitamin D plays a key role in the defense against tuberculosis. Note that it is possible that malabsorption resulting from not following the gluten-free diet could reduce the effectiveness of antituberculosis drugs in those being treated for tuberculosis.

Cancer

In Spring 2008, James, who is 73, came to us with diffuse abdominal pain and weight loss. We investigated his symptoms with upper endoscopy, and a duodenal biopsy showed damaged villi, which indicated that he had celiac disease. James began a gluten-free diet but did not improve. Six months later, a colonoscopy showed that he had colon cancer.

There have been reports of cancer associated with celiac disease, but the connection between the two is not clear. Many of these reports can be explained by physicians discovering celiac disease by chance in patients with a cancer that is causing gastrointestinal symptoms. Still, there is probably a small excess risk of gastrointestinal cancer in celiac disease because of, among other factors, malnutrition of vitamins and ongoing chronic intestinal inflammation.

Most research in cancer and celiac disease has focused on lymphoma, especially non-Hodgkin lymphoma. Early reports seemed to point to an extremely high risk for lymphoma in celiac disease. However, more recent research instead shows moderate (2- to 6-fold) increased risk for lymphoma compared to the general population. Note that this means that most people with celiac disease will *not* develop lymphoma. In a year, 1 in 5,000 individuals without celiac disease develops lymphoma, compared with 5 in 5,000 people with celiac disease. Although this risk is small, there are lymphoma subtypes, such as non-Hodgkin enteropathy-associated T cell lymphoma, that almost never occur in people without celiac disease.

Death

Both adults and children with celiac disease are probably at a slightly increased risk of death. This increased risk is most pronounced in the first year after diagnosis. For children, the risk of dying prematurely because of celiac disease is *extremely* small. The reasons for this small increase in childhood mortality are unclear.

For adults, our research team examined the risk of death in three groups: 29,000 individuals with celiac disease; 13,000 individuals who did not fulfill the criteria for celiac disease but might be in an early stage of celiac disease; and 3,700 individuals with normal small intestinal mucosa but positive blood tests for celiac disease.[4] We found a 39% increased risk of death in individuals with confirmed celiac disease but also an increased risk of death in those in the other two groups. The greatest increase in risk compared to the general population was seen for cancer in all three groups. By five years after diagnosis, the risk of death for patients with celiac disease had improved but had not completely normalized. The reason for this is unclear, but it is important to remember that not everyone who is diagnosed is adequately treated and a portion of those with celiac disease are not on a strict gluten-free diet, both of which may explain this persistent increase in risk of death seen in large studies.

SELF-MANAGEMENT TIPS

☐ Most of the severe complications discussed in this chapter are rare and will not occur. Although 1 in 700 individuals with celiac disease will have sepsis in a 10-year period, so will 1 in 1,700 individuals without celiac disease. Some of these complications are because of genetics, which cannot be changed. Concentrate on healthy habits that you can control.

☐ It is likely that a strict gluten-free diet reduces the risk of developing the complications of celiac disease. However, for most complications, data on the importance of the gluten-free diet are actually scarce. One exception is the importance of the gluten-free diet in pregnant women. In pregnant women with celiac disease, following the gluten-free diet reduces the risk of low birth weight in the offspring.

☐ Those with celiac disease and repeated bacterial infections should consider an immunization against pneumococci.

☐ Don't smoke, get regular physical exercise, see your physician regularly, and eat a healthy gluten-free diet. Learn how to handle stress creatively and fully enjoy your life.

Further Reading

- Barera G, et al. Occurrence of celiac disease after onset of type 1 diabetes: a 6-year prospective longitudinal study. *Pediatrics* 2002;109(5):833–38.
- West J, et al. Fracture risk in people with celiac disease: a population-based cohort study. *Gastroenterology* 2003;125(2):429–36.
- Riches PL, McRorie E, Fraser WD, Determann C, van't Hof R, Ralston SH. Osteoporosis associated with neutralizing autoantibodies against osteoprotegerin. *N Engl J Med* 2009;361(15):1459–65.

- Ludvigsson JF, et al. Coeliac disease and risk of sepsis. *Gut* 2008;57(8): 1074–80.
- Ludvigsson J, et al. Small-intestinal histopathology and mortality risk in celiac disease. *JAMA* 2009;302(11):1171–78.

Acknowledgements

Gratitude goes to Svante Norgren, Johan Svensson, Karin Ekström-Smedby, Karl Michaelsson, and Jan Källman for their feedback on this chapter.

Jonas F. Ludvigsson, MD, is a Swedish pediatrician and epidemiologist. He carries out research on celiac disease at the Karolinska Institute in Stockholm and in Örebro, Sweden. In 2010, he received the Rising Star in European Gastroenterology award from the Association des Societés Nationales Européennes et Méditerranéennes de Gastroentérologie and United European Gastroenterology Federation.

Cancer: Risks and Realities

Richard F. A. Logan, MD, FRCP

J ane is a 50-year-old woman who was diagnosed with celiac disease five years ago. She began a gluten-free diet (GFD) after diagnosis, and within a year her tissue transglutaminase antibody levels returned to normal. However, she recently began having some mild stomach pain. Jane had an upper endoscopy, and the biopsies taken from her duodenum revealed signs of inflammation (more intraepithelial lymphocytes than normal), although the villi looked healthy.

Jane has read that people with celiac disease are more likely to get cancer. She wants to know if this is true, how great her cancer risk is, and whether having increased numbers of intraepithelial lymphocytes increases her risk.

Why Is Cancer Associated with Celiac Disease?

The suggestion that people with celiac disease might have a greatly increased risk of cancer, or of any malignant disease, first arose from research published in the 1960s. At that time, we believed that celiac disease was very uncommon, affecting perhaps 1 in 5,000 people. There were no reliable blood tests to screen for the disease, and diagnosis required biopsies collected using a Crosby capsule. The capsule, attached to a fine tube, was swallowed and then withdrawn after the capsule had been "fired," collecting biopsy samples. This procedure often required admission to the hospital.

As a consequence, the few people who were diagnosed with celiac disease often had many years of low-grade ill health or were diagnosed only when they had severe malabsorption or other conditions associated with untreated celiac disease. Thus, the early studies of malignant disease and celiac disease were based on hospital data and were likely to include more complex cases in very ill people who had been referred to specialists.

In recent decades, several large population-based studies (which attempt to include all cases of celiac disease arising from a defined population) have been published.[1-4] These show that the risks of malignant disease are much lower than originally suggested and may in fact be lower than for the rest of the population for two common malignancies (breast and lung).

Which Cancers?

Four malignant conditions have been clearly shown to occur more commonly in people with celiac disease (Table 1). These are enteropathy-associated T-cell lymphoma (EATL), non-Hodgkin lymphoma, adenocarcinoma of the small intestine, and squamous cell cancer of the upper esophagus.

EATL was the first malignant condition to be clearly associated with celiac disease. Over the years, this name has changed according to which particular cell was thought to be the cause. Although the increase in risk seems very large, this is because it is such a rare tumor. For example, in a recent study from Holland, the number of new cases a year was one for every million Dutch people.[5] It tends to occur in people whose celiac disease has not responded to a GFD or who had undiagnosed celiac disease. This may explain why it occurs 2 to 3 times more often in men than women: More women have their celiac disease diagnosed. It is usually diagnosed within two to three years of diagnosis of celiac disease; sometimes, it is the reason that undiagnosed celiac disease is found.

The increased risk of EATL seems to be greatest in people with very advanced damage to the villi (Marsh III changes). This may explain why people with dermatitis herpetiformis, where the small intestinal changes are generally less marked than in others with celiac disease, have a much smaller increased risk.[6] This may also explain why studies that followed people presumed to have celiac disease based on positive celiac tests done on stored blood specimens showed no increased risk of EATL; these people tended to have less marked small intestinal abnormalities.

In measuring the increase in risk of EATL, it has become clear that people with celiac disease also have an increased risk of other types of lymphoma, generally described as non-

TABLE 1. Risk for Malignant Conditions in Celiac Disease

Malignant Condition	Range of Estimates of Relative Risk*	Lifetime Risk in the General U.S. Population†
Enteropathy-associated T-cell lymphoma	× 25–50	Too few cases to estimate
Any non-Hodgkins lymphoma (NHL)	× 2–6	2%
Adenocarcinoma of the small intestine	× 10	0.2%
Squamous cell cancer of the upper esophagus	× 2–4	0.5%‡
Breast cancer	× 0.3–0.6	12%
Lung cancer	× 0.4–1.0	7%
Any malignant disease	× 1.0–1.3	41%

*Relative risk is the risk in one group compared to the risk in another group. In this case, "× 2" would mean twice as common in celiac disease as in the general population, whereas "× 0.5" would mean half as common in celiac disease as in the general population.
†From National Cancer Institute SEER Cancer Stat Fact Sheet: http://seer.cancer.gov/statfacts/index.html.
‡For all esophageal cancers, including lower esophagus.

Hodgkins lymphoma. These lymphomas account for about 2% of all malignant conditions occurring in the United States. The increase in risk is about two to four times that of the general population, after subtracting for the cases with EATL. There is no evidence that these types of lymphoma result from severe damage of the small intestine or that risk is reduced by following a GFD.

There are two other malignant conditions associated with celiac disease. Adenocarcinoma of the upper small intestine is extremely uncommon in the general population. It appears to be more common in celiac disease but to a much lesser degree than EATL. The risk probably increases with the severity of small intestinal damage and decreases as the small intestine recovers on a GFD.

Squamous cell cancer of the upper esophagus is another uncommon malignancy that appeared to be more common in celiac disease in the past but may no longer be. A risk factor for this malignancy is a long-term deficiency of iron, which used to occur when celiac disease was more difficult to diagnose. No increase in risk of this cancer has been found in several recent studies of malignancy in celiac disease.

The good news is that women with celiac disease have an estimated 40–70% reduced risk of breast cancer. This might not sound large, but considering that breast cancer is the most common cancer in women in the United States and all of the developed world, this translates into a large reduction in the overall risk of malignancy. Why the risk of breast cancer is reduced in women with celiac disease is not yet known, but reduced risk was clearly seen in two large European studies that followed people with celiac disease for several years after diagnosis.[1,2]

The risk of lung cancer may also be reduced in people with celiac disease. This is not yet firmly established, but several population-based studies have found that people with celiac disease are less likely to be smokers than other people.

Risk and Timing of Diagnosis

Most studies have found that the risk of being diagnosed with a malignant condition is highest within a year or two of the diagnosis of celiac disease and that after this period, risk is much lower or not increased at all.[1–3] There are two likely explanations for this finding. The first is that the medical investigation involved in the evaluation of symptoms (such as weight loss) may lead to the diagnosis of both cancer and celiac disease, which are not truly related but appear associated because they were diagnosed around the same time. This is a more common occurrence in populations like the United States where many people with celiac disease are undiagnosed and celiac disease is usually not tested for until people present with severe symptoms. This leads to a thorough work-up, during which both celiac disease and a possibly unrelated cancer may be diagnosed.

The second possible reason that risk of cancer recedes over time is because treatment with a GFD reduces the severity of the inflammation in the small intestine, which reduces the chance that a malignant condition will develop. Although this explanation is probably true concerning development of EATL, it would not explain the reduction in risk of malignant conditions outside the small intestine.

Jane's Outcome

Jane's small intestine is healed, reducing her risk for the most common cancer connected to celiac disease, EATL. For Jane, the increase in the intraepithelial lymphocytes found in her biopsy is not a cause for concern and may be because of any number of benign causes, such as medications or minor inadvertent gluten exposure. We discussed the very good overall prognosis of celiac disease.

I explained that, in general, people with celiac disease who follow the GFD are, with time, just as healthy as anyone else. Although cancer is always scary, as long as Jane does her best with the GFD, she is no more likely to get cancer than anyone else.

SELF-MANAGEMENT TIPS

☐ The risk for cancer in celiac disease is modest and predominantly occurs within the first year or two of diagnosis.

☐ The highest risk of cancer is for EATL, which is related to severity of damage to the small intestine.

☐ The risk of cancer is very small for those who follow a GFD and respond by healing of the small intestine.

References

1. Askling J, Linet M, Gridley G, Halstensen TS, Ekstrom K, Ekbom A. Cancer incidence in a population-based cohort of individuals hospitalized with celiac disease or dermatitis herpetiformis. *Gastroenterology* 2002;123:1428–35.
2. West J, Logan RFA, Smith CJ, Hubbard RB, Card TR. Malignancy and mortality in people with coeliac disease: population based cohort study. *Br Med J* 2004;329:716–18.
3. Viljamaa M, Kaukinen K, Pukkala E, Hervonen K, Reunala T, Collin P. Malignancies and mortality in patients with coeliac disease and dermatitis herpetiformis: 30-year population-based study. *Digest Liver Dis* 2006;38:374–80.
4. Goldacre MJ, Wotton CJ, Yeates D, Seagroatt V, Jewell D. Cancer in patients with ulcerative colitis, Crohn's disease and coeliac disease: record linkage study. *Eur J Gastorenterol Hepatol* 2008;20:297–304.
5. Verbeek WHM, Van De Water JMW, Al-Toma A, Oudejans JJ, Mulder CJJ, Coupe VMH. Incidence of enteropathy–associated T-cell lymphoma: a nation-wide study of a population-based registry in The Netherlands. *Scand J Gastroenterol* 2008;43:1322–28.
6. Lewis NR, Logan RFA, Hubbard RB, West J. No increase in risk of fracture, malignancy or mortality in dermatitis herpetiformis: a cohort study. *Aliment Pharmacol Ther* 2008;27:1140–47.

Richard F. A. Logan, MD, FRCP, is a gastroenterologist and Professor, Division of Epidemiology and Public Health and Nottingham Digestive Diseases Centre, Queens Medical Centre University of Nottingham, Nottingham, United Kingdom.

CHAPTER 47

Bone Disease

Harold Rosen, MD

C ynthia is a 32-year-old woman who was recently diagnosed with celiac disease. Although the diagnosis was made just last month, her symptoms had been troubling her on and off for the past 10 years, and Cynthia and her doctors suspected that she had been living with active celiac disease for a number of years.

Immediately after diagnosis, Cynthia started a gluten-free diet (GFD). Although she is feeling better, Cynthia is concerned about whether her bones have been affected by the disease, especially because her grandmother recently had a hip fracture related to osteoporosis, a severe form of bone loss. Active celiac disease interferes with the body's ability to absorb nutrients from food, so it can potentially disrupt the absorption of calcium and other nutrients necessary for the health and strength of the skeleton. This can lead to thinning of the bones (osteopenia). At her gastroenterologist's advice, Cynthia began taking 1200 mg of calcium with 1000 units of vitamin D daily but has not had further evaluation of her bone mineral density.

Why Bone Loss Occurs

The proper functioning of your muscles and nerves critically depends on how much calcium is available in the blood. This is such a top priority for life that our bodies have evolved a system to regulate the concentration of blood calcium within a very narrow range (8.4–10.2 mg/dl). If we go for a few days without a glass of milk, blood calcium levels do not fall very much. However, if blood calcium levels fall from their usual of 9.0 mg/dl to 8.8 mg/dl because of an absence of dietary calcium, the parathyroid glands (not to be confused with their neighbor, the thyroid gland) sense the slight drop in calcium and make and release more parathyroid hormone (PTH). The role of PTH is to raise blood calcium levels, which it does by ordering calcium to be mobilized from the largest "store" of calcium in the body, the bones. This is the natural way that the parathyroid glands maintain blood calcium levels—at the expense of the bones.

This system is an excellent *short-term* solution for poor calcium intake, because it prevents the muscles, including the heart, from malfunctioning every time we run out of milk in the refrigerator. However, if your calcium intake is poor over the *long term,* this causes a continuous drain of calcium from the bones. Think of your bones as being like your bank account. If you run low on pocket money every once in a while, you can take some out of the bank. If you withdraw money from the bank *every day* for your daily expenses, pretty soon your bank account balance is alarmingly low.

Therefore, the only way to avoid fragile bones is by getting enough calcium from your diet. To do this, you must also take in enough vitamin D, which the intestines require to make use of the calcium in your food. The National Osteoporosis Foundation recommends an intake of 1200 mg of calcium and 800–1000 units of vitamin D for normal, healthy individuals. This is usually enough to avoid depleting the bones of calcium to maintain the desirable concentration of calcium in the blood.

Unfortunately, most people do not take in enough calcium and vitamin D, so over time their bone mineral density declines. How do you get adequate calcium? Most of us get it from dairy foods. A cup of milk or yogurt or an ounce of cheese each has about 300 mg of calcium, so four servings of dairy would give you plenty of calcium. Calcium-fortified juices also have about the same amount of calcium as a glass of milk, so a cup of calcium-fortified orange juice would count as one of the four servings of dairy you need each day. If you eat only two servings of dairy daily, you would get just 600 mg of calcium from food; in this case, you would need to take an additional 600 mg of calcium as a supplement to have the 1200 mg of calcium available to your body. Because very few foods have appreciable amounts of vitamin D, the recommended 800–1000 units of vitamin D usually need to be taken as a supplement.

How Celiac Disease Affects Bones

Like everyone, people with celiac disease need to get enough calcium and vitamin D. But your small intestine may not be absorbing what you need. So, even if you take 1200 mg of calcium and 800–1000 units of vitamin D daily, your body still might be robbing your bones of calcium to maintain the blood calcium levels. Preserving bone density is another very good reason to follow a strict GFD.

Finally, we know that chronic inflammation itself, as is seen in inflammatory bowel disease and rheumatoid arthritis, can lead to low bone mineral density.[1] For all these reasons, the risk of fracture in people with celiac disease is slightly higher than it is for the general population.[2]

Diagnosing and Treating Low Bone Mineral Density in Celiac Disease

When you are diagnosed with celiac disease, the number one priority is to treat the malabsorption of the small intestine with the GFD. Over several months on this diet, your ability to absorb nutrients will improve. At the same time, I recommend that all people with celiac disease take 1200 mg of calcium and 800–1000 units of vitamin D daily, so that after a few months, you will have enough calcium and vitamin D available and a healthy small intestine to absorb them normally. This way, any existing calcium and vitamin D deficiency will be corrected over time, preventing further bone loss, and reversing any bone loss that may have occurred before you were diagnosed.

Not everyone on a GFD completely normalizes their absorption of calcium and other nutrients. This might be because of an inability to heal the intestine completely because of inadvertent gluten exposure or other reasons. Therefore, after you have been on a GFD and taking 1200 mg of calcium and 800–1000 units of vitamin D daily for 3–6 months, it's advisable to have your health care provider check how well you are absorbing calcium. This is done with a blood test to measure the levels of calcium, albumin (a binding protein), phosphorus (which usually falls when PTH is high), PTH, and 25-hydroxyvitamin D (the form of vitamin D that circulates in the blood) and comparing the results to normal (Table 1). In the event that your vitamin D levels are low, you might require higher, prescription-strength doses such as 50,000 units of vitamin D once weekly. In that case, you will need to have your blood checked every six months to make sure that the vitamin D dose is sufficient but not too much; vitamin D excess can occur at very high doses (typically above 10,000 units per day) and can lead to high blood and urine calcium levels, which may cause kidney stones, mental confusion, and problems with heart rhythm.

I don't usually require newly diagnosed celiac patients to have an X-ray measurement of bone density (commonly called a *DXA;* Figure 1). Even if it showed that your bone density is slightly lower than normal, which increases your risk for bone fracture a bit higher than normal, the treatment would still be a GFD and adequate amounts of calcium and vitamin D. In general, bone mineral density testing is recommended for those with celiac disease after one year on a GFD.[3] It is worth noting that this recommendation is controversial because there is no evidence in men or premenopausal women with celiac disease for doing anything other than keeping a strict GFD and making sure vitamin D levels are normal.

It is also important to note that medications like alendronate (Fosamax) have only been shown to be effective in women who have stopped menstruating. In general, women who menstruate regularly maintain fairly stable bone density unless they are deficient in calcium or vitamin D. It may be worthwhile seeing an endocrinologist, ideally one who specializes

TABLE 1. Bone-Healthy Levels of Nutrients

Test	Standard Normal Range	Goal
Calcium	8.4–10.2 ng/dl	8.4–10.2 ng/dl
25-Hydroxyvitamin D	20–100 ng/dl	>30 ng/dl*
Albumin	3.4–4.8 g/dl	3.4–4.8 g/dl
Phosphorus	2.7–4.5 mg/dl	2.7–4.5 mg/dl
Parathyroid hormone	15–65 pg/ml	<65 pg/ml

*Although the normal range for Vitamin D is 20–100 in most labs, growing evidence suggests that levels less than 30–35 are not optimal for bone health.

in bone health, if your blood tests (vitamin D, PTH) do not normalize with treatment or if you are male or a premenopausal woman considering taking an osteoporosis medication.

What Cynthia Did

Cynthia's initial 25-hydroxyvitamin D level was mildly low at 26 ng/dl. After a year on a GFD with calcium and vitamin D supplementation, her repeat level was 42 ng/dl. She elected to have a DXA taken, which showed her bone density was in the normal range. She has continued supplementation with 800 mg of calcium and 1000 units of vitamin D daily and will have another DXA done around the time of menopause.

SELF-MANAGEMENT TIPS

☐ Because of problems with nutrient absorption, celiac disease is associated with lower bone mineral density in many people but the risk of fracture is only slightly increased.

☐ Because of the fact that most people don't take in enough calcium and vitamin D and the potential for continued malabsorption, everyone with celiac disease needs to take calcium and vitamin D supplements.

☐ Vitamin D level should be checked at diagnosis and followed until you reach a normal level of more than 30 ng/dl.

☐ Consider having a bone mineral density test only after vitamin D levels have normalized and you have been on a GFD for one year.

References

1. Fornari MC, Pedreira S, Niveloni S, Gonzalez D, Diez RA, Vazquez H, Mazure R, Sugai E, Smecuol E, Boerr L, Maurino E, Bai JC. Pre- and post-treatment serum levels of cytokines IL-1beta, IL-6, and IL-1 receptor antagonist in celiac disease: are they related to the associated osteopenia? *Am J Gastroenterol* 1998;93:413–18.
2. West J, Logan RF, Card TR, Smith C, Hubbard R. Fracture risk in people with celiac disease: a population-based cohort study. *Gastroenterology* 2003;125:429–36.
3. Bernstein CN, Leslie WD, Leboff MS. AGA technical review on osteoporosis in gastrointestinal diseases. *Gastroenterology* 2003;124:795–841.

Harold Rosen, MD, is Director of the Osteoporosis Prevention and Treatment Center at Beth Israel Deaconess Medical Center in Boston, Massachusetts. In this capacity, he runs bone densitometry; sees patients in consultation for osteoporosis and metabolic bone disease; and teaches students, residents, and fellows.

CHAPTER 48

Skin Manifestations of Celiac Disease

Ludovico Abenavoli, MD, Giovanni Gasbarrini, MD,
and Giovanni Addolorato, MD

We met Mario, a 46-year-old man, three years ago. He had suffered from psoriasis for more than 15 years and was first treated with corticosteroid therapy, with little improvement in his skin lesions. In 1997, Mario was referred to the outpatient dermatology department of our hospital because his psoriasis had not improved and to deal with the side effects of long-term steroid use.

Mario was taken off the steroid therapy and began immunosuppressive therapy with cyclosporine. However, his skin still did not improve, and as the dose of cyclosporine was increased, he developed a common mild form of skin cancer called *basal cell epithelioma*, so the cyclosporine treatment was halted. Mario was then treated with oral retinoids and steroid creams, without any significant improvement. After two years, Mario was losing weight and experiencing abdominal pain, vomiting, and diarrhea. An endoscopic examination with jejunal biopsy showed that his intestinal villi were damaged, which led Mario to a diagnosis of celiac disease. However, Mario never ate completely gluten free, and his psoriatic skin lesions worsened and his gastrointestinal symptoms continued.

In 2006, Mario's dermatologist recommended that he be admitted for skin treatment at our hospital. At admission, Mario had serious, widespread psoriatic skin lesions, iron deficiency anemia, and low blood levels of folate, vitamin B_{12}, and vitamin D. His blood tests also showed elevated levels of antiendomysial antibodies and immunoglobulin (Ig) A and IgG antibodies to gliadin, showing that his celiac disease was active.[1] Mario's duodenal biopsy at his next endoscopy showed that his small intestine was inflamed and that his intestinal villi were totally damaged.

The Skin and Celiac Disease

Dermatitis herpetiformis is a well-known consequence of celiac disease.[2] But in recent years, we have learned that there are other skin conditions created by or associated with celiac disease (Table 1). In general, it appears that intestinal diseases play a role in diseases of the skin. Some immune-mediated skin diseases other than dermatitis herpetiformis have been reported to reverse with a gluten-free diet, in particular

TABLE 1. Skin Diseases (Other than Dermatitis Herpetiformis) that May Be Related to Celiac Disease

Disease Type	Shows Improvement on Gluten-Free Diet
Autoimmune	Alopecia areata
	Cutaneous vasculitis
	Dermatomyositis
Inflammatory	Psoriasis
Allergic	Urticaria
	Atopic dermatitis
	Prurigo nodularis
Miscellaneous	Oral lichen planus
	Aphthous stomatitis
	Chronic ulcerative dermatitis

alopecia areata (reversible patchy hair loss of the scalp and beard caused by inflammation), psoriasis, and aphthous stomatitis (commonly known as oral canker sores).[3] It is likely that chronic stimulation of the immune system by gluten may be a cause of these immune system disorders.[4]

In particular, there is an association between psoriasis and damage to the intestinal lining, primarily the kind of damage caused by celiac disease. Psoriasis is one of the most common chronic and recurrent skin diseases, but it is a complex disease that we don't yet completely understand. Typically, the skin is inflamed, reddened, scaly, and sometimes has pustules.

Studies show that when people with psoriasis are diagnosed with celiac disease and begin a gluten-free diet, their psoriasis improves. When they resume eating a normal diet, the psoriatic lesions become worse. Those with poorly controlled celiac disease, as measured by antibody markers, and psoriasis often require the use of systemic immunosuppressants, such as cyclosporine, or psoralen plus ultraviolet A (commonly called *PUVA*) therapy to treat their psoriasis.

Most of what we know about celiac disease and skin diseases is from case reports rather than large studies, so it is difficult to draw solid conclusions about the cause-and-effect relationship and the mechanisms involved. One area being studied focuses on whether these individuals have abnormal small intestinal permeability. This would allow substances such as the body's own or foreign antigens (which trigger an immune response) to cross the membranes of the intestine, which could begin an antibody-driven immune response and inflammation and eventually lead to malabsorption.

What Mario Did

While he was in the hospital, Mario began a true gluten-free diet. He left a few days later without any medications for his psoriasis, and because Mario strictly followed the GFD, he had rapid improvement of his gastrointestinal symptoms. After two months on the gluten-free

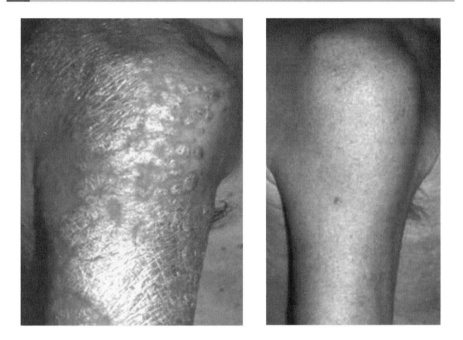

diet, his psoriatic skin lesions disappeared (Figure 1).[5] An endoscopy with duodenal biopsy performed four months after his hospital stay showed a marked improvement of the intestinal mucosa. Another biopsy two months later, after six months of eating gluten free, showed that his villi were normal. At present, Mario is still adhering to the gluten-free diet and is free of psoriatic skin lesions.

SELF-MANAGEMENT TIPS

☐ The effects of celiac disease can be seen in body tissues and organs other than the gastrointestinal system, including the skin.

☐ Eating gluten free can improve or cure psoriasis in those who also have celiac disease.

☐ Those with certain skin conditions (see Table 1) should consider being tested for celiac disease.

References

1. Rostom A, Dubé C, Cranney A, et al. The diagnostic accuracy of serologic tests for celiac disease: a systematic review. *Gastroenterology* 2005;128(Suppl. 1):S38–46.
2. Green PH, Cellier C. Celiac disease. *N Engl J Med* 2007;25:1731–43.
3. Abenavoli L, Proietti I, Vonghia L, et al. Intestinal malabsorption and skin diseases. *Dig Dis* 2008;26:167–74.
4. Lammers KM, Lu R, Brownley J, et al. Gliadin induces an increase in intestinal permeability and zonulin release by binding to the chemokine receptor CXCR3. *Gastroenterology* 2008;135:194–204.
5. Addolorato G, Parente A, De Lorenzi G, et al. Rapid regression of psoriasis in a coeliac patient after gluten-free diet: a case report and review of the literature. *Digestion* 2003;68:9–12.

Ludovico Abenavoli, MD, is Assistant Professor in the Department of Experimental and Clinical Medicine, University "Magna Græcia," Catanzaro, Italy. **Giovanni Gasbarrini, MD,** is Professor and **Giovanni Addolorato, MD,** is Associate Professor at the Institute of Internal Medicine, Catholic University, Rome, Italy.

CHAPTER 49

Anemia and Celiac Disease

Anne Roland Lee, MSEd, RD, LD

Alexia is a 26-year-old woman who was diagnosed with celiac disease just six months ago. Before her diagnosis, Alexia had suffered from diarrhea, abdominal cramps, fatigue, and easy bruising for years. She has always been on the thin side for her height, at about 120 pounds. Once she was diagnosed with celiac disease and started a gluten-free diet (GFD), her gastrointestinal symptoms improved within the first month. The only instruction she received about the diet was an information sheet supplied by her physician. Despite this, Alexia reported that she felt so much better that she "is like a new woman." She has returned to some social activities that she had given up years ago because of her constant fatigue.

However, even though her gastrointestinal symptoms are gone, Alexia's extreme fatigue returned. After waiting two months to see if she would feel better, she went back to the doctor concerned that something else might be wrong. Although her other values were normal, the blood work revealed that she had iron deficiency anemia. Alexia's hemoglobin was 10.0 g/dl (normal is >11.5 g/dl for females and >13.5 g/dl in males), her hematocrit was 25.9 (normal is 35–47 for females and 42–52 for males), and her ferritin was 22 ng/dl (normal is 30 ng/dl or more).

What Is Iron Deficiency Anemia?

Anemia is the most common nutrient deficiency in the world. Simply, it is lack of iron. Although anemia is very common and the symptoms may negatively impact daily life and quality of life, anemia is not usually life threatening.

Up to 10% of all females who are between adolescence and 49 years of age are iron deficient. The rate of iron deficiency increases to 20% in women who are pregnant, and half of all women in underdeveloped countries have it. Another interesting fact is that the rate of iron deficiency in Caucasian women is double that of Hispanic or African-American women.

Anemia may be a result of poor intake of iron-rich foods, blood loss, or impaired absorption of iron. Working out routinely causes some iron loss, but it is a minimal amount and is far outweighed by the overall benefits of a regular exercise routine. However, sustained, intense exercise, such as the training required for a marathon, may increase iron losses to the level of requiring routine supplementation.

Several studies have shown that between 10% and 15% of individuals with iron deficiency anemia are found to also have celiac disease. In fact, most individuals who are newly diagnosed with celiac disease have iron deficiency anemia, although the exact number is not clear.

What Contributed to Alexia's Iron Deficiency

It was entirely possible that Alexia's iron deficiency was the result of long-term decreased iron absorption that is commonly associated with untreated celiac disease. However, Alexia's blood tests showed that she was eating gluten free, and the absence of her gastrointestinal symptoms indicated that her gut was likely healed, or healing. Therefore, Alexia's doctor referred her to me for a dietary consult, and we took a look at how Alexia was eating.

Alexia's Typical Meal Plan

BREAKFAST: gluten-free puffed rice cereal, 1 cup 2% milk, banana, and coffee with 1 tsp. sugar and 1 oz. 2% milk

LUNCH: yogurt, rice crackers, apple, iced tea

SNACK: gluten-free cookies

DINNER: grilled chicken, mashed potatoes, carrots, glass of wine, ice cream

Alexia eats within the gluten-free dietary guidelines. However, a gluten-free dietary pattern, in general, has been shown to be low in several nutrients, including iron.[1-4] It was clear that Alexia's usual food intake was low in iron and fiber and potentially low in B vitamins.

Alexia showed me the diet sheet she had received at diagnosis. Although it presented the basics about how to eat gluten free, it did not instruct her to take a multivitamin, to eat foods high in iron, or to try nutrient-rich alternative grains.

Unfortunately, the standard GFD described on Alexia's diet sheet did not meet the recommended intake for fiber, B vitamins (thiamin, riboflavin, niacin folate), iron, or calcium.[1-4] It was clear that the cause of Alexia's anemia was her diet rather than malabsorption.

Adding Iron to a Gluten-Free Diet

Adding iron-rich foods to a GFD is a bit tricky. Many iron-rich foods are also gluten-containing foods. Most wheat-based cereals, pasta, and breads are enriched with iron and are, therefore, excellent sources of iron. However, gluten-free foods are not required to be enriched. The GFD not only restricts the usual good dietary sources of iron, but also presents other potential nutrient deficiencies that could be reversed by eating iron-rich foods such as beans and grains.

Including nutrient-dense grains, beans, and occasional red meat would significantly improve the nutrient profile of Alexia's diet. One study showed that substituting a grain or grain product with a higher nutrient profile at each meal for a standard gluten-free starch significantly increased important nutrient levels in the diet, increasing protein to 20.6 from 11 g, iron to 18.4 from 1.4 mg, calcium to 182 from 0 mg, and fiber to 2.7 from 5 g. The "alternative diet" provided an improved nutrient profile over the standard GFD.[3] By selecting beans and alternative grains, Alexia would not only increase her iron intake but also increase her fiber, calcium, and B vitamin intake, all nutrients of concern for a young woman on a GFD. For example, if Alexia substituted a gluten-free whole-grain cereal for breakfast, used high-fiber gluten-free bread at lunch, and added brown rice at dinner instead of potatoes, she could increase the fiber in the diet as well as the B complex vitamins. I asked Alexia to consider trying gluten-free oatmeal or a cold cereal of amaranth or millet flakes at breakfast, gluten-free high-fiber brown rice bread at lunch, and side dishes of quinoa, brown rice, or buckwheat pasta with her dinner.

There are two types of iron-rich foods: heme iron and nonheme iron (Table 1). Heme iron is from animal sources and is easily absorbed. Nonheme iron comes from grains, beans, and vegetables and needs the addition of either a heme iron food or an acid-based food to increase the absorption of the iron.

Beans

Pound for pound, beans offer a great source of key nutrients, including iron and fiber, for significantly less money and less fat. In general, beans supply approximately six to seven grams of protein per half-cup serving. This is equal to a one-ounce serving of lean meat. In addition, beans offer some nutrients that animal proteins do not. Beans are a rich source of fiber. Each half-cup serving offers approximately six grams of fiber, which is 25–30% of the recommended daily intake, and it is primarily soluble fiber.

TABLE 1. Sources of Iron in Food

Heme Sources	Nonheme Sources
Clams	Beans
Liver	Grains
Oysters	Pumpkin seeds
Mussels	Potato with skin
Beef	
Shrimp	
Sardines	
Turkey	

Soluble fiber is the type of fiber that, in the intestines, forms a gel-like substance that binds fats. A diet rich in soluble fiber is associated with decreased risks of colon cancer and heart disease and helps reduce LDL cholesterol level. Beans are also very low in fat and contain no cholesterol. Beans also supply phytochemicals, which are plant-based chemicals that play protective roles in the body. Antioxidants are the phytochemicals that help protect the cells from damage and therefore help maintain a healthy immune system. The more colorful the outside of the bean, the richer the source of antioxidants.

Grains

Grains offer several solutions for a person with celiac disease and anemia (Table 2). They are a source of iron. Grains also provide fiber to help relieve potential constipation from iron supplements. They also offer many of the B vitamins that are commonly missing in the standard GFD.

Combining Foods for Maximum Iron Absorption

Not only are beans and grains sources of B vitamins, especially thiamin and folate, but many are very good sources of minerals in addition to iron: phosphorus, magnesium, manganese, potassium, calcium, copper, and zinc to name a few. The one drawback to using a bean or grain to get iron and other minerals is that they are in a bound form. This means that you need to eat the food with either an animal-based protein (such as meat, eggs, or cheese) or a food high in ascorbic acid (vitamin C) to free the iron for absorption. This is as easy as topping buckwheat pasta with tomato sauce (for the vitamin C), eating quinoa with grilled chicken, or adding 3 oz. of a vitamin C–containing beverage to the meal.

Historically, many cultures of people have solved this nutritional issue through food combining. Many dishes combine grains and beans with foods that are high in vitamin C or have

TABLE 2. Nutrients in Grains per 1-Cup Serving

| | Iron (mg) | Fiber (g) | B Vitamins | | | | Protein (g) | Calcium (mg) |
			Thiamin (mg)	Riboflavin (mg)	Niacin (mg)	Folate (mcg)		
Amaranth flakes	0.67	3.6	0.027	0.042	0.992	4	5.91	6
Buckwheat groats	1.34	4.5	0.067	0.066	1.579	24	5.69	12
Millet	1.1	2.3	0.184	0.143	2.314	33	6.11	5
Quinoa	7.865	5	0.017	0.337	2.491	41.5	11.14	51
Rice, wild	0.98	3	0.085	0.143	2.11	43	6.54	5
Rice, brown	1.03	3.5	0.199	0.023	2.594	8	4.52	20
Sorghum	4.225	6.05	0.2275	0.1365	2.81	—	10.85	27

animal protein: Think of traditional tacos with beans and ground meat, quinoa salad with tomatoes, or a Mediterranean fish stew. Eating tomatoes, broccoli, cabbage, collards, kale, peppers, and snow peas with beans provides the ascorbic acid needed. Having vitamin C–rich fruit with the meal will also enhance the release of the minerals in the gut. Foods like cantaloupe, citrus fruits, guava, papaya, and strawberries do the trick and are easy to combine with a bean or grain meal. For example, a marinated bean salad with citrus or papaya chunks would be pleasing to the palate as well to your nutrient needs. A fruit smoothie of berries and silken tofu is a great source of protein, calcium, and iron. Another way to enhance the availability of the bound nutrients is to add animal protein to the dish, such as a bit of ground turkey, beef, or even fish to a bean stew.

Changes that Alexia Made

Based on the nutrient information we discussed, I suggested a simple three-step plan that would help restore Alexia's health.

- Take a daily gluten-free multivitamin and mineral supplement with iron
- Make some simple dietary changes:
  - □ Eat more iron sources: liver, eggs, beef, dried fruits, and alternative gluten-free whole grains.
  - □ Eat iron-rich foods with foods rich in vitamin C or that have high acid content.
  - □ Take an iron supplement with meals, especially with either vitamin C–rich foods or high-acid-content foods to enhance iron absorption.
  - □ Increase fiber (along with water) intake gradually to avoid constipation, but don't eat too much fiber, because it would decrease iron absorption.
- Learn more about the potential side effects of iron supplementation, specifically changes in stool color, constipation, foods that decrease iron absorption, and abdominal discomfort, and work to manage them.

Alexia's Outcome

Alexia returned in six months for a follow-up visit. The good news was that her blood work showed signs of improvement. Her hematocrit increased from 25.9 to 30.4, ferritin from 22 to 28 ng/dl, and hemoglobin from 10 to 12.8 g/dl. Although these are still not in the normal range, the increases are significant and going in the right direction. One reason the values may not have been in the normal range is that Alexia had trouble taking her iron supplement. She felt she managed the multivitamin with iron, but when her doctor recommended that she take an iron supplement once or twice a day, Alexia had some reactions. Typically, iron supplements are large pills that can be difficult to swallow; they can also cause an upset stomach, bloating, and constipation, all of which Alexia experienced. These troubles made her stop taking the iron supplement although she continued with the multivitamin with iron. She also added several iron-rich foods to her diet, but her lunch changed little because it was easier to handle at work. Alexia has also added eggs and red meat to her diet three times per week for the added iron.

Alexia's Richer-in-Iron Meal Plan

BREAKFAST: gluten-free amaranth flakes cereal with 1 cup 2% milk and 2 Tbsp. raisins and coffee with 1 tsp. sugar and 1 oz. 2% milk

LUNCH: yogurt, brown rice crackers, apple, iced tea

SNACK: trail mix with dried fruits and nuts, tomato juice

DINNER: grilled shrimp, quinoa, carrots, glass of wine, ice cream

Because the iron supplement caused Alexia discomfort and her anemia is showing signs of recovery, we decided that Alexia could continue to use only the women's multivitamin with iron. We encouraged Alexia to continue adding nutrient-dense foods to her new meal pattern, to increase her intake of fluids, and to start a daily activity program to aid in the relief of any constipation she might have. Alexia plans to return in another six months for follow up and monitoring of her blood values.

SELF-MANAGEMENT TIPS

☐ The standard GFD is low in iron, fiber, and B vitamins.

☐ Include iron-rich foods to avoid anemia. Iron-rich grains and beans also supply needed fiber and B vitamins.

☐ Try interesting whole grains, such as amaranth, quinoa, and buckwheat, which are nutrient rich.

☐ Learn to combine iron-rich foods with animal protein and foods containing high amounts of vitamin C, which releases iron for absorption.

☐ If tolerance of the iron supplement is an issue, try different formulas or try splitting the tablet into quarters or halves and take them at intervals over a day.

References

1. Dickey, W, Kearney, N. Overweight in celiac disease: prevalence, clinical characteristics, and effect of a gluten free diet. *Am J Gastroenterol* 2006;101:2356–59.
2. Hallert C, Grant C, Green S, et al. Evidence of poor vitamin status in coeliac patients on a gluten-free diet for 10 years. *Aliment Pharmacol Ther* 2002;16:1333–39.

3. Lee AR, Ng DL, Dave E, Ciaccio EJ, Green PH. The effect of substituting alternative grains in the diet on the nutritional profile of the gluten-free diet. *J Hum Nutr Diet* 2009;22(4): 359–63. Epub 2009 Jun 10.
4. Thompson T, Dennis M, Higgins LA, Lee AR, Sharrett MK. Gluten-free diet survey: are Americans with coeliac disease consuming recommended amounts of fibre, iron, calcium and grain foods? *J Hum Nutr Diet* 2005;18:163–69.

Anne Roland Lee, MSEd, RD, LD, is Director of Nutritional Services at Schär USA and an Adjunct Professor at University of New Mexico in the Nutrition Department as well as a doctoral candidate. Her research is on the nutritional adequacy, economic impact, and quality of life issues surrounding the gluten-free diet.

CHAPTER 50

Celiac Disease and Fertility

Ralph Warren, MD, FRCPC, and Ellen Greenblatt, MD, FRCSC

Charlotte and Howard are married, and both are now 35 years old. After three years of marriage, they decided to start a family, and Charlotte stopped taking her birth control pills.

Howard is healthy and athletic, but Charlotte tires easily. She was once told that she had chronic fatigue syndrome. They are nonsmokers. Almost consistently at past annual medical evaluations, Charlotte was found to have mild iron deficiency anemia, which was blamed on menstrual blood losses and a diet low in red meat. She has frequently taken iron pills for several weeks, in addition to a daily multivitamin containing iron, folic acid, and vitamin B_{12}.

After 16 months of trying without becoming pregnant, Charlotte and Howard were referred to a fertility clinic. Testing revealed that neither of them had any reproductive abnormalities. They were told they had "unexplained infertility." Following two unsuccessful attempts at in vitro fertilization, and considerable emotional upheaval and expense, they submitted an application to an adoption agency.

Can Unexplained Infertility Be Explained?

An estimated 16% of American and Canadian couples are infertile, which is defined as the lack of conception following 12 months of unprotected intercourse. In women, ovulation disorders or Fallopian tube dysfunction accounts for 30% of infertility. Male factors, such as sperm deficiencies, account for another 30% of cases of infertility, and a combination of male and female factors, such as low sperm count plus ovulation dysfunction, occur in approximately 30% of couples. The remaining 10–15% of fertility problems are classified as unexplained. However, some portion of this may be because of undiagnosed celiac disease in either the man or the woman. Undiagnosed celiac disease may be present in up to 4% of women with unexplained infertility, higher than the prevalence of celiac disease in the general population (0.5–1%).[1]

Unfortunately, celiac disease is rarely considered as a possible explanation of unexplained infertility. Anatomical and hormonal disorders receive earlier and greater emphasis. Infertility may be the initial and only indication of celiac disease, but more often subtle features are already in place, such as unexplained iron deficiency anemia, irritable bowel syndrome, unexplained osteoporosis, mood swings/depression, or chronic fatigue syndrome.

How Celiac Disease Affects Fertility

Celiac disease may affect fertility through the presence of autoimmune and hormonal factors as well as through nutritional factors because of malabsorption. Iron, folate, zinc, selenium, and vitamin K deficiencies have been implicated in infertility, but precise mechanisms are unclear.[2] Large-scale, well-designed clinical studies would provide answers as well as increase awareness of the connection between undiagnosed celiac disease and fertility problems.

Men and women with undiagnosed celiac disease may have a lower degree of sexual satisfaction and frequency of intercourse that can be corrected after one year on a gluten-free diet (GFD).[3] Hormonal deficiencies, poor semen quality, and reduced sperm counts have also been corrected using a GFD in men with celiac disease.[4] Vitamins A and E and zinc are known to be essential for sperm production. Male fertility may be impaired if celiac-related malabsorption of these fat-soluble vitamins and zinc occurs.

Fertility: An Urgent Issue

Estimates are that most adults have had celiac disease for up to a decade before they are diagnosed. For women facing infertility, undiagnosed celiac disease is an urgent problem that can disrupt life during their reproductive years (Table 1).

Menstruation
Undetected celiac disease may affect the entire span of a woman's reproductive years. Studies from the United Kingdom, Italy, and Argentina have reported delayed onset of menstruation, irregular and skipped menstrual periods, and earlier menopause in women with undetected celiac disease.

- Menstruation may be delayed 1–2 years beyond age 12.
- Irregular and skipped menstrual periods occur more frequently.
- Menopause can begin as much as 5 years earlier, for instance at age 45 instead of age 50.

TABLE 1. Effects of Undetected Celiac Disease on Fertility and Pregnancy

Menstrual Symptoms	Fertility	Maternal Complications	Fetal and Neonatal Complications
Delayed onset of puberty	Decreased frequency of intercourse and recurrent miscarriages leading to fewer children	Pregnancy at a later age	Intrauterine growth restriction
Menstrual irregularities			Premature delivery
Earlier menopause		Increased need for Caesarean section delivery	Low birth weight
			Short duration of breastfeeding

However, women with celiac disease who followed a GFD experienced no increase in these menstrual variations from women without celiac disease.[5-7]

Pregnancy

Women with undetected celiac disease who are pregnant appear to be 2–3 times more likely to suffer recurrent miscarriages.[5-8] A report from the United Kingdom suggests that autoimmune mechanisms may directly affect placental function in women with undetected celiac disease.[9] Risk for miscarriage falls to that of the general population for women on a GFD.

One study found that women with celiac disease tended to have babies at a later age. This surprising trend toward increased fertility with increasing age (age 35–40 years) was found regardless of whether they had treated or undetected celiac disease. There also was a 30% increase in Caesarean section deliveries in these older women. This was likely because of older maternal age itself, with celiac disease activity a potential but uncertain contributor.[10]

Offspring

Several European studies have shown that women with undetected celiac disease were at greater risk of having low–birth-weight babies and babies who had experienced intrauterine growth restriction. The severity of their celiac disease did not seem to play a significant role in the degree of risk, which suggests that these effects are because of celiac-related autoimmune factors rather than malnutrition. There was a dramatic reduction in the incidence of low–birth-weight babies and intrauterine growth restriction after treatment with a gluten-free diet.[5,7,8,11,12]

A large study in Sweden found that infants of fathers or mothers with celiac disease had a much greater chance of having low birth weight and possibly premature delivery. The findings in this study suggest that, in addition to the known genetic role for human leukocyte antigens (HLA types) in permitting the development of celiac disease, there may be non-HLA genetic factors influencing neonatal outcome in couples where either of the parents has celiac disease.[13]

Finally, women with undetected celiac disease, regardless of the severity of their celiac symptoms, tended to breast feed for less time. Those treated with a GFD breast fed 2.5 times longer.[5]

Since 2000, most people diagnosed with celiac disease are in their middle years or older. According to the Canadian Celiac Survey of 2002/2003, most celiac patients were diagnosed between the ages of 30 and 60 years, peaking when in their forties, which is generally beyond reproductive age. Unfortunately, women with undiagnosed celiac disease may receive the explanation for their unexplained infertility only retrospectively, once they are postmenopausal.

Many experts recommend that blood testing for celiac disease be included in the diagnostic protocol of all fertility clinics and implemented by all obstetrician-gynecologists investigating infertility and recurrent miscarriages. Therapy for celiac disease with the GFD clearly increases favorable pregnancy outcomes in women with known celiac disease.

What Happened to Charlotte

Charlotte's anemia worsened, prompting her referral to a gastroenterologist who performed blood tests, one of which showed that she had an immunoglobulin A tissue transglutaminase level of 48 units (less than 20 units is the normal level). She then had an upper endoscopy with duodenal biopsies, the results of which confirmed her diagnosis of celiac disease.

After receiving guidance from a dietitian with expertise in celiac disease, Charlotte began a GFD. She also took daily gluten-free iron and multivitamin supplements. Charlotte's energy level quickly increased, and within four months, her anemia disappeared and her iron stores were replenished. Ten months later she became pregnant. Her pregnancy went smoothly, and she delivered a healthy son weighing 7 lb. 10 oz. without any problems.

SELF-MANAGEMENT TIPS

☐ Infertility may be the only sign of undiagnosed celiac disease.
☐ Any unexplained infertility warrants testing for celiac disease.
☐ Therapy with a GFD increases fertility and prevents pregnancy complications in women with proven celiac disease.

References

1. Collin P, Vilska S, Heinonen PK, et al. Infertility and coeliac disease. *Gut* 1996;39:382–84.
2. Rostami K, Steegers EAP, Wong WY, et al. Coeliac disease and reproductive disorders: a neglected association. *Eur J Obstet Gynecol Reprod Biol* 2001;96:146–49.
3. Ciacci C, De Rosa A, De Michele G, et al. Sexual behaviour in untreated and treated coeliac patients. *Eur J Gastroenterol Hepatol* 1998;10:649–51.
4. Farthing MGH, Edwards CRW, Rees LH, et al. Male gonadal function in coeliac disease: 1. Sexual dysfunction, infertility and semen quality. *Gut* 1982;23:608–14.
5. Ciacci C, Cirillo M, Auriemma G, et al. Celiac disease and pregnancy outcome. *Am J Gastroenterol* 1996;91:718–22.
6. Smecuol E, Maurino E, Vasquez H, et al. Gynecological and obstetric disorders in coeliac disease: frequent clinical onset during pregnancy or the puerperium. *Eur J Gastroenterol Hepatol* 1996;8:63–69.
7. Eliakim R, Sherer DM. Celiac disease: fertility and pregnancy. *Gynecol Obstet Invest* 2001;51:3–7.
8. Gasbarrini A, Sanz Torre E, Trivellini C, et al. Recurrent spontaneous abortion and intrauterine fetal growth retardation as symptoms of coeliac disease. *Lancet* 2000;356:399–400.
9. Anjum N, Baker PN, Robinson NJ, et al. Maternal celiac disease autoantibodies bind directly to syncytiotrophoblast and inhibit placental tissue transglutaminase activity. *Reprod Biol Endocrinol* 2009;7:16.
10. Tata LJ, Card TR, Logan RFA, et al. Fertility and pregnancy-related events in women with celiac disease: a population-based cohort study. *Gastroenterology* 2005;128:849–55.

11. Norgard B, Fonager K, Sorensen HT, et al. Birth outcomes of women with celiac disease: a nationwide historical cohort study. *Am J Gastroenterol* 1999;94:2435–40.

12. Ludvigsson JF, Montgomery SM, Ekbom A. Celiac disease and risk of adverse fetal outcome: a population-based cohort study. *Gastroenterology* 2005;129:454–63.

13. Ludvigsson JF, Ludvigsson J. Coeliac disease in the father affects the newborn. *Gut* 2001;49:169–75.

Further Reading

- Cranney A, Zarkadas M, Graham I, et al. The Canadian Celiac Health Survey. *Dig Dis Sci* 2007;52:1087–95.
- Pellicano R, Astegiano M, Bruno M, et al. Women and celiac disease: association with unexplained infertility. *Minerva Medica* 2007;98:217–19.
- Pope R, Scheiner E. Celiac disease during pregnancy: to screen or not to screen? *Arch Gynecol Obstet* 2009;279:1–3

Ralph E. Warren, MD, FRCPC, is Associate Professor of Medicine (retired), University of Toronto, and consultant in gastroenterology, St. Michael's Hospital and the Toronto GI Clinic, Toronto, Ontario, Canada. **Ellen M. Greenblatt, MD, FRCSC, FABOG (REI),** is Associate Professor, University of Toronto, and Medical Director, Center for Fertility and Reproductive Health Mount Sinai Hospital, Toronto, Ontario, Canada.

CHAPTER 51

Neurologic Manifestations of Celiac Disease

Marios Hadjivassiliou, MD, and David S. Sanders, MD

Barry, a 53-year-old English man, had developed a gradual loss of balance and lack of coordination, called *ataxia,* with occasional falls over a six-month period. This was investigated with a number of blood tests and imaging of the brain, which showed shrinkage of the cerebellum, the balance organ at the back of the brain. Tests for vitamin deficiencies and other causes of loss of balance, including genetic tests, were negative. As there was no family history of a similar problem, he was diagnosed with loss of balance with no cause found.

Unfortunately, Barry's symptoms gradually became worse, and he was referred by his primary care physician to our ataxia clinic in Sheffield, UK. We saw him two years after he first consulted a physician, and at this stage, he was largely bound to a wheel chair. He denied having any gastrointestinal symptoms, such as diarrhea, weight loss, abdominal pain, or bloating. Examination showed abnormal eye movements (nystagmus) and clumsiness with the use of his arms and legs. He was able to bear weight, but it was impossible for him to walk without holding onto at least one person. Barry walked with a very broad-based gait, his legs spread apart. He had normal muscle strength and normal sensation. A repeat brain scan showed further shrinkage of the cerebellum.

Additional investigations included blood tests for celiac disease and gluten sensitivity, specifically for immunoglobulin A and G antigliadin, endomysial (IgA-EMA), and tissue transglutaminase (IgA-tTG) antibodies. All of these tests were abnormal (see Chapter 4 on blood testing). Barry was therefore diagnosed as having gluten ataxia. He was referred for an upper endoscopy with duodenal biopsy. This test confirmed his diagnosis of celiac disease.

Neurologic Problems and Celiac Disease

Traditionally, we think of gluten sensitivity as a disease of the small intestine, which makes sense given that, historically speaking, the symptoms are generally confined to the gastrointestinal tract. (See the Introduction for definitions of celiac disease and gluten sensitivity.) But in the last 15 years, more support has built for the concept of gluten sensitivity as a systemic disease with diverse manifestations and targets affecting nearly any part of the body. Similar to the skin lesions in dermatitis herpetiformis (see Chapter 9 on dermatitis herpetiformis), neurological manifestations can be very prominent even in the absence of intestinal damage.[1]

A large variety of problems can occur because of the autoimmune response to gluten that are not obvious because they do not involve the intestinal tract. This is an important observation because two thirds of people with neurological complaints because of gluten sensitivity have no significant intestinal damage and would not meet standard diagnostic criteria for celiac disease.[2] Even in those who have intestinal damage, gastrointestinal symptoms are typically not prominent, as in Barry's case.

The most common neurological manifestations are gluten ataxia[3] and gluten neuropathy.[4] Gluten neuropathy refers to damage of the nerve endings in feet and hands resulting in loss of sensation. Patients describe a feeling of walking on a thick carpet, numbness, tingling, and sometimes weakness and loss of sensation in feet and hands.

Additional manifestations include headache with brain abnormalities seen with imaging, muscle disease, and spinal cord disease. The majority of such patients do not have any bowel symptoms. Episodic, often severe headaches can be common in individuals with gluten sensitivity, who may also have abnormal magnetic resonance imaging (MRI) brain scans.[5] The link to gluten sensitivity is suggested by the fact that the headaches tend to resolve after beginning a strict gluten-free diet (GFD).

The age at onset of all neurological manifestations tends to be in the early 50s. It is common to observe additional autoimmune diseases, such as hypothyroidism, type 1 diabetes, and pernicious anemia, in patients or in their first-degree relatives (see Chapter 44). We are still learning about the ways in which gluten sensitivity can lead to neurologic damage. However, it is clear that the immune system in people with gluten sensitivity is abnormally overactive when they consume food containing gluten. Such overactivity is not limited to the intestine and can show itself with damage to many different parts of the body. Although neurological symptoms may be related to vitamin deficiencies, in individuals with gluten sensitivity, neurological manifestations are often immune mediated. Nerve, muscle, and brain tissue biopsies show evidence of inflammation around arteries in the brain's balance center and/or the peripheral nerves in the hands and feet as well as muscle.[2]

Testing for Neurologic Manifestations

People with these types of symptoms are likely to consult neurologists, who may not consider gluten sensitivity as the source of neurological problems or test for it using the appropriate antibodies. In addition, the specific tests indicative of inflammation of the bowel because of celiac disease—IgA-EMA and IgA-tTG—may not be accurate for making the diagnosis of gluten-related neurological manifestations, particularly in people without intestinal damage. Typically for celiac disease, IgA class antibodies are the most accurate (see Chapter 4 on blood testing). However, for neurological manifestations, IgG antibodies may be more important. Our practice is to test for IgA-tTG, IgA-EMA, and both IgA and IgG antigliadin antibodies.

If any of these antibodies are positive, we then perform a duodenal biopsy. If the biopsy shows damage consistent with celiac disease, the patient clearly needs to go on a GFD for life. On the other hand, even if the biopsy is normal, if the test for a gluten-related antibody is positive and no other cause for neurological dysfunction has been found, we still recommend a strict GFD with regular monitoring. Neurological manifestations usually show improvement after a year on strict GFD with evidence of elimination of the antibodies.[6,7]

Because the traditional celiac blood tests are often not accurate for the detection of neurological manifestations of celiac disease, new tests are being developed. tTG6 is found mostly in the brain but is closely related to the tTG2 found in the intestine. Antibodies to tTG2 are the basis of the standard IgA-tTG test for celiac disease. Individuals with antibodies primarily against tTG6 may not trigger a positive celiac IgA-tTG test. This is comparable to dermatitis herpetiformis where people may form antibodies to tTG3 (tTG3 is found in the skin, not the intestine) which cause inflammation (see Chapter 9). Although testing is not yet clinically available, antibodies against tTG6 may become a useful marker for the neurological effects of the disease in the same way that antibodies against tTG2 have become a useful marker for the intestinal damage.[8]

Treating Neurologic Manifestations

Unlike the small intestine's absorptive cells, the brain cells of the cerebellum have no ability to regenerate. A strict GFD can stop cell death, but it cannot reverse severe damage. This makes it extremely important to suspect, diagnose, and treat gluten sensitivity at the earliest opportunity. However, the GFD, if used early enough, can result in some improvement in cells that are damaged but not yet lost. Note that, although bowel symptoms tend to improve soon after beginning the GFD, improvement in the neurological symptoms takes about a year. Studies have shown such improvement for cases of gluten ataxia or gluten neuropathy.[6,7] The improvement was independent of the presence of intestinal damage at diagnosis.

If neurological deterioration continues despite closely following a GFD (usually associated with persistent positive antibodies), the patient needs education about the importance of the GFD and consultation with a dietitian to uncover sources of inadvertent gluten ingestion. If the progression continues despite a confirmed strict GFD with no presence of antibodies, this may call for the use of immunosuppressive treatment (see Chapter 43 on refractory celiac disease). Such cases are rare, and most people respond to the GFD.

What Barry Did

Barry began a GFD and has been followed closely. He has not gotten any worse, and his brain scan remains the same without any further shrinkage four years after his diagnosis of gluten ataxia. Repeat testing showed that all the celiac antibodies are now negative. Unfortunately, Barry hasn't improved either, and he remains disabled by the damage to his balance that had already occurred. Earlier diagnosis and treatment may have resulted in a better outcome for Barry.

SELF-MANAGEMENT TIPS

☐ Gluten sensitivity includes a spectrum of disorders and can present with manifestations outside the gut.

☐ Neurological manifestations are common and may be present even in the absence of any gastrointestinal symptoms or intestinal damage.

☐ Patients with loss of balance or neuropathy should be routinely screened for gluten sensitivity.

☐ Development of neurological manifestations in individuals already known to have celiac disease is usually associated with not following the GFD and requires counseling by a celiac dietitian.

☐ Treatment of gluten-related neurological issues should be a multidisciplinary effort between a neurologist, gastroenterologist, and dietitian, all skilled in celiac disease.

References

1. Hadjivassiliou M, Gibson A, Davies-Jones GAB, Lobo A, Stephenson TJ, Milford-Ward A. Is cryptic gluten sensitivity an important cause of neurological illness? *Lancet* 1996;347:369–71.
2. Hadjivassiliou M, Sanders DS, Grünewald RA, Woodroofe N, Boscolo S, Aeschlimann D. The neurology of gluten sensitivity. *Lancet Neurol* 2010;9:318–30.
3. Hadjivassiliou M, Grünewald RA, Chattopadhyay AK, et al. Clinical, radiological, neurophysiological and neuropathological characteristics of gluten ataxia. *Lancet* 1998;352: 1582–85.
4. Hadjivassiliou M, Grunewald RA, Kandler RH, et al. Neuropathy associated with gluten sensitivity. *J Neurol Neurosurg Psychiatry* 2006;77:1262–66.
5. Hadjivassiliou M, Grünewald RAG, Lawden M, Davies-Jones GAB, Powell T, Smith CML. Headache and CNS white matter abnormalities associated with gluten sensitivity. *Neurology* 2001;56:385–88.
6. Hadjivassiliou M, Kandler RH, Chattopadhyay AK, et al. Dietary treatment of gluten neuropathy. *Muscle Nerve* 2006;34:762–66.
7. Hadjivassiliou M, Davies-Jones GAB, Sanders DS, Grünewald RAG. Dietary treatment of gluten ataxia. *J Neurol Neurosurg Psychiatry* 2003;74(9):1221–24.
8. Hadjivassiliou M, Aeschlimann P, Strigun A, Sanders DS, Woodroofe N, Aeschlimann D. Autoantibodies in gluten ataxia recognise a novel neuronal transglutaminase. *Ann Neurol* 2008;64:332–43.

Marios Hadjivassiliou, MD, is a Consultant Neurologist and Honorary Reader in Neurology, Royal Hallamshire Hospital, Sheffield, United Kingdom. **Professor David S. Sanders** is Consultant Gastroenterologist and Honorary Professor in Gastroenterology, Royal Hallamshire Hospital and the University of Sheffield, Sheffield, United Kingdom.

CHAPTER 52

Liver Disorders in Celiac Disease

Alberto Rubio-Tapia, MD

When Marina, a 50-year-old woman, came to see me, she had been through six months of feeling unwell, with fatigue, joint pains, bloating, persistent diarrhea, and involuntary loss of 10 pounds. Marina was a professional chef, but her past medical and family histories were unrevealing, with no recent international travel.

Marina had normal temperature, pulse, and blood pressure, and she looked tired but not acutely ill. When palpated, she didn't have pain in her abdomen, and her liver and spleen felt normal. But her blood work revealed a different picture. Marina had anemia (hemoglobin 11 g/dl) but with normal white cell and platelet counts. And her liver function tests were abnormal: Total bilirubin was 0.7 mg/dl (normal is 0.1–1 mg/dl), aspartate aminotransferase (AST) was 150 units/L (normal is 8–48 units/L), alanine aminotransferase (ALT) was 200 units/L (normal is 7–55 units/L), and alkaline phosphatase (ALP) was 180 units/L (normal is 39–100 units/L). Celiac blood test for immunoglobulin A tissue transglutaminase antibodies (IgA-tTG) was 250 units (normal is less than 20 units).

An upper endoscopy showed that her small intestine had abnormal wrinkles (known as scalloping) and loss of circular folds in the lining of the duodenum. Intestinal biopsy specimens showed some loss of absorptive villi and inflammation. Further blood tests revealed gamma glutamyltransferase was 24 units/L (normal is 1–45 units/L), suggesting that the source of the high ALP was from the bone rather than the liver.

For this reason, we also looked at her bone health. Calcium was 7 mg/dl (normal is 8.4–10.2 mg/dl), phosphorus was 2 mg/dl (normal is 2.7–4.5 mg/dl), 25-hydroxyvitamin D was 18 ng/ml (normal is >30 ng/dl), albumin was 4 g/dl (normal is 3.4–4.8 g/dl), and parathyroid hormone was elevated at 90 pg/ml (normal is 15–65 pg/ml). Thyroid stimulating hormone level was 2 mIU/L (normal is 0.3–5.0 mIU/L). Bone densitometry showed thinning of the bones (osteopenia) without osteoporosis. A diagnosis of celiac disease with secondary osteomalacia (a softening of the bone also known as rickets in children) and possible celiac hepatitis was established. Marina was instructed to follow a strict gluten-free diet (GFD) and take supplemental calcium and vitamin D. (See Chapter 47 for more about bone disease in celiac disease.)

What Is Celiac Hepatitis?

Liver problems in celiac disease can range from a mild alteration of liver chemistry without any symptoms to severe liver failure. The most frequently seen type of liver problem is called *celiac hepatitis*. It is detected by elevated liver transaminases (AST and ALT), a condition known as *hypertransaminasemia*. In addition to liver chemistry, liver architecture is usually abnormal in celiac hepatitis, but the changes are mild and/or nonspecific.[1,2] However, unlike other types of hepatitis, the abnormalities of this condition are totally reversed by a GFD.[1-4]

Abnormal liver chemistry, especially hypertransaminasemia, is common in untreated celiac disease, affecting 40% of adults and 60% of children at the time of diagnosis.[1,3] Hypertransaminasemia is usually mild to moderate (elevation of enzymes less than 5 times the upper limit of normal).[1] It can be the only clue that someone has celiac disease. Celiac disease may also be the cause of chronic "unexplained" hypertransaminasemia in up to 9% of the cases.[1]

Because celiac disease may also be associated with other chronic liver diseases, especially those of autoimmune origin (Table 1), it's critical for everyone diagnosed with celiac disease to have their liver function checked.[4] Liver function tests reveal how well the liver is producing the protein albumin and clearing a blood waste product, bilirubin. Liver chemistry tests also measure enzymes that liver cells release in response to damage or disease such as AST, ALT, and ALP.[2]

In addition to the conditions listed in Table 1, case studies have revealed that celiac disease is sometimes, although rarely, associated with a few other liver diseases, namely primary sclerosing cholangitis and unexplained liver failure.

Case studies have also noted the development of celiac disease after antiviral treatment of hepatitis C virus infection.

TABLE 1. Liver Disorders Associated with Celiac Disease

Type of Liver Disease	Percent of Patients with This Liver Disease Who Have Celiac Disease	Percent of Patients with Celiac Disease Who Have This Liver Disease
Unexplained hypertransaminasemia, reversible after a gluten-free diet, "celiac hepatitis"	9%	40%
Primary biliary cirrhosis	1.3–7%	0.17%
Autoimmune hepatitis	4–6%	0.3%
End-stage liver disease of diverse cause (mostly autoimmune) before liver transplantation	3–4.3%	0.05%
Nonalcoholic fatty liver disease	3%	0.03%

From References 1 and 3.

Cause of Liver Injury in Celiac Disease

The reasons why liver damage may occur in celiac disease are poorly understood. This may be because of a predisposition to liver damage conveyed by "shared" genetic factors, such as human leukocyte antigen genes.[4] The same genes that are necessary for the development of celiac disease (see Chapter 6 on genetic testing) may increase the risk of other liver disorders, and vice versa.[1,4] Also, the effects of abnormal intestinal absorption on the whole body and/or other yet undefined mediators induced by gluten exposure may together play a role.[4]

Finding Liver Damage

Nonspecific symptoms such as feeling unwell or fatigue are common; however, most people with celiac hepatitis have no symptoms or signs of liver disease. Physical examination is usually normal. The presence of "hepatic signs" such as jaundice (discolored skin and eyes that appear yellowish color), ascites (abdominal swelling), hepatomegaly (enlarged liver), splenomegaly (enlarged spleen), or encephalopathy (abnormal thinking because of liver damage) suggests either an alternative diagnosis or an additional type of chronic liver disease.[1] Hepatic signs can be present in patients with advanced liver disease (cirrhosis) and celiac disease.

You may need additional laboratory or imaging studies (e.g., ultrasonography with different views of the liver) to evaluate the overall health of your liver or to investigate other causes of liver disease. A biopsy of the liver—a procedure in which a small sample of liver tissue is removed for microscopic analysis—is often required when the symptoms or liver abnormalities suggest the possibility of coexistent chronic liver disease or cancer or when the liver abnormalities do not return to normal after following a GFD for at least a year.[2]

Treating Celiac Hepatitis

Strict GFD is the most effective treatment for celiac hepatitis.[1–4] In fact, liver function returns to normal after one year on the GFD in most people with celiac hepatitis. To avoid recurrence of liver damage and prevent other celiac disease complications, it's crucial to avoid all foods that contain gluten for life.

Marina's Outcome

Marina met with a dietitian who provided her with information that helped her eat well and gluten free. Marina started to feel better in just a few days after starting a GFD, and her symptoms and diarrhea completely disappeared after a few weeks. After six months on a strict GFD, her celiac and liver chemistry tests returned to normal. That improvement confirmed the diagnosis of celiac hepatitis. Although ALP can be a nonspecific marker of liver injury, in Marina's case, the abnormal elevation of this enzyme was more likely explained by bone disease (osteomalacia) brought on by vitamin D deficiency, a well-known complication of celiac disease in adults.

References

1. Rubio-Tapia A, Murray JA. The liver in celiac disease. *Hepatology* 2007;46: 1653–58.
2. Rubio-Tapia A, Murray JA. Liver involvement in celiac disease. *Minerva Med* 2008;99(6): 595–604.
3. Ludvigssson JF, Elfstrom P, Broome U, Ekbom A, Montgomery SM. Celiac disease and risk of liver disease: a general population-based study. *Clin Gastroenterol Hepatol* 2007;5(1):63–69.
4. Volta U. Pathogenesis and clinical significance of liver injury in celiac disease. *Clin Rev Allergy Immunol* 2009;36(1):63–70.

Alberto Rubio-Tapia, MD, is Assistant Professor of Medicine in the Division of Gastroenterology and Hepatology of the Department of Medicine of the Mayo Clinic College of Medicine in Rochester, Minnesota. Dr. Rubio-Tapia is also a member of the Celiac Disease Research Program and the Gastrointestinal Research Unit at the Mayo Clinic.

CHAPTER 53

Future Treatments for Celiac Disease

Daniel A. Leffler, MD, MS, and Detlef Schuppan, MD, PhD

One of the most common questions we get during clinic visits and lectures is, "When will a pill for celiac disease be available?" This simple question has no simple answer. In fact, we have to ask even more questions to understand why this is so.

Why Isn't There Any Medication for Celiac Disease?

Until very recently, the medical community has suffered from two misconceptions, which together have ensured that few scientists spent time researching celiac disease treatments. First, we believed that celiac disease was very rare. Second, we believed that the gluten-free diet (GFD) was essentially a perfect treatment for celiac disease that would bring (nearly) all patients back to perfect health without any side effects. It's difficult to blame people for not spending large amounts of time and money on a problem that we thought we had solved in the 1950s!

But we now understand that celiac disease is very common: It's estimated to affect about 1% of the people in the United States, most of them undiagnosed. And we now see that the GFD is not the perfect therapy: Many people never completely heal their intestines and have intermittent symptoms, and many experience significant economic and social hardships in following the GFD. Only in the last few years has celiac disease finally begun to catch the attention of the medical and scientific community. Many people are working hard to find solutions that will help people with celiac disease. The wide variety of food products now marked "gluten free" is just one sign of this.

A number of very substantial barriers remain, however, before we have a "celiac pill" on the market. One of the most important is deciding how to test whether a celiac disease treatment really works. No treatment has ever been approved for celiac disease, so there is no precedent for knowing what the United States or European drug regulatory agencies will accept as proof of effectiveness.

Ironically, the fact that the GFD is a really good treatment makes it difficult to show that another treatment is helpful. In other diseases, like ulcerative colitis, you can test whether a medication reduces number of bloody, loose stools, abdominal pain, or hospitalizations. Most people with *treated* celiac disease, on the other hand, rarely have significant symptoms, and most recurrent symptoms occur because of inadvertent gluten exposure and generally quickly resolve after getting back on the gluten-free diet. We haven't yet designed a study that can prove, in a typical group of patients with celiac disease, that a drug is as good as a GFD or is worth taking in addition to a GFD.

Also, the "side effects" of the GFD are social, economic, and to some extent nutritional. These are much harder to measure, and often considered less important, than the typical medication side effects of rash, liver problems, or upset stomach. For this reason, the safety profile of medications for celiac disease will have to meet a standard for safety that few medications on the market currently reach.

What Might the First Celiac Medications Be Able to Do?

The most promising medications developed so far are not replacements for the GFD. The two types of treatments closest to approval are drugs that either tighten connections between intestinal cells (called *tight junctions*) so that gluten cannot get through or enzymes that break down gluten in the stomach before it can reach the intestine. Either drug may be effective against low-level gluten exposure, up to a few hundred milligrams such as what would be found in sauces or medications or even grams (a cookie or cracker) of gluten per day, but at this point it seems unlikely that either could allow people to eat a regular diet.

Is There Any Hope of a Cure for Celiac Disease?

A cure for celiac disease—defined as something that allows people to eat a totally regular diet—is probably a long way off. However, we are learning a great deal about how the immune system works and is able to recognize some proteins as safe and identify others as dangerous and trigger a response to them. One of the most interesting possibilities is a sort of desensitization, such as a "reverse vaccination" for celiac disease. Usually, vaccines are designed to teach the immune system to recognize a virus or bacteria so that, if you are exposed to it in the future, you can fight it off effectively. It might be possible to do the opposite: Teach the immune system to ignore (not react to) a protein like gluten. We are many years away from being able to do this approach, which has promise not just for celiac disease but also for a range of food and environmental allergies.

Is Anyone Working on Treatments for Refractory Celiac Disease?

Thankfully, refractory celiac disease and its most severe form, intestinal T-cell lymphoma, is a rare disorder (see Chapter 43). However, effective and safe treatments are completely lacking. The small number of patients affected and the multiple subtypes make finding treatments difficult. The current options have been adopted from treatments of cancer or inflammatory bowel disease, which are obviously very different from refractory celiac disease (Table 1). Investigators around the world are beginning to work together in new ways to share

TABLE 1. Potential Nondietary Therapies for Celiac Disease

Therapy	Mode of Action	Clinical Candidate	Status
Zonulin antagonist	Tightens barriers between intestinal cells	AT-1001	Phase II
Oral enzyme therapy	Breaks down gluten before it can cause damage	M. Xanthus Prolyl Endopeptidase	Phase I
		Germinating Barley Prolyl Endopeptidase	Phase I
		A. Niger Prolyl Endopeptidase	Phase I
TTG inhibitor	Prevents gluten from being converted to an active, more toxic form in the intestine	KCC009	Preclinical
IL10	Anti-inflammatory	N/A	Preclinical
Anti-IL15	Anti-inflammatory	HuMax IL15	Preclinical
		MutIL 15 Fc	Preclinical
Anti-IFNγ	Anti-inflammatory	Fontolizumab	Preclinical
Integrin antagonists	Anti-inflammatory	Multiple	Preclinical
CCR9 antagonist	Anti-inflammatory	CCX282-B	Preclinical
T-cell–silencing agents	Anti-inflammatory	N/A	Discovery
HLA-DQ2 blockers	Prevents gluten from binding to white blood cells so the immune system cannot be activated	N/A	Discovery

ideas and test new treatments. Because there are currently no good therapies for refractory celiac disease, we would expect any therapy that works to be approved quickly. Such therapies are on the horizon but proof of their effectiveness will be difficult because of the low numbers of patients. One promising therapy is bone marrow transplantation from another person for intestinal lymphoma.

Detlef Schuppan, MD, PhD, is Professor of Medicine at Harvard Medical School, Boston, Massachusetts, and the University of Munich, Germany. He is Director of Research at the Celiac Center at Beth Israel Deaconess Medical Center and serves on the board of multiple international gastroenterology associations. He has been a leader in the field of celiac disease for many years and was responsible for first identifying the role of tissue transglutaminase in celiac disease. Dr. Schuppan has published more than 300 papers, and his current work focuses on the immune mechanisms underlying both celiac disease and liver disease.

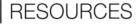

Support Groups

Celiac Organizations

Find a list of celiac organizations in countries around the world and links to their Web sites at http://celiacdisease.about.com/od/theceliactraveler/a/IntlSocieties.htm.

United States
American Celiac Disease Alliance
2504 Duxbury Place
Alexandria, VA 22308
Phone: 703-622-3331
Email: info@americanceliac.org
www.americanceliac.org

American Dietetic Association (not strictly celiac related)
120 South Riverside Plaza, Suite 2000
Chicago, IL 60606
Phone: 1-800-877-1600
www.eatright.org

Celiac Disease Foundation
13251 Ventura Boulevard, Suite 1
Studio City, CA 91604-1838
Phone: 818-990-2354
Email: cdf@celiac.org
www.celiac.org

Celiac Sprue Association USA, Inc.
PO Box 31700
Omaha, NE 68131-0700
Phone: 877-272-4272
Email: celiacs@csaceliacs.org
www.csaceliacs.org

Gluten Intolerance Group of North America
31214 124th Avenue SE
Auburn, WA 98002
Phone: 206-246-6652
Email: info@gluten.net
www.gluten.net

The Healthy Villi–New England Support Group
225 School Master Lane
Dedham, MA 02026
Phone: 888-4-CELIAC or 617-262-5422
www.healthyvilli.org

National Foundation for Celiac Awareness (NFCA)
124 South Maple Street, Second Floor
Ambler, PA 19002
Phone: 215-325-1306
Email: info@celiacawareness.org
www.celiacawareness.org

Canada
Canadian Celiac Association
5170 Dixie Road, Suite 204
Mississauga, ON L4W 1E3 Canada
Phone: 800-363-7296/905-507-6208
Email: info@celiac.ca
www.celiac.ca

Andorra
ACEA-Celíacs d'Andorra
http://www.celiacsandorra.org

Argentina
Argentina Celiac Association
http://www.celiaco.org.ar

Australia
The Coeliac Society of Australia
http://www.coeliac.org.au

Brazil
Associação dos Celíacos do Brasil
http://www.acelbra.org.br

European Coeliac Societies—umbrella organization
www.aoecs.org

India
Celiac Society for Delhi
www.celiacsocietyindia.com

Israel
The Israeli Celiac Association
www.celiac.org.il

New Zealand
Celiac New Zealand
www.coeliac.co.nz

Russia
Saint-Petersburg Coeliac Society
www.celiac.spb.ru

North American Allergy Organizations

Allergy/Asthma Information Association
295 The West Mall, Suite 118
Toronto, Ontario M9C 4Z4
Phone: 800-611-7011
Email: admin@aaia.ca
www.aaia.ca

American Academy of Allergy, Asthma & Immunology
555 East Wells Street
Suite 1100
Milwaukee, WI 53202-3823
Phone: 414-272-6071
Email: info@aaaai.org
www.aaaai.org

Food Allergy & Anaphylaxis Network
11781 Lee Jackson Highway, Suite 160
Fairfax, VA 22033-3309
Phone: 800-929-4040
E-mail: faan@foodallergy.org
www.foodallergy.org

North American Digestive Disease/Disorder Organizations

American Gastroenterological Association
4930 Del Ray Avenue
Bethesda, MD 20814
Phone: 301-654-2055
www.gastro.org

American Neurogastroenterology and Motility Society
45685 Harmony Lane
Belleville, MI 48111
Phone: 734-699-1130
Email: admin@motilitysociety.org
www.motilitysociety.org

Children's Digestive Health and Nutrition Foundation
1501 Bethlehem Pike
PO Box 6
Flourtown, PA 19031
Phone: 215-233-0808
Email: cdhnf@cdhnf.org
www.cdhnf.org or www.celiachealth.org

International Foundation for Functional Gastrointestinal Disorders
PO Box 170864
Milwaukee, WI 53217-8076
Phone: 888-964-2001 or 414-964-1799
E-mail: iffgd@iffgd.org
www.iffgd.org

National Digestive Diseases Information Clearinghouse
2 Information Way
Bethesda, MD 20892–3570
Phone: 800–891–5389
TTY: 1–866–569–1162
Email: nddic@info.niddk.nih.gov
www.digestive.niddk.nih.gov

North American Society for Pediatric Gastroenterology, Hepatology, and Nutrition
PO Box 6
Flourtown, PA 19031
Phone: 215-233-0808
Email: naspghan@naspghan.org
www.naspghan.org

The Importance of Advocacy

Andrea Levario, JD

At the beginning of this decade, celiac disease was considered to be a rare condition in the United States, estimated to affect about 1 in 10,000.[1] Few people had ever heard of it, and there was little research being done to learn more about the condition. And while the course of treatment is strictly linked to diet, the food industry was not focused on increasing the number of gluten-free products.

In February 2003, the landscape for individuals living with celiac disease changed dramatically with the publication of a landmark study on the prevalence of celiac disease in the United States.[2] Research revealed that the actual prevalence of celiac disease is 1 in 133. This shed light on the needs of the millions yet to be diagnosed. This estimate placed celiac disease above type 1 diabetes and Parkinson's and Alzheimer's diseases in terms of numbers of Americans affected. The most urgent concern was the availability of safe, gluten-free products. Unlike Canada or countries in Europe, the United States lacks uniform labeling for gluten-free foods. Newly diagnosed patients were already struggling to identify safe food products at the supermarket.

Although raising awareness of celiac disease has always been a top priority among the clinicians specializing in celiac disease and the celiac community, awareness alone cannot deliver many of the desired results—funding for research, clinician education, and improved food labeling and insurance coverage, to name a few. Awareness alone cannot effect change in public attitudes and policies; it must be teamed with advocacy.

In general, the core mission of many disease-related organizations, like the Juvenile Diabetes Research Foundation and the Crohn's & Colitis Foundation of America, is to find cures. To reach this goal, the nonprofit groups sponsor research and advocate increased Federal funding of disease-related research at the National Institutes of Health. In communities across the country, individuals, with guidance from their national groups, speak out in town halls and other appropriate public meetings to heighten awareness and advocate for changes in public policy or law. Not only does this educate policy makers, it also puts a human face on the disease and demonstrates why changes are warranted.

Millions of individuals have shared their experiences and the challenges of living with a chronic or life-threatening medical condition with policymakers, and it has changed all of our lives. Women older than age 50 are now screened for breast cancer, babies are tested at birth for phenylketonuria, and antiretroviral drugs have changed the lifespan of people with HIV. The achievements brought by advocating on behalf of a community can be measured in lives saved, advances in medical treatments, and even cures.

In their statement, the panelists of the National Institute of Health's Consensus Development Conference on Celiac Disease specifically highlighted access to an advocacy group as one of the key elements in managing those affected by the disease.[3] They emphasized the importance of support groups, physicians, dietitians, patients, and their families working collectively with a common purpose. They advised that this would place the community in the best position to educate, advance research, and advocate for individuals with celiac disease. Their message was that advocacy brings change.

In 2003, the American Celiac Disease Alliance (www.americanceliac.org/advocacy.htm), known at that time as the American Celiac Task Force, outlined an advocacy strategy focused on adding information about allergens to food labels. Every segment of the community—support groups, food manufacturers, researchers, and physicians—identified ways in which they could educate lawmakers. Letters were sent and calls were made to share key information about celiac disease as an inherited condition, along with personal stories. Patients with celiac disease, family members, and friends delivered a clear, consistent message.

Fewer than 40,000 individuals were diagnosed with celiac disease in 2003, whereas the number of individuals with food allergies topped 10 million. Because celiac disease also involves an immune-mediated reaction, partnering with food allergy organizations, which were also advocating for clear allergen statements, made perfect sense. Working alongside established and well-known groups provided credibility and created a greater sense of urgency for Congress to act. A mere 18 months after the prevalence study was released, the Food Allergen Labeling and Consumer Protection Act was signed into law. This requires the top eight allergens, including wheat, to be clearly listed on food product labels. In addition, it requires standards to be developed for labeling products "gluten free." The latter provisions were incorporated in direct response to the concerns presented by patients with celiac disease, and the relatively unknown community of celiac advocates earned recognition for its efforts in the landmark legislation.

The celiac community's initial efforts succeeded because it was able to show how inconsistent and incomplete food labeling affects the daily lives of those with celiac disease. They understand the value of educating policymakers and food manufacturers about this lifelong disease. I want to underscore the importance of these efforts and the importance of continuing them.

Beyond product labeling, there are other significant issues for individuals with celiac disease. These include being able to obtain health or life insurance and working to ensure that Federal dollars will fund all facets of disease research, including studies of related autoimmune disorders and potential treatment protocols. Similar advocacy efforts will be required in each case; the path and approach have already been charted.

Education is the starting point for advocacy. Many policymakers know very little about celiac disease. Who better to educate them than those who live with celiac disease? Thanks to the Internet, patients, family members, and friends can send a letter to their representatives and senators in a matter of minutes. Share your story and the facts about celiac disease.

Urge them talk about celiac disease during May, National Celiac Disease Awareness Month. Without letters such as these, the food labeling law might never have passed. Closer to home, individuals can work with local support groups to provide information to restaurants and encourage them to offer gluten-free meals. If a school or church has a health fair, volunteer to attend and distribute information and answer questions. In each of these settings, individuals have the opportunity to educate and advocate about celiac disease. For change to occur, voices must be heard. Be sure to add yours.

References

1. Fasano A. Current approaches to diagnosis and treatment of celiac disease: an evolving spectrum. *Gastroenterology* 2001;120(3):636–51.
2. Fasano A, Berti I, Gerarduzzi T, Not T, Colletti RB, Drago S, et al. Prevalence of celiac disease in at-risk and not-at-risk groups in the United States: a large multicenter study. *Arch Intern Med* 2003;163:286–92.
3. NIH Consensus Development Conference on Celiac Disease. *NIH Consens StateSci Statements* 2004; 21(1):1–22.

Advocacy Resources

- American Celiac Disease Alliance (www.americanceliac.org). This is the national advocacy organization for celiac disease in the United States and represents the entire community.
- THOMAS Library of Congress (http://thomas.loc.gov). This site provides online access to Federal legislative information dating back to 1989 (101st Congress). Obtain copies of bills, track legislation, and find House and Senate schedules.
- U.S. House of Representatives (www.house.gov) and U.S. Senate (www.senate.gov). Identify your congressional district and your representative and senator in Congress.

Andrea Levario, JD, is Executive Director of the American Celiac Disease Alliance. She has more than 20 years of experience in public policy and advocacy, having worked on Capitol Hill, for the federal government, and for nonprofit organizations. She is also the parent of a child with celiac disease.

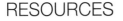

Staying Gluten Free in Health Care Facilities

Ronni Alicea, RD, MBA

Aslip in the shopping mall parking lot landed Mike in the local hospital emergency room. Hours later, he would learn that he needed total hip replacement and then several weeks in a skilled nursing center and rehabilitation facility for physical therapy. His undiagnosed celiac disease had led to osteoporosis. Marcie just heard the great news: She is pregnant. Now she is looking ahead, and her concern is trust. Will she have gluten-free options available when she is in the hospital around the time of labor and delivery?

Whether planned or unplanned, stays in health care facilities are challenging, especially when managing a special diet is added to the experience. Although this chapter focuses on short-term stays, the same issues apply to residential care facilities. The key is being prepared to educate your health care providers about your needs. Although health care professionals are familiar with celiac disease and gluten-free eating, they may not have significant experience or training.

Prepare Info about You

It's always wise to compile and keep updated a list of the medications and supplements you routinely take and a brief medical history that includes the fact that you must eat gluten free. This is especially helpful in case you are not able to answer questions. Give a copy to your emergency contact and keep another copy in your wallet and/or car glove compartment.

Include in this information your individual reaction to gluten ingestion. For example, does gluten exposure cause you to experience confusion, nausea, or diarrhea? It may not be clear to medical personnel whether your symptoms are from a virus, reaction to new medication, food-borne illness such as salmonella, or gluten ingestion. A restaurant card that has basic diet information is also useful.

Using "Facility Speak"

Tammy, who has type 1 diabetes and celiac disease, found herself in the emergency room after spraining her ankle during an after-work softball match. She declined the graham crackers offered as a snack to relieve her low blood glucose and, after describing her gluten-free diet, was offered a rice-based cereal bar containing malt. Malt is in many of the products that are advertised as "wheat free," but wheat free doesn't necessarily mean gluten free; malt often comes from barley. Tammy had to be specific in asking for carbohydrates that do not contain gluten, such as fruit juice or rice cakes and cheese, instead of the usual snacks.

When you are admitted, whether it is to the emergency room, another department in the hospital, or a long-or short-term care facility, request that your diet order be "gluten-free diet" (GFD) and that the allergy section state "wheat, rye, barley, and oats." Certified gluten-free oats are not stocked in most health care food service inventories. This will alert three key departments—dietary, nursing, and pharmacy—about your need to avoid the gluten protein found in many foods. Even then, you may be limited to plain meals in the first few days after an admission if the facility does not have many GFD orders. They may have planned gluten-free menus but need to order some of the specialized food items.

Three Key Players in Keeping You Safe

If you have a planned admission, you have three calls to make a week before the admission. For unplanned admissions, ask for their phone extensions so you or a family member can make contact.

Food Service Director
The food service director manages the kitchen. Introduce yourself, ask whether a gluten-free menu is available, and explain that you will need to stay completely gluten free. The great news is that now many health care food distributors have gluten-free foods identified and available, although it may take extra time to order and receive them.

Every food service kitchen staff understands what food allergies are, even if they have not made a GFD specifically, so this is an effective way to present celiac disease (although celiac disease is not a food allergy; see Introduction). The challenge is to help them understand that gluten is in seemingly unrelated food items, such as soup base and scalloped potatoes, in addition to the obvious bread and pasta. Keep in mind that they want to understand how to keep you safe but may need time and help.

We commonly use the words *cross-contamination* when describing gluten-free food production. Food service employees are generally taught this food safety term in the context of preventing food-borne illnesses, such as *E. coli,* and proper thawing of frozen foods. Techniques include using separate cutting boards and utensils when handling and preparing meat, fish, chicken, and vegetables and separating raw and cooked items.

Staff will usually need to be told that this idea applies to keeping food gluten free. Use the term *cross-contact.* This term may more clearly communicate that food that is safe for you cannot touch anything with gluten. Gluten-free bread cannot go through the toaster with the white, rye, and whole wheat bread and that regular and gluten-free pasta cannot be drained in the same colander. Breaded chicken cannot touch your chicken breast even when cooked thoroughly; gluten-free bread needs to warm or toast in the oven by itself; and a hamburger patty will be unsafe if it is accidentally placed on a bun that is later removed.

Ask that staff follow the same protocol as food allergy management when preparing your food trays. Offer the following resources. The Dietary Managers Association has several articles on food service issues (search for gluten free at www.dmaonline.org). An education piece and sample menus can be found at www.celinalfoods.com.

Facility Dietitian

The facility's registered dietitians in the clinical nutrition department are your most active advocates in the facility. They will make sure that you are nourished and devise a comprehensive plan to meet your health care goals in a gluten-free way. They will arrange with the nursing staff for you to have gluten-free snacks and even arrange gluten-free personal hygiene products if needed. Request to be placed at "high nutrition risk" at check in and to the admitting physician and nurse so that the registered dietitian visits you promptly.

The facility's dietitians have been integral in planning its menus, and GFDs need expert planning, without which they may be lacking key nutrients.[1] Although this may not be as important for a three-day hospital stay, meals during a longer stay have to meet all your nutrient needs. Many kitchens manage GFDs by eliminating gluten-containing foods without properly substituting the carbohydrates, vitamins, or minerals found in the unsafe meal item.

Facility diet manuals generally contain information on foods that are allowed or not allowed on the GFD. In-depth information for dietitians is available in the *Nutrition Care Manual* and the Evidence Analysis Library of the American Dietetic Association (www.eatright.org).

Patient Services Advocate

The person you want to speak with in your third call is less well defined and the department name may be different. You may get connected with the Social Services or Social Work Department.

Consider Mike, who suffered a mild stroke and hip fracture and subsequent hip replacement. He needed several departments to understand GFD basics in order to eat safely, including the emergency department, the surgical floor, and the postoperative area. His assessments included swallowing skills, where crackers are commonly used, and occupational therapy for independent cooking and dining. Then he was discharged to a skilled nursing facility for additional rehabilitation.

At the skilled nursing facility, Martin wanted to socialize and participate in the daily activities, such as birthday celebrations, religious services, and crafts during his rehabilitation stay. All of these activities were vital for his successful rehabilitation and required planning for gluten-free options. He worked with the facility's Social Work Department and found that communication and training on his part allowed him to determine his own choices and get quality care.

Extra Support: Getting and Giving

If you find that the facility is just not getting your GFD correct and the staff is resistant to education, please alert your local ombudsman. Under the Federal Older Americans Act, every state is required to have an ombudsman, who will investigate your complaints and be your advocate. Facilities should have the local phone number posted in plain view. Visit www.ltcombudsman.org and jot the number down or call the Ombudsman Resource Center at 202-332-2275. I sincerely hope you never need it.

In our busy life we can all use more friends. If you have a few hours please consider volunteering in a health care facility. There is always need for someone to call bingo numbers or read to the visually impaired. Maybe they have a resident with celiac disease? You will feel great and will learn how to be a better advocate for yourself.

SELF-MANAGEMENT TIPS

- ☐ Hospitals and other medical facilities are complicated institutions that often will not have good, nutritionally sound gluten-free food options readily available.
- ☐ If your hospitalization is planned, such as elective surgery or labor and delivery, call ahead to speak with the food service representative, dietitian, and patient service advocate. You may even consider choosing a medical facility based partially on their experience/expertise with celiac disease.
- ☐ If you are hospitalized suddenly, ask to speak with the dietitian on duty as soon as possible to help arrange a GFD.
- ☐ Carry information about your dietary needs with you at all times, and give a copy to your emergency contact.

Reference

1. Thompson T, Dennis M, Higgins LA, Lee AR, Sharett MK. Gluten-free diet survey: are Americans with celiac disease consuming recommended amounts of fiber, iron, calcium and grain foods? *J Human Nutr Diet* 2005;18:163–69.

Ronni Alicea, RD, MBA, is a consultant dietitian based in Somerset County, New Jersey. She writes and speaks to professionals, foodservice workers, and consumers on managing the gluten-free diet in health care facilities. Ms. Alicea founded Celinal Foods to help residential care providers assure safe and nutritious gluten-free lifestyles as needed.

GLOSSARY

acetyl glucoseamine: a glyconutrient made by the body that appears to have anti-inflammatory properties and has been suggested for use in multiple inflammatory disorders, including inflammatory bowel disease

alanine aminotransferase (ALT): a chemical released into the blood with some forms of liver damage

alkaline phosphatase (ALP): a chemical released into the blood with some forms of liver or bone damage

alopecia areata: hair loss

anemia: a decrease in the number of red blood cells in the body. Most commonly, individuals with celiac disease are anemic due to either bleeding from the gastrointestinal tract, poor absorption of iron (a necessary component in making red blood cells), or a combination of the two.

antibody: proteins made by the immune system that bind to other proteins and molecules, which allows the immune system to attack them

anticholinergic: a type of medication that can slow down the gastrointestinal tract, often causing dry mouth or sleepiness

arthralgia: joint pain

arthropathy: inflammatory joint disease

aspartate aminotransferase (AST): a chemical released into the blood with some forms of liver damage

ataxia: decreased coordination, usually due to a nerve problem that can cause difficulty walking

autoimmune diseases: diseases in which the immune system attacks healthy parts of the body; examples are celiac disease, thyroid disease, vitiligo, rheumatoid arthritis, and type 1 diabetes mellitus

biopsy: small piece of tissue removed from a part of the body (skin, small intestine, etc.) for close examination under a microscope

cell surface markers: proteins on the surface of cells; there are many kinds and have many functions

chemokines: chemicals released by the immune system with various functions, such as increasing or decreasing inflammation

chromosome: a long, coiled piece of DNA (genetic material); changes in number or size of chromosomes is associated with many diseases, including Down syndrome and some cancers

collagenous sprue: small intestinal disease often related to celiac disease in which excess connective tissue (collagen) forms under the lining of the intestine, leading to malabsorption

colonoscopy: procedure in which a long, thin tube is introduced through your rectum into your colon and sometimes to the small intestine; biopsies may or may not be taken

comorbid: a medical condition that accompanies another medical condition

C-reactive protein: nonspecific blood measure of inflammation, not usually elevated in celiac disease

Crohn's disease: type of inflammatory bowel disease that can affect any part of the gastrointestinal tract

cytokines: chemicals released by the immune system with various functions, such as increasing or decreasing inflammation

dental enamel hypoplasia: defects in the hard, protective coating on teeth

direct immunofluorescence: a microscopic technique used to look for specific proteins

Down syndrome: disorder of chromosomes that is associated with a spectrum of presentations

duodenum: the first part of the small intestine, which is attached to the stomach

electrolyte imbalance: abnormal amounts of important minerals and chemicals in the blood

endomysial antibody (EMA): measured in blood to detect celiac disease; for technical reasons, EMA testing has largely been replaced by tTG testing

endoscopy: medical procedure involving introduction of a tube with a microscope; examples include EGD and colonoscopy

epidemiology: study of the health of populations

epilepsy: seizure disorder

epithelial cells: special cells that line surfaces of the body that are exposed to the environment; examples include skin, intestine, and saliva gland

esophagogastroduodenoscopy (EGD): procedure in which a long, thin tube is introduced through your mouth into your stomach and small intestine; biopsies may or may not be taken

excipient: inactive substance used in medications or supplements

ezymatic hydrolysis: type of body reaction in which a chemical breaks down another substance

fibrosing alveolitis: a lung disease causing scarring, also known as pulmonary fibrosis

follicular keratosis: dark bumps on the skin, usually only a cosmetic problem

gamma-glutamyl transferase (GGT): chemical released into the blood with some forms of liver damage

genetic alleles: different forms of a gene performing a specific function

gliadin: alcohol-soluble part of gluten

glossitis: condition in which the tongue is inflamed, covered with ulcers, and is tender and painful

gluten: the major protein found in wheat; related proteins in rye and barley are called secalin and hordein, respectively

gluten challenge: medically supervised exposure to a specific amount and duration of gluten, used to evaluate for celiac disease in cases where the diagnosis is uncertain

glutinen: acid- and base-soluble part of gluten

hematocrit: the part of the blood made up by red blood cells

hemoglobin: the protein in red blood cells that carries oxygen

Hirschprung's disease: disease resulting from lack of nerves in some or all of the colon, causing distention and constipation

hyposplenism: poor spleen function, which can increase risk/severity of infection; the spleen filters blood, removing damaged cells and helping to clear infection

IgA-tTG antibody: the most common blood test used to diagnose and monitor celiac disease

ilium: the third and last part of the small intestine, which is attached to the colon

immune-mediated reaction: reaction causing an immune reaction

immunoglobulin: proteins made by the immune system that bind to targets and cause an immune reaction; also known as antibodies

immunosuppressive therapy: treatment that suppresses immune system function; examples include 6-mercaptopurine, azothioprine, prednisone

interleukins: chemicals released by the immune system with various functions; there are many interleukins which can either increase or decrease inflammation

intraepithelial lymphocytes: white blood cells found in the lining of the small intestine

intrauterine growth restriction: birth weight or fetal growth that is low for gestational age

irritable bowel syndrome (IBS): chronic gastrointestinal symptoms that are not caused by a identifiable physical or autoimmune problem

jejunum: the second or middle part of the small intestine

kefir: fermented milk drink

latent celiac disease: condition in which there is positive celiac antibody, such as tTG or EMA, but no intestinal damage

leaky gut/intestinal permeability: disorder in which the intestine no longer tightly controls the passage of substances across the intestinal lining in either direction; a common result of many types of intestinal damage

lymphocytes: common type of white blood cell; divided into two major catagories: T-cells and B-cells

leukocytes: white blood cells, includes lymphocytes (T-cells and B-cells) and monocytes, macrophages, neutrophils, eosinophils, basophils, and dendritic cells

Marsh lesions: named for a pathologist who divided intestinal damage into a different classes. Marsh 1 has increased intraepithelial lymphocytes; many things can cause this lesion. Marsh 2 has increased intraepithelial lymphocytes and deep crypts but normal villi; this is the least common lesion but can indicate early or partially healed celiac disease. Marsh 3 has increased intraepithelial lymphocytes, deep crypts, and damaged villi; divided into classes a, b, and c, with some, most, or all villi damaged, respectively.

methemglobinemia: disorder, often caused by drugs, that leaves the hemoglobin in red blood cells unable to carry oxygen

myalgia: muscle pain

neoplasm: cancer, malignancy

neuropathy: nerve damage, often causing numbness, tingling, or pain

osteopenia or osteoporosis: slight or severe decrease, respectively, in bone mass that can be due to many causes

peroxidase autoantibodies: autoimmune reaction to peroxidase associated with auto-immune thyroid disease

phenylketonuria: genetic disease in which people lack specific enzymes that break down specific types of protein

polyphenol: a plant chemical with antioxidant properties

prokinetics: medications that speed up the movement of the gastrointestinal tract

prolamins: proline- and glutamine-rich storage proteins found in grains; many grains contain prolamins but are not closely enough related to gluten to cause inflammation in celiac disease

pulmonary hemosiderosis: disease in which there is chronic bleeding into the lungs, causing iron deposits

quercetin: a food component known as a bioflavonoid with anti-inflammatory and anti-oxidant properties

ROME criteria: criteria used for diagnosing irritable bowel syndrome, generally employed in research studies

sarcoidosis: chronic inflammatory disorder causing clusters of white blood cells to form in tissues; affects almost any organ but most common in the skin, lungs, or liver

short-chain fatty acids: type of fat made up of small molecules that is used by the colon and some other cells as a major source of energy

silent celiac disease: celiac disease with intestinal damage but no apparent symptoms or nutritional abnormalities

Sjogren's syndrome: chronic autoimmune disease in which moisture-producing glands such as saliva and tear glands are destroyed

steatorrhea: abnormally high amounts of fat in stool that typically cause the stool to float and appear greasy; often, fat globules can be seen in stool

sulfones: chemical that contains sulfur

thrombocytosis: overproduction of platelets (cells in the blood responsible for forming blood clots)

tissue transglutaminase (tTG): common enzyme in the body that is important in inflammation and making connective tissues; a central factor in celiac disease

tuberculosis: infection, usually of the lungs

Turner syndrome: disorder of chromosomes that is associated with a spectrum of presentations.

ulcerative colitis: type of inflammatory bowel disease affecting only the colon

villous atrophy: loss of absorptive surface of the small intestine in celiac disease and a small number of other diseases, including infections; the countless, tiny, finger-like projections that increase the surface area of the intestine and aid in the absorption of water and nutrients are lost, leading to a flat intestinal surface and malabsorption

vitiligo: autoimmune disease targeting melanocytes (the cells that produce skin pigment), leading to patches of white skin

white blood cells: cells that make up the immune system

Williams syndrome: disorder of chromosomes that is associated with a spectrum of presentations, including heart problems and developmental delays

zinc carnosine: antioxidant that has been shown to protect the intestine from damage due to aspirin and similar drugs and chemotherapy and potentially is useful in liver disease

INDEX